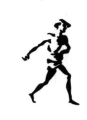

Women

with photographs by Harry Langdon
Introducing Prime Time Workout

JANE FONDA

Coming of Age

with Mignon McCarthy

SIMON AND SCHUSTER · NEW YORK

DESIGNED BY EVE METZ
PRODUCTION MANAGER: RICHARD L. WILLETT
PHOTO EDITOR: VINCENT VIRGA
ILLUSTRATIONS BY BARBARA SHOCK
MECHANICALS BY IRVING PERKINS AND ASSOCIATES
PRIME TIME WORKOUT CHOREOGRAPHY BY CAROL GARABEDIAN
HAIR BY BARRON
MAKEUP BY JEFF JONES

MANUFACTURED IN THE UNITED STATES OF AMERICA
COMPOSITION BY AMERICOMP, BRATTLEBORO, VT.
PRINTED AND BOUND BY THE BOOK PRESS, INC., BRATTLEBORO, VT.
10   9   8   7   6   5   4   3   2   1

Library of Congress Cataloging in Publication Data

Fonda, Jane, date.
    Women coming of age.

    Bibliography: p.
    Includes index.
    1. Health.   2. Exercise for women.
    3. Middle-aged women—Health and hygiene.
I. McCarthy, Mignon.   II. Title
RA778.F68   1984   613′04244   84–14099

ISBN: 0-671-46997-5

Permission to print the following is gratefully acknowledged:

Excerpt from *Break of Day*, by Colette, copyright 1961, Martin Secker & Warburg, Ltd., reprinted by permission of Farrar, Straus & Giroux, p. 9;

Quotations by Maggie Kuhn, Founder and National Convener, Gray Panthers, pp. 19 and 147;

Excerpt from *On Golden Pond*, film script by Ernest Thompson, p. 21;

Quotations from personal interview with Randi Gunther, Ph.D., pp. 34 and 115;

Quotations and biographical information from personal interview with Julie Jordan, pp. 75–76;

Quotations and biographical information from personal interview with Hazel Washburn, pp. 79–80;

Excerpt from *The Mirror Crack'd*, film script by Jonathan Hales and Barry Sandler, pp. 102–103;

Quotation from "An Unsentimental Journey," by Grace Paley, *Ms.*, February 1978, p. 106;

Quotation from personal communication with Estelle Ramey, M.D., p. 139;

Quotation from "The Sexual Lives of Women Over 60," by Carol Tavris, *Ms.*, July 1977, p. 147;

Quotation from *Growing Older, Getting Better*, by Jane Porcino, Ph.D., published by Addison-Wesley, 1983, p. 155;

Quotation from *The Controversial Climacteric*, by P. A. Van Keep, W. H. Utian, and A. Vermeulen, published by MTP Press, 1982, p. 169;

Quotation and biographical information from personal interview with Patricia M. Walters, p. 235–36.

Women Coming of Age

CONTENTS

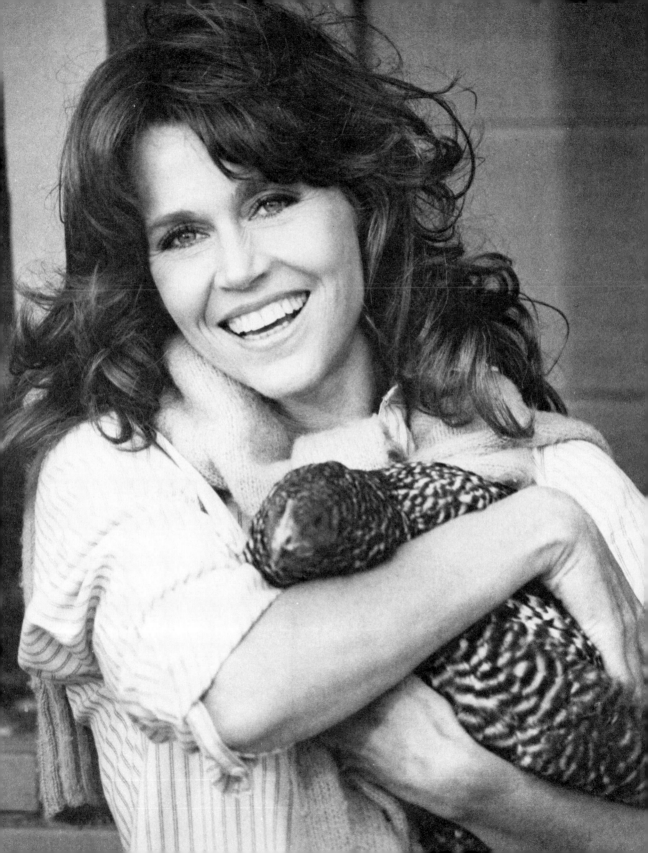

PART ONE

Women in Midlife

Whenever I feel myself inferior to everything about me, threatened by my own mediocrity, frightened by the discovery that a muscle is losing its strength, a desire its power, or a pain the keen edge of its bite, I can still hold up my head and say to myself, "Let me not forget that I am the daughter of a woman who bent her head, trembling, between the blades of a cactus, her wrinkled face full of ecstasy over the promise of a flower, a woman who herself never ceased to flower, untiringly, during three quarters of a century."

Colette
Break of Day

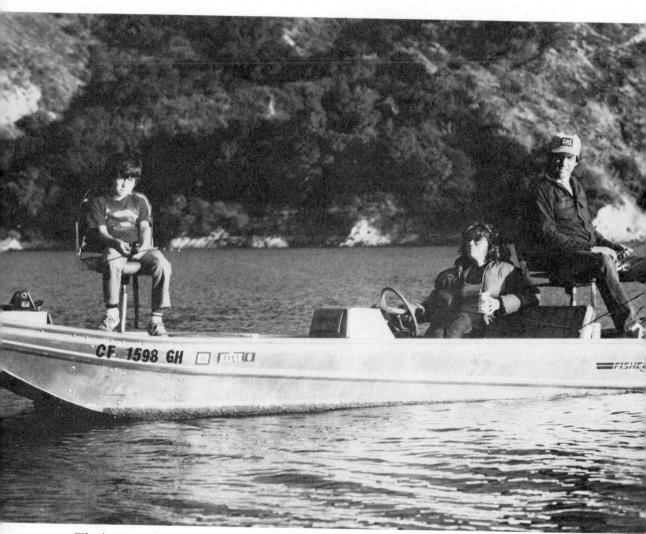

That's me with Troy and Tom fishing on Lake Cachuma in the hills above Santa Barbara.

CHAPTER 1

FROM MY OWN EXPERIENCE

WHEN I FINISHED my first Workout Book, I swore I'd never do it again. I'm not a writer. For me, sitting in front of a piece of blank paper trying to figure out how words should follow one another is more frustrating than the most difficult scene I've ever had to face as an actress. I find myself bad-tempered, snapping at noisy children, shouting at rowdy dogs, and ferociously finding a million things to do to avoid facing that damned empty page. Yet here I am again, four years later, putting the final touches on another manuscript.

Between books, in those intervening years, I've become a woman consciously middle-aged. This and all that's led toward it has been what ultimately brought me back to the trials of the writing table. There were the physical signs of my own aging. And there was the illness and death of my father which handed down to me the role of elder.

I think Nature began having its way with me sometime in the years approaching my mid-forties when the first truly noticeable signs of getting older began to appear. At this writing I am forty-six and the lines on my face show up on film despite the skillful lighting of even the cleverest cinematographer. Strands of gray now lace my hair. My back, which I broke while diving as a teenager, has let it be known it needs pampering. Long evenings spent sitting in the bottom of some old outboard motorboat, watching my husband outsmart the bass, sends my sacroiliac shrieking all the way to the chiropractor. A bump on my little finger turns out to be arthritis, and I say to myself, "Ah, Fonda, it's finally happening. You're a middle-aged broad!"

But I don't feel "middle-aged," with everything that's supposed to mean. I can run farther, stretch deeper, climb steeper, lift heavier,

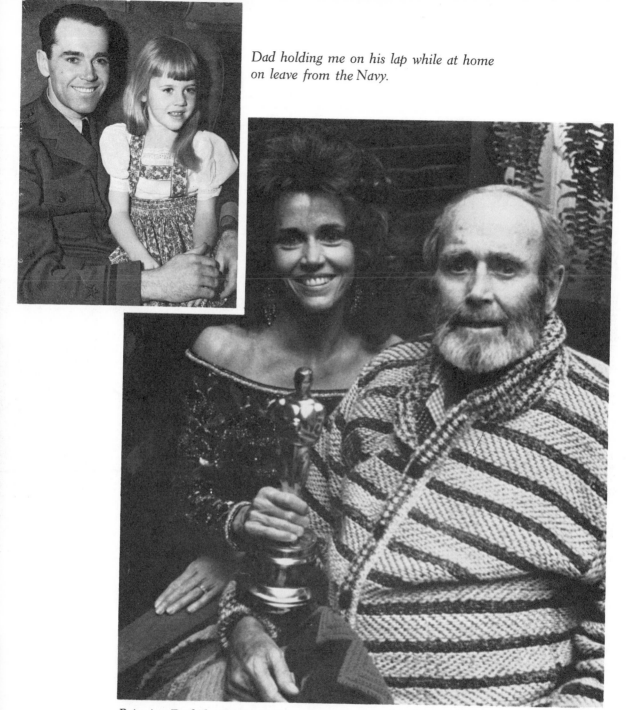

Dad holding me on his lap while at home on leave from the Navy.

Bringing Dad the Oscar for his performance in On Golden Pond.

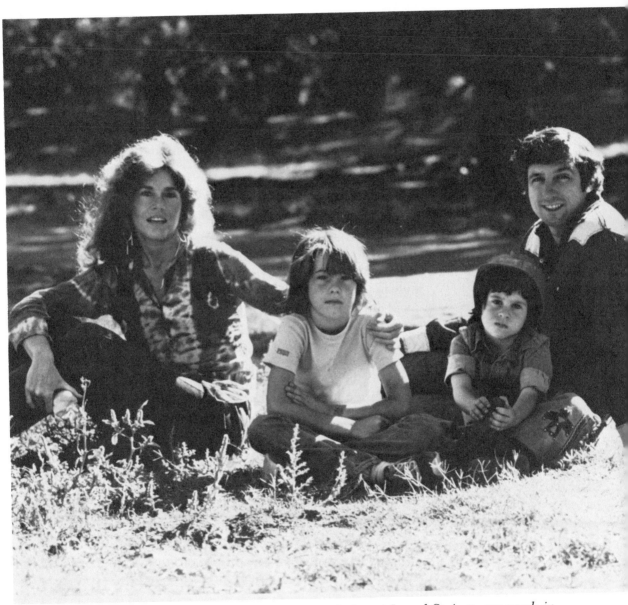

Me, Vanessa, Troy, and Tom a number of years ago relaxing at Laurel Springs, our ranch in Santa Barbara.

stand taller, and dance longer than when I was twenty. Back then in the "olden days," as my son likes to call it, I *was* young. Now, I *feel* young.

Might I not be exempt from aging? Maybe I can escape time's crusty clutches? But then there's my back again and that bump and all the rest staring back at me in the mirror, and I'm forced to admit that, strong and fit as I may be overall, I'm still a woman in midlife, challenged by that fact and scared by it as well.

The passing of my father placed all of this into a far deeper context. While living, our parents are the barriers between us and mortality. When they pass on, we step up to the head of the line. Being with my father during the months of his decline shattered any childhood illusion of living on forever. I realized then, sitting at his bedside those many days, that it was not so much the idea of death itself which frightened me as it was being faced with the "what ifs" and the "if onlys" when there's no time left, arriving at the end of the third act and discovering too late it hasn't been a rehearsal.

Suddenly time itself became exquisitely precious. Time spent with my father. My own time remaining. I felt the need to project myself into the future, to visualize who I want to be and what I want my life to be at its close. I realized that I have only one life, and unless some miracle occurs it's more than half over. I've wasted time during the first half, started down wrong paths, taken some things for granted. Now I'm entering a new phase with a new gift—the gift of experience. I have my past, all that's come before, to learn from. With this I can rechart a course for the time that remains, based not on myth and romance but rather on reality and self-knowledge. There must be no "if onlys" about the things that really matter— my children, my husband, my friends, my community, my hopes for our country and for world peace. I must begin now to frame a philosophy that will encompass the latter part of my life. Of course, this means being braver for the second half, willing to take leaps of faith, to make choices and take chances that couldn't be taken when children were dependent and when I had less experience.

In my mind I've already laid the first brush strokes toward a picture of the woman I would wish myself to be in the twilight of my life. I see an old woman walking briskly, out-of-doors, in every season. She's feisty. She's not afraid of being alone. Her face is lined and full of life. There's a ruddy flush to her cheeks and a bright curious look in her eye because she's still learning. Her husband often walks with her. They laugh a lot. She enjoys simple things. She likes to be with young people and she's a good listener. Her grandchildren love to tell her stories and to hear hers because she's got some really good ones that contain sweet, hidden lessons about life. She has a conscious set of values and the knack to make them compelling to her young friends.

With that kind of image emerging to draw me forward, in which I oftentimes see my father too, I say to myself, Okay, Fonda, if that's how you want to see yourself at eighty, how are you going to make sure you get there? How are you going to live your life in your forties, fifties and sixties to lead you toward that vision? How will you steer your course between the dangers and the opportunities of this new phase?

Getting Prepared

If I've learned anything over the years, it's that when confronted with a new situation, one does best to face it with as much information as possible. I learned this deceptively simple lesson from the births of my two children. The first was for me a lonely and frightening experience, one I went through unrehearsed, *unprepared.* I was swept along, passively, in a sea of pain. The second birth was completely the opposite. My husband, Tom Hayden, and I studied birthing with Femmy DeLyser, childbirth educator and the author of the *Workout Book for Pregnancy, Birth, and Recovery.* With Femmy's help, I was *prepared* for what lay in store. Along with Tom, I planned for the birth, visualized it, and exercised for it. The pain was no less, the process was no faster—that can be a matter of one's genes or heredity—but the preparation meant not losing control. It gave me the ability to ride atop rather than be submerged by the pain. The nature of the experience was completely transformed.

Now, a dozen years after my last child was born, I'm entering another period of profound change. Midlife. One part of me relishes the new maturity it brings. One part is also frightened—so hard to let go of children, of the success that came with youth, of old identities when new ones aren't yet clearly defined. But I know that the same principle of preparation I learned in childbirth will see me through—first, by my *being physically stronger* and, equally impor-

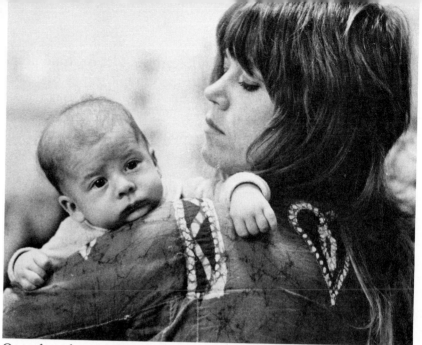
One of my favorite Troy pictures. He still makes this face.

tant, by *understanding what is happening to me and knowing how to respond.* I can let myself be blindly propelled into midlife, backing into it with my eyes squeezed shut, praying it will be all right. I can wing it, groping in the dark. Or I can enter with my eyes open. I can take charge and seek out what I need to know in order to make informed decisions in the many changing areas of my life.

What, I wondered, can women in midlife realistically expect of themselves physically? Is continued fitness, sexuality, and vitality possible? Do we have special nutritional needs now? Can we slow the aging process? Is there an equivalent to the childbirth breathing technique to ease us through the transition into midlife?

In seeking answers to these questions, I came to understand that midlife holds a very particular set of physical and psychological challenges for women and that these are affected by how we eat, move, view ourselves, and live our lives. I also began to feel the need for a workout more solicitous of my hips and back, a workout that still challenged me but one slightly slower paced, with movements that flowed and didn't jar my joints.

So I decided to write another book that would address all of these concerns.

The first Workout Book was conceived as a complete health and fitness book—for everyone. The new book I envisioned was to go deeper into one phase of life. Yet, in many ways I knew this would also be a book for *all* women, of every age, because each of us is affected by what it means to be an aging woman in this society. I hoped men too would want to read it, not only to better understand women at midlife but also to learn about their own physical changes, which, with the exception of menopause, are identical to ours.

I wanted this to be a practical book that would say everything I had wanted to know myself. I wanted it to provide a concrete program for midlife well-being. And I wanted to communicate to other midlife women my conviction that aging doesn't have to be negative.

After embarking upon the project, I soon realized that unlike my first book, for which I was able to draw largely from past experience, the writing of this was to carry me into my future. I had my intuition and my ideas about it, yes, but no body of finished knowledge on which to stand. A great deal of research would have to be done.

To help me in this task, I turned to my friend, Mignon McCarthy. Mignon had been studying for her Ph.D. in Literature at Stanford University before becoming Executive Director of the Campaign for Economic Democracy, the California organization that my husband and I are part of. She combines great intelligence and political and social concern with a belief like mine in the importance of physical fitness. I knew her participation in the writing of this book would enable me to cast my net wide and to draw together everything known about the midlife woman.

Most surprising to us was the discovery that while a great deal is known about women's reproductive health, knowledge about the many other aspects of our health is scanty at best. Further, most research on aging has been done *by* men and *with* men as its subjects. The country's longest-running study on aging, for example, has followed the normal aspects of aging in men since the 1950s. Not until twenty years into the project, at the end of the 1970s, were women included. "Women have been badly neglected in terms of studying the aging process," asserted the National Institute on Aging (NIA), now a sponsor of this research. "Neither the Legislative nor the Ex-

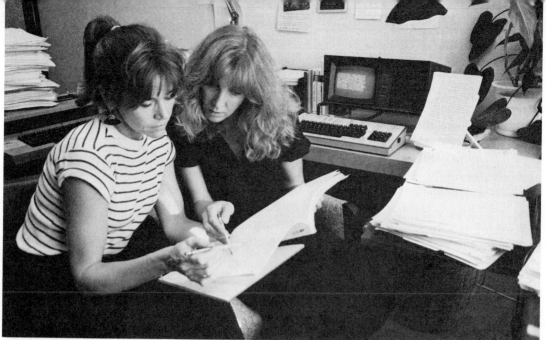

Me, Mignon, and our Kaypro computer at work on this book.

ecutive branch has made a comprehensive study of the problems of midlife women."

In spite of these first findings, we persisted and probed, reading everything we could get our hands on, going down many different paths. We began to come upon small pockets of new studies being done by dedicated researchers across the country, many of them midlife women themselves. In addition to this fledgling research, we met many individuals and groups of women who shared with us their frustrations and successes, their stories tragic and comic, and their hard-won understanding of this period in their lives.

The result is the book before you—and my new Workout program called Prime Time. Writing it has been my own way of preparing for midlife, embracing it *con gusto*. My hope is that it can help you to do the same.

2

NEW FRONTIER

*We who are older have nothing to lose! We have
everything to gain by living dangerously! We can be
the risk-takers, daring to challenge and change systems, policies, lifestyles, ourselves.*

Maggie Kuhn
Founder, Gray Panthers

TO BE A MIDLIFE WOMAN in our society is, in many respects, to be a
pioneer. The middle years of life for women represent virtually un-
charted territory—and it is those of us now in or approaching midlife who will draft its maps. We have to clear a path through the
debris of outworn yet still harmful myths that obscure the real
promise of this new period in our lives.

Few of us have anyone to point the way. None of the women who
peopled my earlier life shed any positive light on what was to come
at this later stage. My mother chose to take her own life when she
was younger than I am now. Her doctor told me that among the
many phantoms shadowing her world was the fear of youth's passing. Your mothers, like mine, may have also come upon these years
fearfully. Perhaps they were uncertain of the tools needed in this
new phase, which may have seemed to them the far edge of life.

We are the transition generation.

Those of us in midlife today are at the heart of a major redefini-
tion of "middle age" as the women before us have known it. For
those who will follow us, our daughters and their generation, the
middle years will be fundamentally transformed. What has been a
dreaded and shunned phase of life will become for them a highly
valued and productive time. For us, in the epicenter of this change,
a massive shift in our notion of midlife is already repositioning this
period from its former place near life's end to one vitally at life's
center.

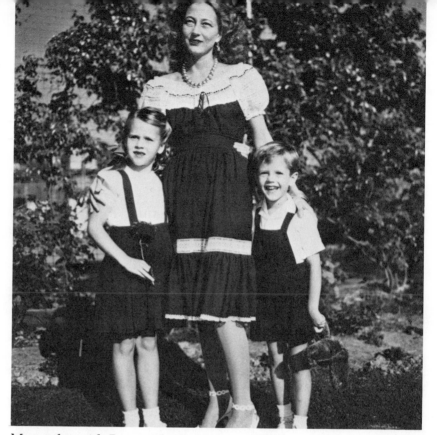

My mother with Peter and me. This was taken to send to Dad overseas during the war so he could have a recent photo of us.

When does midlife begin—at forty, at forty-five? Does it end at sixty, at sixty-five? Such numbers seem so arbitrary, so inadequate to account for all the variations experienced by individual people. And early midlife is clearly very different from later midlife. Mindful of these limitations, I have come to think of midlife as a diverse span of three decades—fifteen years on either side of menopause, which generally occurs around the age of fifty. I include ages thirty-five to thirty-nine because our bodies do begin to change even as early as thirty. These changes may not be visible in our early thirties, but if we can acknowledge them we will allow ourselves time to prepare, to ease ourselves more comfortably into the next stage.

But, oh, what cries of protest we hear from younger women who rebel at the thought that they can be considered middle-aged! And no wonder. Our society is not kind to women as we grow older. We've been prized for our ability to reproduce and for a sexual at-

NORMAN THAYER
Middle age means the middle, Ethel, the middle of life. People don't live to be a hundred and fifty.

ETHEL THAYER
We are at the far edge of middle age, that's all.

NORMAN
We're not, you know. We're not middle-aged. You're old and I'm ancient.

ETHEL
Oh, pooh. You're in your seventies and I'm in my sixties.

NORMAN
Just barely, on both counts.

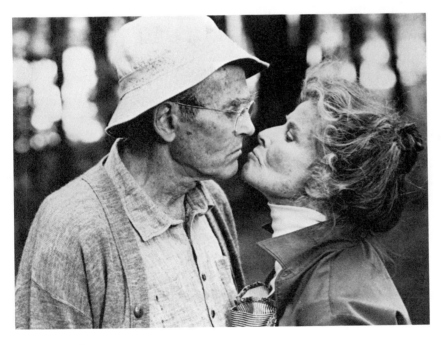

Henry Fonda
Katharine Hepburn
On Golden Pond

tractiveness based on youth. Hence, we've faced double trouble when, reaching midlife, we leave both youthful and fertile years behind. We've found ourselves to be healthy survivors in a culture that rejects us and that does not want our full participation.

THE MYTHS

Our generation inherits a whole mythology of aging that prescribes an early obsolescence for women, heaving us over the hill at forty, removing us from the flowing mainstream of life. We are to have no worthwhile contribution to make to our society. We are to believe it's too late to fulfill or to reshape our life's goals, whatever they may be. We are led to expect an inevitable and swift decline in our physical, psychological, and intellectual well-being which means becoming unhealthy, emotionally bereft, and mentally dull.

With this kind of future before her, a woman's fear of aging begins early. I've seen it close to home among the young girls who

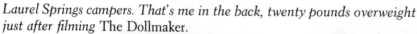

Laurel Springs campers. That's me in the back, twenty pounds overweight just after filming The Dollmaker.

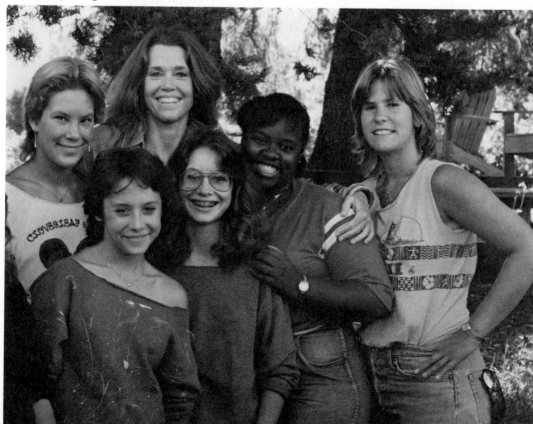

come to the children's camp Tom and I have run for the past eight years. Last summer when I said my age aloud amidst a group of campers, for example, several of the teenagers winced and whispered to me that I shouldn't let on how old I was because I didn't *look* forty-six. Of course, they viewed their advice as complimentary. I was tempted to respond with an updated version of Gloria Steinem's now-famous retort, *"This* is what forty-six looks like!"

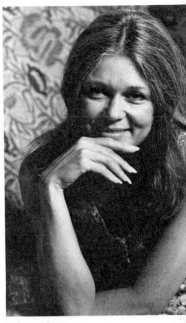

Gloria Steinem.

It saddened me that these young women already viewed midlife as something to hide from, believing they were at that moment in the best years of their lives. Yet, most of us probably wouldn't want to go back now to those earlier years. We prefer where we are today. I like being able to look back—at twenty-five-cent movies with news-reels, a world free of fast-food chains, an era with no TV when people actually talked to one another, a time when we respected and trusted our country's leadership and no child ever wondered if there would be a tomorrow.

I wouldn't want to give up these memories. Nor would I want to relinquish all I've learned along the way in exchange for being young again. By midlife, most of us know ourselves better, like ourselves better, understand our bodies and what pleases us better. We're more self-confident and less dependent on the approval of others. We're less inhibited and potentially feel ourselves to be more excit-ing sexual partners—and we seek that in others. But, my, isn't it a well-kept secret? And it will remain so as long as we unwittingly buy into society's negative attitudes, leaving the young ones no distant future to look forward to.

Often, the fear of being discarded for "younger models" in our jobs and in our relationships with men pressures us into denying our age—not only to others but to ourselves as well. But when we take up the exhausting burden of denying our age, we are also denying who we are. To the extent we succeed in passing as younger, we abandon where we've been. We rob ourselves of genuine pride in the years we've really lived. And we separate ourselves from the women who may show signs of aging more quickly, at a time when closeness with other women can give us strength, solace and valida-tion. Our lives end up consisting of three phases: being young, *pre-tending* to be young, and old age. The whole rich middle period is lost. As an actress, I can tell you Act Three can be pretty shaky when Act Two is missing.

A Double Standard

For a man, the middle years are his prime, a time when he is more likely to be at the peak of his career. His self-worth and his sexuality derive from his full participation in life. These are not tied to the state of his physical being or, more narrowly, to his reproductive organs as they are for us. His attractiveness is not in question. His sexuality is above suspicion.

While a woman's face, like her body, is valued as long as it remains smooth and unchanging, a man's lines are the product of experience. The changes in his appearance become *additions* to who he is as a person, whereas those same changes in us become *liabilities*. Paul Newman gets silver hair and becomes distinguished. I get gray hair and am told I'd best dye it. My pal Redford gets furrows and character lines. I get wrinkles and crow's feet. It ain't fair!

SALLY FORTH — by Greg Howard

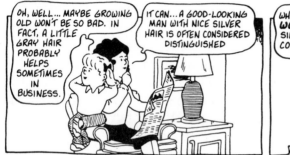
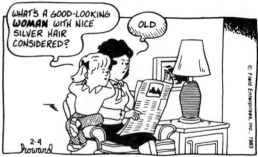

Cultural Missing Persons

For me, as a film actress, middle-age holds a special set of challenges and anxieties. What I have to offer in my work is not at all separate from me, as would be the case if my talents lay in some other field like sculpting or medicine or management. My creative "product" is my very self—the characters and emotions I create with my body, my face, my eyes, my hands. What you see is what you get. This puts me in a precarious position at age forty-six, since until quite recently American producers and writers have seemed to think that American audiences don't want to see a woman with wrinkles, at least not in a leading screen role where she might be re-

24

quired to be sexual and dynamic and where her character would be pivotal.

In the world of movies and television, the most important image-making institutions of our society, active, strong, independent midlife women have been virtually invisible. We've been cultural missing persons. The Screen Actor's Guild (SAG) helped to document this after a ten-year study in the 1970s of prime time and children's weekend television programming: positive portrayals of women begin to disappear from television as women reach forty. The presence of powerful, sophisticated, sexy men over forty, on the other hand, begins to increase. Most women on TV are *under thirty;* most men *over thirty-five!* (How often do we see an older man paired with an older woman?) Our absence in the media only serves to deepen an already ominous view of aging in the minds of our children and ourselves. The heaviest TV-viewers, SAG found, are the most likely to believe that women become old very early in life and to think there are few older persons in general in our society! On television, SAG concluded, "A man is for all seasons, but a woman only for spring."

Well, I'm autumn and I'm mad! Several options are open to me. I can retire. Or, I can attempt to maintain the image of "an attractive woman in her late thirties"—I get offered a lot of those. Or I can own up to the fact that I don't really want to go backwards. I'm not interested in playing younger women even if I *could* be made to look that age. I would find it constricting to have to bring myself back to my thirties. I want to play *my own age,* with everything that means. I'm interested in the character of women who are where I am now.

Those of us who are midlife actresses have to forge new identities, and at the same time convince those same writers and directors, the ones who see only pre–thirty-five, that there are *a lot* of midlife women out there who would flock to see good films about women of their age.

Fortunately, many of us who are mature actresses have already become producers. This increases the likelihood that we will be the first generation of actresses to give a cultural face and voice to midlife women, correcting society's blind spot, proclaiming via the mass media, the creator of the popular consciousness, that there does indeed exist a vibrant, sensual, appealing, *lined* woman's face between

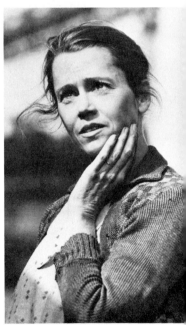

Me as Gertie Nevels in The Dollmaker, *the realization of a twelve-year dream that began when I first read Harriet Arnow's novel.*

the prettiness of youth and the special beauty and character of a woman in her seventies and eighties.

TURNING POINTS

All of the myths and misperceptions about middle-aged women in this society are on a collision course with new realities. Some may already be familiar to you:

- There are more of us than ever before.

- We're entering the middle years physically stronger than ever before.

- And all of this is occurring at the same time that women of all ages are reexamining their place in society and discovering the real potentials that exist for them.

Growing Strong

We have reached a period of unprecedented transformation in our society. We are moving from a culture of mostly young people to one whose majority consists of midlife and older people. There are also more women than men. Consider these points:

1. People born during the baby boom following World War II are now entering their middle years. *Forty million* of them are women.

2. Because young people are having fewer babies, the middle-aged represent a larger and larger *proportion* of our society. Midlife women alone are approaching a remarkable 20 percent of the *entire* population, giving us the potential for enormous influence in the marketplace, in politics, and in society as a whole—far into the twenty-first century.

3. Midlife and older people, with women in the majority, are not only the largest, but the *fastest growing* segment of American society. This flourishing group will represent over 50 percent of the population by the turn of the century.

4. In this country a woman born in 1900 was expected to live to be about forty-seven, the age I am now. At that time, life's midpoint was less than age twenty-five. The lives of most of us then would have ended *during* our reproductive years. Today, the average woman is expected to live to age seventy-eight, the average man seventy-one—an increase of thirty years for most of us!

5. Because of improved nutrition, sanitation and health care, people are living longer everywhere. The aging of the American population is only part of a global phenomenon that will mean a *doubling* of the number of people over sixty worldwide in just twenty years.

6. Excellent health is now possible well into our old age. Many of the chronic diseases and physical disabilities we now encounter when we survive into our later years are *not* the inevitable companions of aging and are for the most part *preventable*.

7. Although we still do not know why women continue to outlive men, we do know that we have longer, healthier lives. We must challenge the cultural assumption that we're supposed to become old around the midpoint of our lives.

Not so long ago, the outer limit of middle age was considered to be around fifty, coinciding with the average age of menopause. Now, midlife is commonly thought of as a much longer time period—extending years beyond menopause. And menopause, while still a central event, is no longer the single determining factor it once was. It takes its place alongside the other equally powerful dimensions of a woman's midlife, which now spans the last of the childbearing years and the beginning of the postreproductive years.

Most of us will have one-third of our lives left to live after menopause.

This fact, among others, is shaking up the tradition we're heir to—of womanhood based foremost on fertility and motherhood.

Our childbearing years make up *less than half* of our life span and the years we actually spend with children at home much, much less than that. This new reality should enable a woman to see herself whole, not defined solely by her uterus or by her relationship to children or to a partner. An expanded midlife may mean expanded identities as well.

Changing Roles, New Risks

Like many of you, I grew up in the 1950s, a time of very prescribed and limited roles for women. The "feminine mystique" was at its peak after World War II when many of our generation married. We learned an idealized version of family life in this decade of togetherness and "Momism," neither of which necessarily translated into the real joys of mothering or true family closeness.

Though women, in fact, began increasingly to work outside the home, we were supposed to be perfect mothers and dedicated homemakers—exclusively. Marriage was to be the pivotal, preeminent event in a woman's life. I recall a sense of being out of it as I approached the end of my sophomore year in college when, unlike so many of my friends, I had no engagement ring on my finger and no subscription to *Bride's* magazine. I was frequently a bridesmaid at the weddings of my friends and, though a wiser inner voice told me to wait, I often feared I'd be doomed to a lonely life on the fringe, with little chance of winning the security, normalcy and other expected rewards of marriage.

In those days, if we prepared at all for our futures, it was only for the first half of our lives. We were raised as though life stopped at forty, after which everything was somehow just an incomprehensible blur. We thought a lot about getting married, but not a lot about what happened after that. The roles of wife and mother, of which we had only a vague but glorified notion, were to last for life. And the concept of women influencing their society was totally foreign. For me at least, the idea that a woman could change anything was limited to diapers, linens and the furniture arrangement.

I'll wager most of us assumed that by our early forties we would own our own homes, send our husbands off to work every morning,

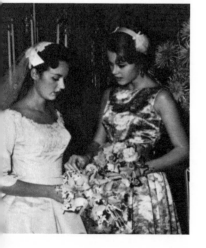

That's me on the right as a bridesmaid.

and be helping our daughters or daughters-in-law through their first pregnancies. But now, through massive transformations in the family and in marriage, only the exception fits this mold of lifelong wifehood and motherhood—though the stereotype understandably persists in our minds as the norm. Today only one family in six fits our long-held concept of the American nuclear family—a working, breadwinning father and a full-time homemaking mother, raising two or more children.

Now, *well over half* of women in midlife work outside the home and more of us are supporting our families, with or without partners. More of us are also facing a greater part of our lives on our own—one out of four midlife women is single. Many of us who married early will have divorced or separated by the time we enter our midlife—one out of three marriages, at the least, now ends in divorce. Some of us will experience the death of our partner as we move toward the later years. And some of us will delay marrying until midlife or decide not to marry at all. Whatever the circumstances, being single in midlife is an increasingly commonplace and accepted way of life.

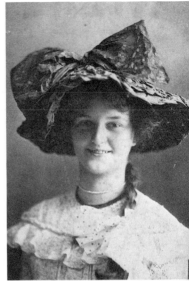

My maternal grandma, Sophie Seymour, as a young girl.

These new patterns of marriage and singlehood bring new patterns of mothering too. More women are arriving at midlife as single mothers raising their children alone—most with fragile financial resources, 30 percent with incomes *below* the poverty line. Women are also having their children later, which means a longer period of mothering in midlife. Women like myself who waited until their thirties to have children will still be raising them in midlife. I will probably be in my early fifties before my first child leaves home. My maternal grandmother already had teenaged grandchildren at that age.

Just decades ago, women expected their lives to be very much like those of their friends and contemporaries. Now, given the assemblage of paths before us, we're infinitely more diverse, as varied as the colors of leaves in autumn. I see this in the many midlife women I talk with across the country—like Doris, a forty-year-old woman from Cleveland who told me, "I've been working since I was twenty and never felt I could afford to take time off till now to have a child. I'm about to have my first." Or Mary, a never-married single woman in her mid-thirties, about to make a major move in careers and also to buy her own home in Los Angeles. "I never thought it would

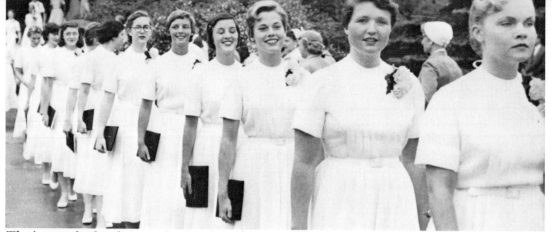

That's me, third in line, graduating from Emma Willard School in Troy, New York. (I designed the dresses.)

happen this way," she said. "But I've saved up and finally am about to realize the dream of having my own place." Or my friend Susan in New York, a woman in her fifties who has just become a new grandmother and also recently launched a new business as an art dealer. "I decided to turn my apartment into a gallery for women's paintings. I love being on my own."

We are not who we were prepared to be in the 1950s— neither is the world the one we expected. "We're becoming the men we always wanted to marry," says my friend Steinem. A broader vision of what it means to be a woman in this society is taking form—just look, on the political frontier, to the history-making nomination of a woman, Congresswoman Geraldine Ferraro, for Vice President of the United States. The notion of a woman's place will never be the same.

Nothing has prepared us for the profound potential in these immense changes. And nothing has prepared us for the possible pain that may be inflicted by the reshaping of the traditional contours of marriage and family. Nevertheless, we're emerging at midlife strengthened, with a new sense of ourselves.

We are learning that developing new roles within and outside of marriage, beyond the strictures of the "feminine mystique," may be good for us—critical to both our psychological and physical health. "The more women become involved away from the household," says the National Institute on Aging, "the better they are doing." Our entry into the world of work, outside the home, is perhaps among the most important elements of our changing status and our changing well-being.

Nine-to-Five

It was women over thirty-five who broke the barriers against married women working outside the home when they entered the paid work force in large numbers during the Second World War. Since that time, midlife women have played an increasingly important role in the American economy. Now nearly 60 percent of us are employed and half of all women who work outside the home are in their middle and later years.

Work has become a large, important part of our lives. Most of us will spend at least *thirty years* in the paid labor force—longer by far than we spend raising our children, longer than we may spend in our marriages. Even with interruptions of our paid employment due to childraising responsibilities, a woman's overall money-earning work life will average only ten years less than a man's. It requires the same planning and care as any other central aspect of our lives—and the determination to succeed in spite of obstacles.

At my office. I don't like desks.

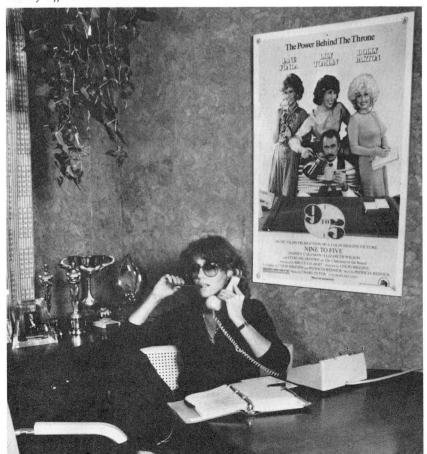

The myths we encounter as women in midlife follow us into our work lives. Still commonplace, for example, is the erroneous belief that achievement and productivity, so fundamental to a man's sense of well-being and happiness, are for us not so important. A midlife woman's work outside the home has been perceived as "busywork" to compensate for too much time on her hands, even though, as for men, the *overriding* reason most of us enter the work force is economic. We've been encouraged not to take our jobs seriously as careers or as life goals, but rather to view them as superfluous transitory activities. We've been taught to conspire against ourselves by developing blind spots when it comes to recognizing our own very real accomplishments in the world of work—outside *or* inside the home.

These harmful misperceptions translate to more tangible difficulties when women try to enter or re-enter the job market during their middle years. As early as thirty-five, a woman is likely to meet up with the Dracula Complex of business—the need for fresh, that is, young, blood. In spite of existing age discrimination laws, this tendency permeates hiring *and* promotion practices, telling us that as workers, we're already old. Midlife women, like all working women, also remain a cheap labor pool for business—last hired in good economic times and first fired in hard times—concentrated in dead-end occupations, such as clerical and service work that traditionally offers only the lowest pay. According to the U.S. Department of Commerce, a midlife woman still earns *less* than her male counterpart in a comparable job with comparable experience even when she's taken no time out to raise children. True to the double standard, a man's salary stays on an upward slope throughout his life while a woman's slides downward, and the two levels never even intersect because he starts out higher. A young woman who begins her work life making 76 cents to a man's dollar will end it as an older woman making 53 cents to his dollar—*barely over half of what her male equivalent earns.*

Getting Better

Yet, notwithstanding the continuing barriers to real equal-employment opportunities, midlife women are in the work force to stay. Our increasing presence and contribution in the economic arena will better fortify us to change the negative working conditions for women and ultimately for men as well. And working outside the home appears to be beneficial to our overall well-being. It was expected that exposure to the stress of the workplace would be harmful, but the reverse has been the case for women. Since the 1960s, for example, our rate of heart disease, the most notorious of stress-related illnesses, has *decreased* rather than increased, even though our numbers in the paid labor force are higher than ever.

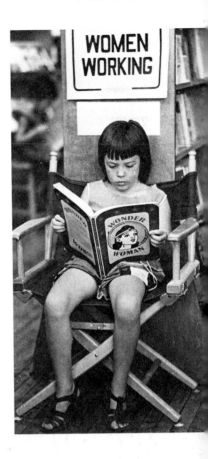

In a small Massachusetts town called Framingham, nearly half the population has been involved for decades in one of the most unique ongoing heart studies in the country. A group of midlife women were followed for a period of ten years to observe the health effects of working. The study found that women who had worked outside their homes for more than half their adult lives were *not* significantly more likely to develop heart disease than women who worked inside the home. The report went further. If any vulnerability to stress in the workplace does exist for midlife women, it appears to lie not in working itself but rather in the *kinds* of work women do. The clerical and sales worker was found to be subject to the most stress of all midlife women working outside the home—not the professional white-collar or even blue-collar worker who might have greater relative freedom of movement or responsibility. The clerical worker who also had children at home was the most likely of all to develop a stress-related problem. Juggling job, housekeeping, the mothering responsibilities more often than not remains the woman's problem alone rather than one shared with a partner, an employer, or policymaker. Our country's criminal negligence in the area of child care leaves the working mother doing double duty— and probably overtime—to make sure bills are paid and food is on the table.

Amazingly, with all these pressures, employed women in general are still more likely to report their health as excellent or good. Women who are exclusively homemakers, on the other hand, seem to experience more chronic illnesses like allergies, asthma, ulcers, and diabetes. All of the evidence so far says we're getting better as our spheres of activity and self-determination enlarge.

According to several important studies, there has also been an unprecedented increase over the last thirty years in the psychological well-being of midlife women. In 1975 the National Center for

Health Statistics reported extraordinary improvements in the mental health of women over forty, compared with an earlier study in 1960. In another example, the Midtown Manhattan Study of midlife women in New York back in the 1950s reported over 20 percent as "psychologically impaired." Remarkably, the same research repeated twenty years later in the 1970s found only 8 percent with psychological difficulties. (During this same time, the mental health problems of men remained unchanged at 9 percent.)

This is good news! Previously, serious depression was considered to be part and parcel of women's growing older. Now this frightening specter is lifting. Of course, some midlife women still experience depression, as women may at any time of life. We spoke about this with therapist Randi Gunther, a woman in her forties who also sees many women of our age in her practice. Dr. Gunther believes that depression in midlife occurs when a woman begins to feel acutely the *limits* in her life, especially in regard to the traditional roles. We may feel an important sense of satisfaction and mastery in the private realm of motherhood and marriage, she explained, "but there's so much of us left over after what the expectation is that women don't know where to go with who they are."

Abiding by what she thought was her part in the social contract, the woman who has chosen the traditional route exclusively is apt to experience a great deal of difficulty when her children leave home, or when her marriage is no longer intact—or both. A woman who has singlemindedly devoted herself to mothering, for example, is more likely to feel deeply bereft at the departure of her children during midlife—left with what, regrettably, has been called "the empty nest." With her life's sole anchor gone, this woman may feel completely adrift, without direction. Rather than experiencing this transition positively, with the important task of nurturing com-

---

It's not responsibility that kills, it's the lack of control. The driver isn't under as much pressure as the passengers.

Estelle Ramey, M.D.
Professor of Physiology and Biophysics
Georgetown University Medical School

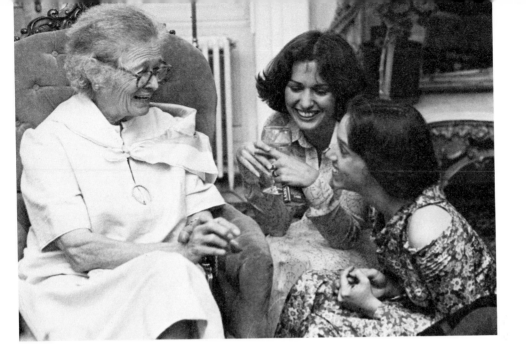

pleted and the possibility emerging of new, more mature relationships with her children, family and friends, she feels at a dead end, with no confidence that she can begin to define her future. At any age, what the traditional homemaker may share with the clerical working mother is the heightened vulnerability that comes from a lack of power or from the hurtful limits of their assigned roles.

Everything is telling us that breaking the boundaries of these old limits, when possible, and taking charge of our lives is in our best interest. As one role contracts, another may expand. And the new risks bring with them new rewards, giving us a strong degree of protection against the myths of aging that have assigned impossible, unsatisfying scripts to mature women and—ultimately—to mature men as well.

Ours is the first generation of women to be better prepared for midlife. Our consciousness about ourselves is changing. We've got the numbers, the health, and the knowledge to make us better able to meet whatever difficulties this phase may bring. We're in a stronger position than ever to seize its many opportunities as well—daring to fail, daring to excel. Our actions, like stones tossed into a pond, will ripple to every inlet of society. As we shape our own futures, positively, so do we help to transform the experience that is midlife.

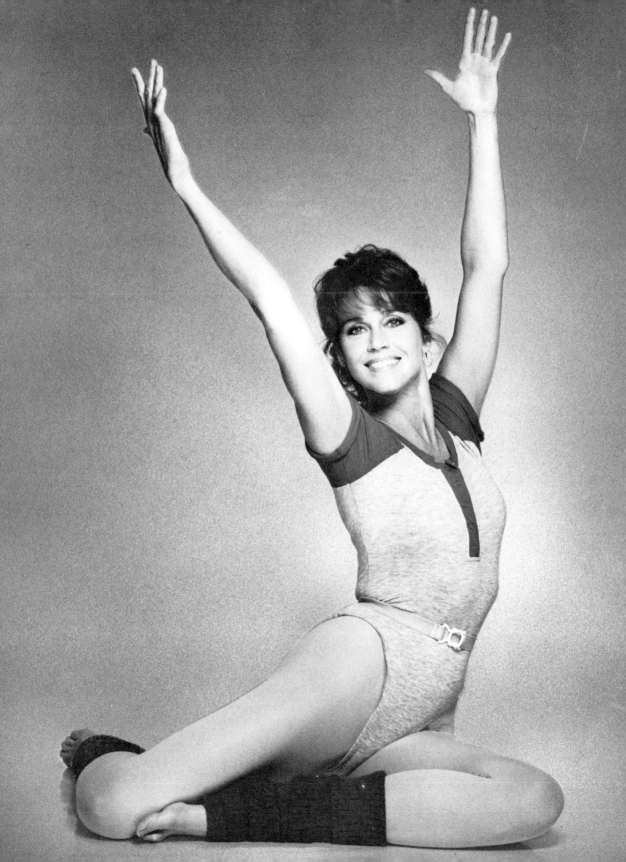

PART TWO
The Body Mature

CHAPTER 3

THE PROCESS OF AGING

SOMEWHERE IN OUR THIRTIES AND FORTIES we begin to come face-to-face with our own aging. My knees talk back to me now after a strenuous hike. I know I risk straining the tendons in my hips if I do especially vigorous aerobics when I'm tired or not wearing support-ive cushioned shoes. The skin around my eyes will be lined and slightly swollen after a night of partying or a fat-rich dinner, things for which I would not have had to pay a price only a few years back. I remember walking through my kitchen early one morning and see-ing reflected in the chrome of my toaster the face of a haggard, puffy-eyed, *definitely* no-longer-youthful person. "Who's that?" I started to wonder, till with shock I realized it was me.

We've all had those moments—coming upon ourselves unpre-pared, seeing ourselves at our worst in instants of nonrecognition—signs of the inevitable that slowly accumulate until we are forced to confront that we are getting on.

In all my probings of the biological reasons for getting older, I've found that the process of aging is, to a large degree, *negotiable*. The point we all need to grasp, finally, is that we have considerable room to modify our experience of aging. Genetics plays a part. The chro-nology of our years can't be changed. But these are only two among many factors that determine just how we age and how long we live. The disease and the decrepitude that have previously made the idea of aging intolerable are *not* inevitable. Rather, they are often the re-sult of the *misuse* and the *disuse* of our bodies.

For better or worse, all that's come before begins to add up in midlife—our eating habits, our exercise patterns, whether we smoke, the way we've generally lived our lives. If we've been living in the fast lane, ignoring our own physical and psychological needs, we'll be aging in the fast lane as well, speeding toward the stereotype of declining vitality in midlife.

But rarely is it too late to switch tracks. We each have the ability to *slow* the aging process. It's even possible that we can physically *improve* with age. If we're not at our maximum level of fitness, which few of us are, there is actually room to make ourselves healthier and in some cases stronger than in our early adulthood. As one scientist observed, we may literally have to "swim against the current of senescence" in our own bodies, but getting better with time is not a myth. The performances of athletic, artistic, and intellectual champions in their forties, fifties, sixties and beyond—Katharine Hepburn, Billie Jean King, Lillian Hellman, Margaret Mead and Martha Graham, to name a few—give us a measure of what's possible.

The potential for a long vigorous life exists for each of us if we choose it. What I hope to provide for you is the wherewithal to intervene in your own behalf with the downward slope of aging. Negotiating a better deal for yourself, as any lawyer worth her salt would advise, requires familiarizing yourself with the basics. Some aspects of the aging process are nonnegotiable, but most will yield—to realistic strategies of nutrition and exercise.

WHAT IS AGING?

Very simply, aging means that over time our bodies gradually lose their reserves, the capacity to cope with constant stimuli and change, to maintain equilibrium despite the body's internal and external demands. A thirty-year-old will bounce back fast from a cold, for instance, but a sixty-year-old will recover more slowly. As we age, there is a decline, however slow, in how well our bodies are able to keep everything in balance—true even for the most fit among us. This needn't mean we actually experience this as an ebbing away of vitality. Remember, we're talking about reserves, the play of the system. If we keep ourselves healthy, we'll also feel healthy well into midlife and beyond. Eventually, at the far end of our lives, the reserve capacity of our bodies will drop below the level necessary to sustain us. Of course, a serious disease or sudden accident can always stop everything prematurely. If we live to an old, old age, however, there will be a point when our measure of vitality will not be sufficient to meet life's challenges, from sudden changes in weather to a lingering viral infection, all the expected and unexpected events that in earlier years would have placed no extraordinary stress upon us. The process of aging will then be completed.

This change in our reserve capacity begins early, roughly between the ages of twenty-five and thirty. Up to this time, the body's ongoing processes of breakdown and renewal essentially equal each other. After young adulthood, this balance shifts. The body's rate of self-restoration begins to lag behind the normal damage that occurs inside our cells. Abnormal damage, such as that caused by smoking or toxins in the air, water, and food, can widen this gap even further. Aging begins with a growing deficit of repair work to be done.

What causes this to happen? An *exact* answer continues to elude us. Some researchers believe we may have an "aging clock" that signals the aging process to begin, a programmed message possibly in the brain or maybe coded genetically into the body's trillions and trillions of cells. Finding such a clock would mean scientists might be able to reset it. But even the likelihood of its existence remains an unknown.

That awesome possibility aside, most aging experts now believe there may be *many* causes of aging, none of which offers a complete explanation in and of itself. We appear to age as the result of a number of different overlapping aging mechanisms that have relatively random beginnings in the tiniest parts of ourselves—the cells of the body.

The cell is the basic unit of life that constitutes the major tissues and organs of the body. Surrounded by its own membrane, every cell is bathed in water and needs oxygen and food to function. At any one time, some cells are old, some new, some in need of repair, some in mint condition. Each has its own age and will renew itself at its own rate.

Some of our body's cells, like those of the skin, are forever new. They divide and replace themselves over and over throughout our lives. Another type of cell does the same, but only intermittently and slowly, possibly dividing only fifty times during our lifetime. These are the cells found, for example, in the tendons, ligaments, and cartilage of the joints. Then there are the cells that are never replaced but, instead, continuously repair and regenerate themselves from birth onward. These are the longest-lived cells in the body, located in the muscles, heart, brain, nerves, and kidneys. "Such an old cell is very much like an old city," according to one lyrical gerontologist. "Whereas the town as a whole may go back centuries, most of its buildings have been destroyed and reconstructed many times."

At any time during the life span of a cell, the opportunity exists for our bodies to generate healthy new cells naturally or to improve old ones. This, in fact, is largely why we can intervene positively in the aging process. Still, over time these miniature biological factories will undergo changes that we can only slow down or postpone. Ultimately, several kinds of damage begin to occur which alter the internal structure and operation of the cell. These changes determine when and how our bodies age.

Biological Errors

The scientific technicalities I want to talk about next may be difficult to wade through, but please bear with me here. The more you understand the underlying mechanisms of aging, the more you'll understand and be motivated to accept the program that I want to present later in this book.

One of the major causes of aging is believed to be a matter of haphazard, genetic errors taking place inside the cell. These microscopic mistakes pile up, cascading eventually into an avalanche of cellular flaws and, therefore, an increasing number of imperfect cells in the body.

This phenomenon involves two of the most important molecules of life located in the nucleus of every cell: DNA (deoxyribonucleic acid), which stores the master blueprint for the whole body, and RNA (ribonucleic acid), which translates DNA's thousands and thousands of programmed orders to the cell. DNA's directives may become blurred over time. Chemical misunderstandings may occur as the genetic message is transcribed from DNA into RNA, and then from RNA into the body's enzymes and other proteins—the raw building and repair materials of the body. Something gets lost in this chain of protein synthesis or manufacture, just as the copy of a copy of a copy loses the sharp definition of the original.

Normally, the cell can repair such errors. But its ability to repair itself well begins to be affected, and at the same time other kinds of damage may overload the whole repair apparatus. Because of all of this, it becomes more difficult for the increasingly vulnerable cell to utilize life-sustaining nutrients and to eliminate its waste products. The cell eventually loses its capacity to maintain or re-create itself in its ideal form.

Biochemical Handcuffing

Another related and important aging mechanism also affects the healthy operation of the cell. With age, there is a tendency for unwanted chemical bondings to take place between chains of molecules outside the cell in the body's abundant connective tissues—the fibrous proteins that provide the scaffolding for every cell and that make up the largest part of our skin, blood vessels, cartilage, tendons and ligaments.

It's normal and in fact necessary for cross-links to form in connective tissue as we're growing up. These bonds are essential in providing structure and strength, while also preserving tissue elasticity. It appears that as we age, however, there is a tendency for the process of cross-linking to continue. Strands of connective tissue become increasingly bound together and, as a result, more rigid and inelastic. The signs of this biological handcuffing gradually emerge in the progressive wrinkling of the skin, stiffening of joints, loss of muscle elasticity, and impaired eye focus. In addition to these classic features of aging, the tiny capillaries leading to the cells become strangled by the tightening tissues around them and the blood vessels themselves become increasingly rigid. The easy flow of oxygen, water, and other nutrients to the cells is thus impeded and, slowly, we begin to lose healthy cells.

Our knowledge of why cross-linking continues as we age is incomplete. It is believed to occur largely as an indirect result of oxidation, the chemical process of oxygen combining with other elements. We can see the effects of oxidation all around us when iron rusts, rubber cracks, and butter goes rancid. Inside our bodies, unseen by us, oxidation occurs every minute of every day. It's an essential aspect of metabolism. But oxygen is both boon and bane. The oxidative process is known to sometimes generate highly reactive by-products that can cause the undesirable chemical bonds of cross-linking—in connective tissues, as we just discussed, and possibly also within the cell itself, resulting in the kind of cellular errors believed to be involved in aging. These destructive substances randomly produced by internal oxidation can also damage the cell membrane.

The body has strong natural defenses against such abnormal oxidation. We have several built-in enzymes that work exclusively both to prevent and to repair its harmful effects. Sometimes, however, these protective enzymes are unable to keep up with the rate of damage, especially so if abnormal oxidation is accelerated by environmental oxidants coming from outside of the body—cigarette smoke, air pollution, pesticides, radioactivity, and excessive exposure to the sun and to alcohol.

Antioxidants

To a certain extent we may be able to slow down the effects of abnormal oxidation, giving our bodies a chance to catch up on repair. I want to leap ahead for a moment, while all of this is still fresh in our minds, to talk about some of the first steps. One obvious place to start is *to avoid environmental toxins as much as we can.* Another may be *to emphasize certain nutrients in our daily diets.* The National Institute on Aging (NIA) has expressed the need for more information on how nutrition may be used *therapeutically,* if at all, to slow the aging process. Nutritionists are finding, for example, that particular vitamins, minerals, and amino acids play a protective role against the unwanted internal oxidation and cross-linking I've just described. These substances inhibit such oxidation in various ways but principally by allowing themselves to be oxidized in the place of vital cells and tissues. We've seen such antioxidants at work in grapefruits that don't go brown once cut or in raisins that remain edible for long periods of time. The natural vitamin C of these fruits protects them from the oxygen in the air which normally causes fresh food to decay.

Everyday nutrients known to be antioxidants include vitamins C and E—the most potent—as well as the B vitamins thiamine (B_1), pantothenic acid (B_5), and pyridoxine (B_6), the bioflavonoids, and the minerals zinc and selenium, which enhance the action of E and C. Selenium, in fact, is an essential part of one of the antioxidant enzymes.

Vitamin E is thought to be the best antioxidant vitamin. It helps to protect the all-important membrane of every body cell from the damage of oxidation. This membrane is the cell's first defense barrier and gatekeeper, admitting all nutrients and hormones, expelling all waste products. If oxidation occurs, holes can develop in this cellular envelope, impairing its function and causing the cell to leak, shrink, and eventually to collapse.

Second only to vitamin E in its antioxidant effects is *vitamin C.* Both vitamin C and vitamin E act to enhance each other's effectiveness.

Are we to conclude that significantly increasing our intake of the antioxidants would intervene positively in the aging process? Some nutritionists believe so; others strongly disagree. The fact is that we don't yet know for certain. Until we do, I believe we should at minimum be sure these nutrients are abundant in the food we eat, since their presence may help to minimize the aging effects of oxidation and to reinforce the body's own internal defenses and ability to repair itself.

Fresh foods are full of the antioxidant vitamins and minerals. So eat plenty of vegetables, fruits, and unprocessed whole grains. It is also a good idea to cut down your intake of the polyunsaturated fats like vegetable oils. While not implicated in heart disease the way saturated fats are, polyunsaturated fats can increase the internal process of oxidation and therefore should be consumed sparingly. A well-balanced diet low in *all* fats is always best for us. (See the chapter called "Eating for the Long Run," to read more on these nutritional topics.)

WHAT TO EXPECT

Aging occurs unevenly in different people, just as it does in the different cells within. Each of us goes through the process in our own way and at our own pace. The aging changes to our cells slowly translate to larger changes in the tissues, organs, and systems of the body. These parts of the body will become, accordingly, less efficient over time, which means more energy will be required to carry out normal functions and to maintain the body's vital balance. The specifics of how this manifests itself, and when, is difficult if not impossible to chart. It's relatively easy to predict physical changes in children at certain ages, but by midlife the full range of who we are, physically and otherwise, is infinitely more complex. As the first head of the NIA remarked, "[Biologically] a group of ten-year-old children will not vary much from child to child, but in an eighty- or ninety-year-old the variance is just tremendous."

Keeping the possibility of vast differences in mind, let's begin to look at the effects of aging by outlining several general aging markers that all of us can expect sometime down the line. These are pretty much the *nonnegotiable* aspects of normal aging.

- The *hair* begins to thin and to lose its pigment, turning gray and eventually becoming white at a pace largely determined by heredity.
- The *skin* begins to lose its elasticity.
- The *eyes* can't focus as well on things close up.
- The walls of the *blood vessels* become more rigid.
- The *cartilage* of the joints begins to lose water.
- The *kidneys* filter out foreign material from the blood more slowly.

From this point, every other aspect of the aging process becomes less predictable. It will be easier to proceed by talking about what aging is *not* or doesn't have to be—and the things that can make a difference.

- **Aging is not a straight downhill dive after thirty,** a message I hope I've already imparted.

Members of the U.S. rowing team.

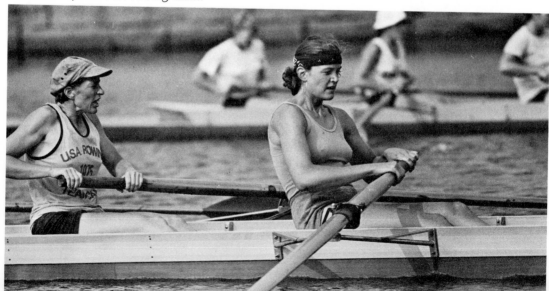

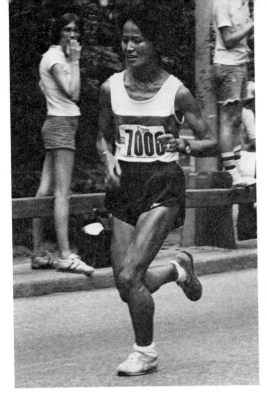

Miki Gorman set the over-40 record in the marathon in 1976.

There are changes to the active tissue of our muscles which can mean a slowing down of *metabolism*, hence an increase of fat tissue. And there are changes to our musculoskeletal system that affect our *joints, our backs and our bones*. And there are changes to our *skin*, in addition to the loss of elasticity.

There are also changes in the *digestion, absorption, and ultilization* of nutrients, as well as the *excretion* of waste products. There are changes to the *cardiorespiratory system*, the *nervous system*, and the *immune system*. Those to the immune system may themselves be a cause of aging.

All of these changes, the tendency toward lowered efficiency and decreased function, can be minimized by a program of good nutrition combined with consistent regular activity.

There is now firm evidence that shows a striking similarity between those changes normally associated with aging and those caused by inactivity—a phenomenon I can't emphasize enough. A leg immobilized in a cast will appear to age *forty years*—in just six weeks! The bones shrink, the muscles atrophy, the skin thins, and the circulation slows. A leg exercised, on the other hand, will show just the reverse of these effects. The bones get stronger, the muscles are strengthened, the skin thickens, and the circulation improves. What this so eloquently tells us is that if we *use it*, we don't have to lose it. Our bodies are not like machines that wear out from use. Rather, the dynamic organs and tissues of our bodies have the extraordinary ability to adapt to challenge. When we use them, when we ask them to do work, they develop an increase in function in a way that can significantly counter the changes that occur with growing older—no matter what our age.

• **Aging is not a loss of intelligence or the beginning of senility.** One of the greatest gains in the science of aging has been to shatter the myth of senility as the inevitable and normal consequence of aging. Even though we seldom expect senility in midlife, that's when we usually begin to start worrying about it.

The twelve billion nerve cells of the brain and nervous system are irreplaceable and as susceptible as any others in the body to the internal cellular changes and cross-linking that I have described. But the widely held belief that we experience steady attrition of brain cells, with a corresponding decline in intelligence and memory, has been effectively challenged.

The aging brain doesn't become exhausted. To the contrary, like a muscle, the brain has to be exercised. Mental sweat is good for its health. The brain, in fact, uses a great deal of energy, accounting for one quarter of our body's basal metabolism. With age, our learning ability can remain intact. We can actually become better at thinking conceptually. Where we may experience a change is in the speed of transmitting messages throughout the nervous system. This can mean a slowing down in our reaction time and maybe even memory time by about 15 percent by the time we're in our seventies or eighties, but it does not mean we are any less intelligent.

Regarding senility itself, only four percent of women and men over the age of sixty-five develop what would be called *real* senility. When it does occur, senility results largely from the serious confusion and forgetfulness caused by Alzheimer's disease or from small localized strokes that block the flow of blood to the brain—and sometimes a combination of both. Unfortunately, many older persons are misdiagnosed as senile. Other conditions can produce a pseudosenility or change in mental ability that mimics true senility: depression, a less vigorous blood and oxygen supply due to poor circulation, and the tendency for fewer key brain chemicals (called neurotransmitters) to be produced with age. Each of these conditions, if discovered, is treatable.

• **Aging is not a disease.** The changes that take place as we grow older are a normal part of life. But there does exist a relationship between aging and disease that is important to know about. The chronic diseases associated with the middle and later years are really examples of the aging process out of control. Such illnesses as heart disease, cancer, diabetes, and cirrhosis all have multiple causes and usually begin inside us years before they surface. Each involves a lessening of organ function and reserves that's similar to that of aging, but vastly accelerated.

Let's take a look at what happens to the heart, lungs, and blood-vessel network, one of the most complex systems of the body. I don't choose this example randomly. Though on the decline, heart disease is still our country's number one killer (number two for mid-life women, number one for older women). Also, how well the cardiorespiratory system functions is one of the best clues to our overall fitness, and it is a system of the body upon which we can have a major effect. Understanding its importance, including what can go wrong, is essential to understanding the importance of aerobic exercise.

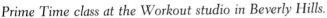

Prime Time class at the Workout studio in Beverly Hills.

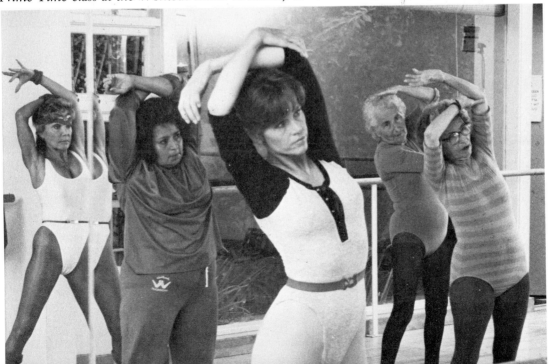

49

The cardiorespiratory system is our pipeline to the cells. It is responsible for delivering blood, which contains oxygen and nutrients, to every cell in the body and for carrying away carbon dioxide and other waste products. It supplies the muscles with the oxygen essential for burning calories for energy. It forms the basis of our aerobic power, usually called our *maximum breathing capacity,* or more colloquially in athletic circles, our "VO_2max" (V for volume, O_2 for oxygen). This is one of the most critical measures of our body's performance—how much oxygen we take in, how much blood is pumped and with what degree of ease throughout the body, and how well oxygen is taken up and utilized by the muscles and other cells of the body. These dynamics are the master key to our vitality.

With age the heart, lungs, and circulatory system gradually begin to lose some of their efficiency. After thirty, there is an average decline of about one percent a year in our maximum breathing capacity. The lungs hold and expel less air and become less elastic. The heart muscle thickens and becomes more rigid, as does the whole blood-vessel network. Each stroke of the heart pumps less blood. Hardened and narrowed arterial passageways cause the heart to work harder to move blood from the chest to the head, arms and legs. As the heart pushes the blood more forcefully through the circulatory network, our blood pressure tends to rise.

All of this is normal and needn't mean a loss of health, provided we treat ourselves well, with proper diet and exercise. If not, these aging changes can escalate into a number of chronic problems. The normal loss of elasticity in the arteries, known as arteriosclerosis, may accelerate into atherosclerosis if fatty plaque begins to cling to arterial walls. When this happens, the easy flow of blood through the circulatory network to the cells is obstructed, forcing the heart to overwork, escalating the natural rise in blood pressure associated with age into chronic hypertension. Hypertension compounds the whole problem because it creates lesions in the blood-vessel walls, which make even more inviting resting places for fatty deposits. Enough clogging can cause a blockage within a blood vessel or within the heart itself that can result in a heart attack, or if the brain is involved instead, a stroke. Atherosclerosis, hypertension, heart attack, and stroke are all interrelated and are each potentially fatal. Combined, they account for *half* of all the disabling health problems in women and men alike.

There is a genetic factor that can predispose us to heart disease. But certain risk factors more within our control are now known to be equally, if not more, significant:

- Inadequate exercise
- Poor diet—especially too much sugar, salt, refined and fatty foods, and too little fiber
- Excess body weight
- Excessive alcohol intake
- Smoking
- Toxins in the environment

These same risk factors are essentially at the root of every other major chronic disease as well. Not surprisingly, they have also been linked to the causes of fast aging!

If you modify your risk factors you can prevent, slow down, and in some cases even reverse the degenerative changes associated with both aging and disease. The changes we experience due to the passage of time alone have *much less* impact than those we set in motion ourselves by excesses and deficiencies in our everyday lives.

The chapters that follow will provide you with plenty of specific information about the skin and aging, how to maintain a healthy weight, and how to take care of the structural glue that holds everything together—our joints, our backs, and our bones—in short all you need to know to stay healthy and energetic through midlife.

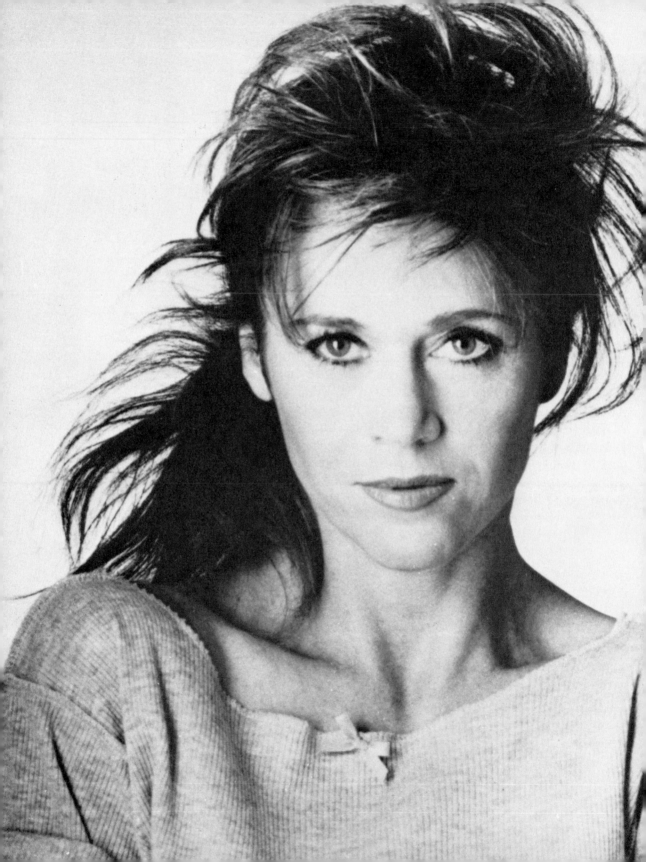

CHAPTER 4

THE SKIN

THE SKIN IS OUR BODY'S ENVELOPE, the wrapping that delivers us to the world. Though we all pay lip service to the dictum "don't judge a book by its cover," we tend to judge a person's age and state of health by the quality of her skin. If as we grow older we expect to be able to keep our skin just as it was in our youth, we'll be doomed to frustration. If, on the other hand, we understand how the skin functions in midlife and adjust our goals and life-styles appropriately, we'll be surprised how much better we can look.

A few basics first. The skin is composed of two layers. The innermost is the dermis, which contains the nerve endings, blood vessels, sweat glands, oil glands, and hair follicles. The outer is the epidermis, the layer of our skin that's constantly renewed. Cells on the underside of the epidermis continuously divide and slowly migrate to the surface, where they dry out, flatten, and die, and are then washed, rubbed, or blown away. Both the dermis and the epidermis are supported by a deeper layer of fat cells and a network of collagen and elastin fibers that give our skin its strength and elasticity. Collagen is the body's most abundant protein and the principal support not only of the skin but also of the blood vessels and connective tissues of our cartilage, tendons, and ligaments.

Certain changes occur in this infrastructure of our skin as part of the natural aging process. To some extent there is nothing we can do about them but they can certainly be slowed and minimized.

1. **Drying**—The sweat and oil glands that are important natural moisturizers for the skin slow down with age, largely as a result of hormonal changes, especially after menopause. With less moisture and oil, in addition to years of accumulated exposure to the elements, the skin dries.

2. **Wrinkling**—Some people think this dryness causes wrinkles. That is not exactly the case, although dryness certainly accentuates

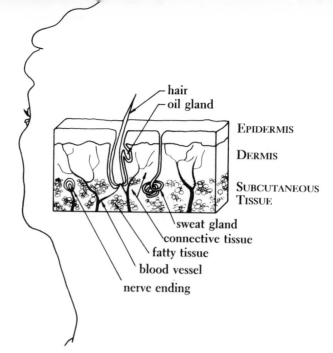

hair
oil gland

EPIDERMIS

DERMIS

SUBCUTANEOUS
TISSUE

sweat gland
connective tissue
fatty tissue
blood vessel
nerve ending

The Structure of the Skin

them. Wrinkles are primarily caused by the aging process known as "cross-linking" discussed in the previous chapter. As a result of cross-linking, unwanted bonding occurs between molecules in the skin's collagen and elastin, which then shrink and tighten. As a result, the skin gradually toughens and loses its elasticity and we begin to notice wrinkles and sagging.

3. **Sagging**—The skin's underlying cushion of fat cells also shrinks as we get older. And because the skin itself is less elastic, it can't so easily conform to the face's smaller dimensions. Like a balloon from which some air has escaped, excess skin begins to sag.

4. **Thinning**—With age, fewer skin cells are produced and there is little turnover in collagen. The skin becomes thinner as a result.

Drying, wrinkling, sagging, and thinning—all are inevitable aspects of aging. But let's take a look at the things we do which cause them to occur prematurely and faster than need be.

What Hurts

If we look at the soft, white, fine-pored skin on our behinds and underarms, compared with our faces and the backs of our hands, we will see that what damages our skin most is not so much age as exposure to *sun, smog, wind,* and *cold.*

As a former sun-worshipper it pains me to say it, but skin enemy number one, the prime offender in the wrinkle department, is the *sun.* Sun not only dries out the skin but is one of the main causes of cross-linking.

To be perfectly honest, I had often been warned about sun-damaged skin. But I liked the feel of warm sun on my body and the look of a tan, so I let the words of warning go unheeded. Alas, the shortsightedness of youth! Every summer I began with the hurtful burn which I would then cultivate into a deep tan. Ah, how great I looked for those few months. But as I hit forty, I began to notice that as the tan faded with summer's end, my skin would break out and new wrinkles would appear on my face and "liver spots" on my hands. After several years of this there was no mistaking it. I was paying for three months of tan with nine months of increasingly weathered-looking skin. The results were cumulative and apparently irreversible. I could do little to turn back the clock. The damage had been done. The best I could do was try to hold the line, not let it get worse.

Added to these very visible bad effects was the possibility of an invisible danger—skin cancer. There's growing evidence that skin cancer is on the rise, a phenomenon that dermatologists attribute to our excessive exposure to the sun. It is the sun's ultraviolet radiation, they say, which does long-term damage to the skin. The most

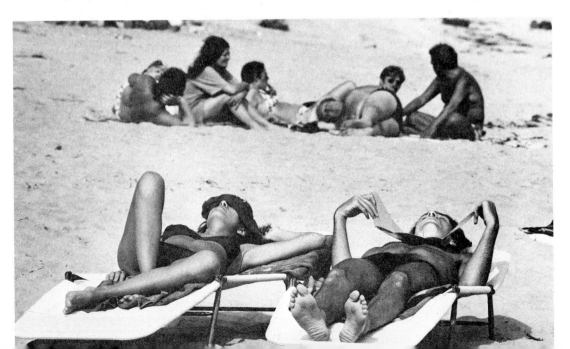

dangerous rays are the shorter ultraviolet B (UVB) rays, most intense between 11 A.M. and 3 P.M. But we now know that the longer UVA rays, present all day, can also lead to skin cancer—even though they are less harmful in terms of sunburn. Both types of ray, especially UVA, can alter the genetic material in the cells of the skin. Over time, the sun's rays dry out the skin's collagen and elastin. They also accelerate cross-linking in these same connective fibers, making them brittle and inelastic.

When you lie for hours unprotected in the sun, cells in the epidermis swell. Blood vessels dilate, causing the pain and redness of sunburn. Cells of melanin, the pigment which determines our skin color, rise to the surface in order to absorb ultraviolet light before it can penetrate deeper layers of the skin. This is the beautiful tan we spend so many hours cultivating. It is actually the skin's way of shielding itself, and therefore a sign that your skin is vulnerable to damage. First comes the burn, then the tan, followed by wrinkles, liver spots, and, if you continue to expose yourself, damage to the skin's genetic DNA material, which can lead to skin cancer.

There are three types of skin cancer. The first two—*basal-cell carcinoma* and *squamous-cell carcinoma*—are clearly caused by ultraviolet light. They are also highly curable by surgery. *Melanoma*, the lethal cancer which attacks 15,000 Americans a year and kills 45 percent of them, is also suspected of being related to sun exposure. The cancer might not appear right away, but when it surfaces it is the result of accumulated damage since childhood. You should be sure to check your skin at *least* once a year either with a partner or alone using a full-length mirror. Look for any growth that has color. It could be red, white, blue, brown, black or gray. Be aware of whether a mole's size has changed or if it bleeds. Any of these signs should send you to a doctor quickly.

I have completely given up lying in the sun because I don't want to be a statistic. I realize now that I am at risk for skin cancer because of years of sunbathing, but I can minimize that risk by stopping now. I do not want to die from vanity. And to tell you the truth, I'm quite happy to have all that time previously spent in pursuit of a tan available to do other, more interesting things.

Not that I don't ever go out in the sun. On the contrary—I'm a jogger, I take long walks, I ski, and I love the out-of-doors. But I

Me and Troy trying to look professional. Christmas 1983, Sun Valley, Idaho.

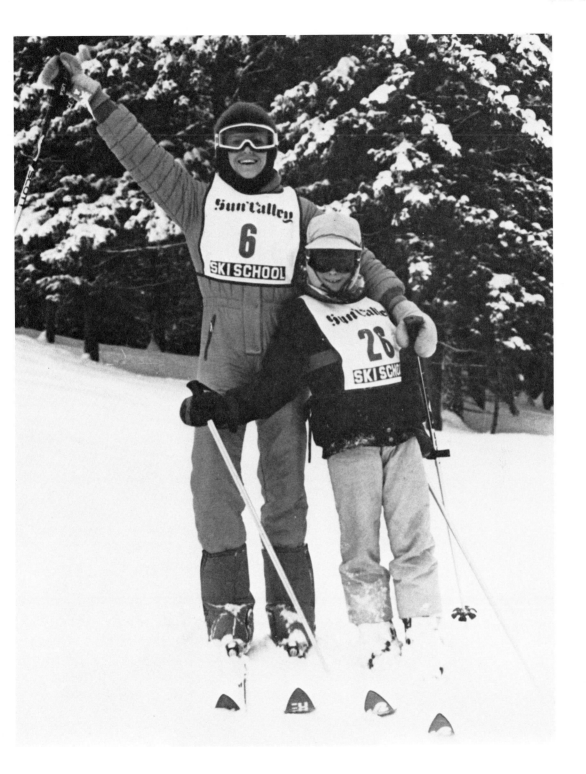

never leave the house without having put on a good sunscreen. We oughtn't forget that the sun is good for us. Without it, there would be no life on earth. It provides heat for us, and if harnessed properly, could be a major energy resource. The sun helps provide vitamin D, especially important to us in midlife to keep bones strong. But while we respect its value, we must take necessary precautions to guard against the sun's dangers. The best protection is to use a high-potency sunscreen, which absorbs or scatters ultraviolet light. Your sunscreen should contain the chemical PABA (para-aminobenzoic acid), the ingredient responsible for screening out the sun's rays.

Sunscreens don't block out the sun completely; rather, they simply filter out the most harmful ultraviolet beams. You should also be aware that ultraviolet light can penetrate haze, light clouds, or fog. It is reflected off sand, water, and snow, so a big hat or umbrella may not provide you with the full protection you need. Ultraviolet light can even zap you under water and penetrate lightweight clothing.

Sunscreens are now rated according to their sun protection factor (SPF); the higher the number, the more protection your sunscreen will provide. The following guide will help you choose the right sunscreen for your particular skin.

Skin Type	Sun Factor
1. Very fair. Always burns, never tans.	10–15
2. Fair. Usually burns, sometimes tans faintly.	6–12
3. Sometimes burns, usually tans.	4–6
4. Almost never burns, always tans.	2–4

If you have oily skin or suffer from acne, you'll want a liquid sunscreen with an alcohol base. If your skin is dry, find yourself a cream-based sunscreen which also serves as a moisturizer. Apply the sunscreen to any exposed area of the skin and don't forget to cover your nose, lips, chest, back of the hands, and if your hair isn't covering them, the rims of the ears and back of the neck. These are the places that absorb the most radiation.

Sunscreens also double as good protection against everyday conditions hard on the skin: air pollution—unavoidable for most of us—that really takes its toll; and wind, cold, and dry air (inside or out) that pull moisture from the skin. A sunscreen or good moisturizer will trap the water in and seal the toxins out. Inside the house, a humidifier or even a pan of water placed near a radiator will help maintain the humidity in overheated rooms that otherwise are so drying to the skin.

In addition to the sun, *alcohol* and *tobacco smoke* are major causes of the cross-linking process that damages connective tissue in the skin's support system. In addition, both impede blood circulation in the skin. Alcohol dilates facial blood vessels. Little webs of broken capillaries are the visible penalties of heavy drinking. Smoking constricts blood vessels, which means less blood, less oxygen, and fewer nutrients get to the skin. Wastes are eliminated sluggishly; more toxins build up. Make a point of noticing the skin of midlife people who continue to smoke and drink a lot and you'll see middle-aged faces with old-aged skins. In fact, the signs begin even before midlife.

If you are not yet ready to give up smoking and drinking, at least fortify yourself by emphasizing in your diet the vitamins they destroy and that help to protect you from the damage they cause—vitamins A, C, E, B_1, B_5, and B_6. But make no mistake. The only true antidote is to go easy on alcohol and to say goodbye to cigarettes.

Chronic dieting is another all-too-frequent practice that will lead to dry and sagging skin. While skimping on calories most dieters are also skimping on the vitamins, minerals, amino acids, and enzymes that are essential to healthy skin. No one can stay on a diet permanently. The continued stretching and relaxing of the skin as one's weight goes up and down taxes even the youngest skin. Imagine its effects on our less-elastic midlife skin. Sagging is the inevitable outcome. In addition, even the tension and anxiety that accompany frequent dieting will show on your face. I cannot recommend strongly enough the importance of finding and maintaining your *natural* weight. Keeping it constant and balanced at this time in life is critical.

MY SKIN REGIMEN: AN INSIDE JOB

I'm often asked what "beauty secrets" I practice, what creams and lotions are best to buy in the search for the perfect cosmetic formula for smooth, youthful skin. I think women are surprised when I respond that I have no special secrets—of that kind. It's not that I haven't tried virtually everything. Believe me, as an actress, I have. But after many, many years, I've found no basis to advertising promises that we can have beautiful skin by using just the right skin care product. Of course, proper cleansing and moisturizing are essential, and some products are better than others; I'll talk about all of that later. But for me, the truest, most reliable beauty potion is regular vigorous exercise combined with good nutrition. These are the most important, effective things you can do for your skin.

If your budget is limited, you'd do better to invest your money in a regular, sweaty, speed-up-your heartbeat exercise program than in a lot of expensive hormonal creams, masks, facials, and the like, whose effect will be at best temporary and superficial. Exercise, on the other hand, increases the circulation and brings a rich flow of nutrients and oxygen through the blood to the skin's cells.

Consistent, strenuous exercise appears to retard every aspect of the skin's aging that we've discussed, including sagging and the loss of elasticity. It can rejuvenate unhealthy worn-out skin. The whole process of normal cell breakdown and production is tuned up and the connective tissues become stronger and less vulnerable to damage. If you've ever been in a dressing room with a group of professional dancers changing clothes, as I have, you've probably been struck by the quality of their skin. I first noticed this when I studied ballet in my early twenties. I made a point of noticing dancers' skin and found almost all of them had beautifully even skin tone. Subsequently, of course, doctors have given a scientific explanation to my observation: dancers, like athletes, have more collagen in their skin—it's thicker! During a workout, the skin's temperature can rise from 86 to 90 degrees or more. This is thought to stimulate an increase in the production of collagen cells, which together with the other positive effects of exercise, thickens the skin—making it firmer, less wrinkled, better toned.

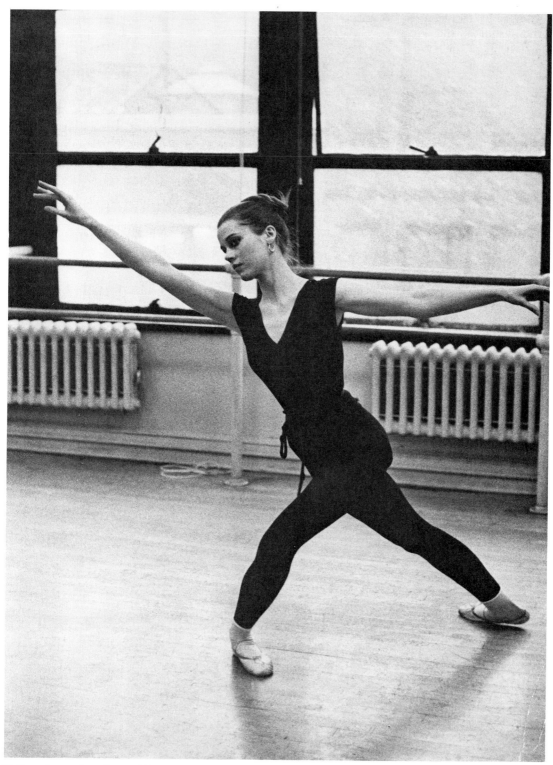

Ballet class when I was 20.

I've noticed definite changes like these in my own skin since I began a more vigorous, systematic workout program and since my eating habits have improved as well. My skin is also much less dry. I used to have to slather myself head-to-toe with moisturizer after every bathing. Now, only occasionally do I need a body lotion, and with proper care rarely suffer from facial dryness. Exercise is a natural from-the-inside-out moisturizer as sweat glands kick into action. Sweating also helps to cleanse the pores, ridding the skin of toxins and wastes. Because of this and the healthy circulation that results from exercise, my skin is clearer, with good color. Now I have less need of a makeup base. In fact, I make a point of using only a tinted moisturizer, if anything, since a thicker base tends to accentuate lines.

On days when I don't look as well as I'd like, instead of covering up the problem with makeup the way I used to, I now work out or run. It's the best facial I can give myself. Even if it means getting up at 4 A.M., I never go before the camera without having put myself

Me and Mignon running with the dogs.

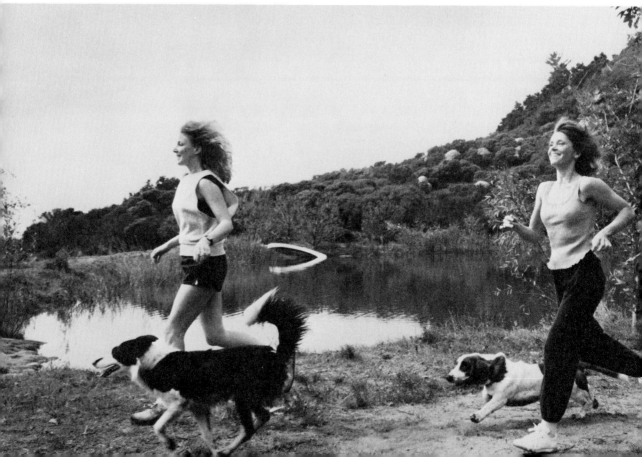

through my paces. What I've lost in tautness, I make up in glow.

What I feed my skin, in addition to the oxygen it gets from exercise, is equally important. The skin is our largest organ, nourished from the inside through the bloodstream. Like the rest of the body, it needs proteins, carbohydrates, fats, vitamins, and minerals. Exercise ensures their speedy delivery to the skin, but it's up to us to regulate the quality of these nutrients.

Deficiencies can result in dryness, skin eruptions, sallow complexions, and other abnormalities. A well-balanced diet of the types of foods we discuss in the chapter called "Eating for the Long Run," will pay off for our skin. In addition, I recommend that the midlife woman emphasize the following pro-skin superstars:

Vitamin A—Helps replenish skin cells. A deficiency will result in dry, rough, splotchy skin.

Vitamin B Complex—Helps prevent scaling and cracking of the skin.

Vitamin C—Aids in rejuvenating the skin, because it is necessary for the manufacture of collagen, the protein that supports the skin and gives it elasticity.

Vitamin E—As an antioxidant, may help to protect skin cells against the damage of abnormal oxidation. Also helps in healing the skin.

Water—When talking about inside-out skin care, we have to make special mention of the skin's best friend: water. Six to eight glasses a day, please. It will help flush out toxins and moisturize the skin.

Facial Exercises

Many women ask me what I think of facial exercises. After all, if I'm strongly advocating working out, I must think specific exercises are good for the face as well. But the face works in a different way from the rest of your body's skin. Because of that, it's probable that facial exercises actually are harmful to midlife and older skins. When you think about it, our faces probably get more exercise naturally than most parts of us. Every time we chew, smile, or talk it's a regular facial workout. If exercising these muscles helped eliminate wrinkles, we'd all be smooth as babies.

The Muscles of the Face

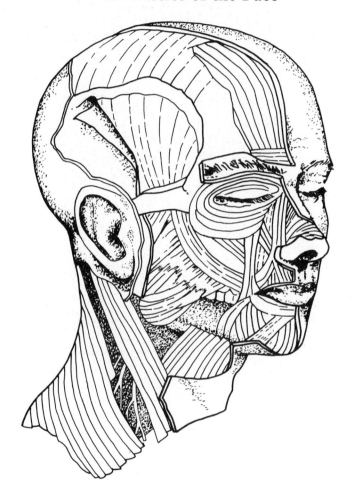

If we could peel back our skin, we would see a latticework of muscle . . .

The stretching and straining of facial muscles and collagen fibers may exaggerate already existing lines. Unlike the skin on the rest of the body, facial skin is attached directly to many separate bands of muscle beneath it. If we could peel back the skin, we would see a latticework of muscle that enables us to move our face into the most diverse and subtle of expressions. As the skin loses its elasticity with age, the lines created when these muscles move become increasingly permanent.

For heaven's sake, this doesn't mean you should curb your laughter, your winks, and your full range of expression. But when you're reading, working, thinking, or watching TV, try to avoid tensing your face into unconscious grimaces. Every now and then check to see if you're pulling the corners of your mouth down, frowning or puckering your lips. These unconscious and unnecessary habits will definitely institutionalize a fine, thin line into a deep furrow.

The muscles of the neck and lower jaw are a different matter, however. Exercising them *can* help to prevent lined necks and double chins. You'll find specific exercises for these areas included later in the Prime Time Workout.

THE OUTSIDE

While proper nutrition and exercise are the best long-term approaches to skin care, it is also important to incorporate into each day a few fundamentals of good cleansing and moisturizing, including an occasional scrub and mask or facial. Improper or inadequate cleansing and moisturizing can age the skin as rapidly as poor diet, smoking, alcohol, and environmental toxins. Too frequent washing, hot water, and strong soap and detergents, for example, can irritate the skin and remove the essential natural oils that protect the skin and hold in moisture.

First, *cleansing.* Abrasive and detergent soaps which are made from synthetic chemicals are more effective in removing dirt and grime, especially in hard water, but they don't discriminate between unwanted grease and the natural surface oils that prevent moisture from evaporating from our skin. Because we tend to have drier skin at midlife, a milder, neutral or slightly acidic soap made from natural fats and oils is recommended. And everything we put on our faces, including soap, should be unscented and unmedicated. Elizabeth Arden, Clinique and Germaine Monteil each make an excellent soap for super-sensitive skins. These are relatively expensive but last for months and months. For general purpose soaps a recent study showed Dove, Emulave, Aveenobar, Purpose, and Dial to be the mildest (and I would add Neutrogena).

My skin tends to be thin and dry, though much less so since I began to exercise regularly and maintain a balanced, healthy diet. As is the case with many women, the skin around my nose and chin tends to be more oily than my forehead, cheeks and the skin around my eyes, due to a larger number of oil glands. As a result, I restrict my use of soap to these areas. I use my fingertips to massage mild soap over my chin and nose and then rinse off with warm (not hot) water and pat dry. I do this gently because pulling and stretching your skin whether in washing, rough drying, or just playing with your face weakens the connective tissue. Every so often if my skin seems in need of a heavier cleansing and is not too dry, I will wash my entire face with a mild soap, always using my hands, not a washcloth.

Some skins are too dry to use even the mildest soap. For these, a cleansing cream is the answer to removing dirt without removing natural oils. Some of these, which I use occasionally, wash off in warm water. Other thicker creams and vegetable oils are removed with cotton, *pure* cotton. (If you use vegetable oils such as almond, sesame or avocado, buy them in small amounts and keep them refrigerated so they won't turn rancid.) Cover your face and neck with the oil or cream, then take pure cotton balls or hunks of absorbent cotton dipped in warm water and gently wipe off the cleanser. Never use dry cotton or facial tissues on your face and neck to remove makeup. Both pull the skin too much, and facial tissues are made from wood pulp, which can be irritating to sensitive skin.

If hard water in your area tends to leave a soapy film on your skin or if your pores seem enlarged and your skin isn't the very dry type, you can go over your face and neck with a cotton ball soaked in astringent. You may want to do this just in the oily areas between the brows and around the nose and chin. The astringent temporarily closes your pores. I'm especially fond of Caswell-Massey's Cucumber Face Lotion. I also use their Cucumber Cold Cream as a makeup remover. (You can order these through the mail. See the Resource Guide at the back of the book for Caswell-Massey's address.)

Worn-out cells on the surface can give your skin a dusty, dull look and slow down the migration of new cells to the surface. There are three ways to help remove this layer of dead cells from the face:

—a complexion brush made with natural bristles
—a small loofa complexion sponge
—a scrub

Either the complexion brush or loofa sponge (I use both) could be used once every week on oily skin and once or twice a month on dry skin—but don't use either on extremely sensitive dry skin. Rub lightly in a small circular motion, then rinse your face with warm water or let the shower wash away the loosened dead cells.

You can also use a scrub to give yourself a deeper cleansing. I use one every two or three weeks depending on how much time I have and the state of my skin. Before using the scrub, I steam my face for five minutes by leaning over a pot of steaming water with a towel draped over my head to contain the steam. I usually put a bag of chamomile tea in the water. I pat some, but not all, of the moisture off my face and then I put a good layer of scrub all over my face, leaving about one inch free around the eye area. Afterwards, my skin sparkles and tingles and yours will too. This is the scrub I like to use:

CORNMEAL SCRUB

Moisten a cup of finely ground cornmeal (uncooked). Rub the meal in circular motions with your fingertips all over your face and throat. This will loosen the dead skin cells, remove dirt, help prevent blackheads, and smooth the skin. Remove the scrub with cotton balls dipped in cool (not cold) water.

The ideal time to apply a mask is right after the scrub. If you don't go on to do a mask, be sure to apply a moisturizer after you scrub. A good mask will stimulate and nourish the skin and close up the pores. You can make your own mask like this one made out of wheat germ which is especially good for stimulating and nourishing dry skin. I think it gives a nice glow to the face and reduces the size of the pores.

WHEAT GERM MASK

Soften 1 tablespoon *raw* wheat germ in 1 tablespoon distilled water. Mix together with 1 teaspoon egg yolk (save the rest of the yolk for another mask by refrigerating in a covered container). Beat wheat germ, water, and yolk till a smooth paste is formed. Then pat the mixture on the entire face (except eyelids). Keep applying the paste until there is a thick coating. Allow to dry (twenty minutes). To remove, carefully loosen the dried mask with a dampened washcloth, rinsing the cloth in warm water so that you are always applying a clean cloth to your face. When all the mask is gone, splash cold water on your face, pat dry, and follow with a moisturizer.

Now, for *moisturizers*. People with a tendency to oily skin should use a water-based moisturizer, just as they should an alcohol-based sunscreen. Dry skin requires an oil-based moisturizer and a cream-based sunscreen. The cosmetician at your pharmacy or department store should be able to tell you which is which. Whether your skin is dry or oily, try to find a product you can use as both moisturizer and sunscreen as I do. I have used several, including Almay's Skin Saver and PabaPlus. I don't recommend the new creams we read about containing, for instance, estrogen, collagen, vitamins, and hydrolyzed protein. These are expensive and their efficacy is unproven scientifically.

If you apply a moisturizer while your face is slightly wet it will make your skin even more supple. This method seems literally to trap moisture in the skin. The tap water in Santa Monica is extremely hard, so I keep an atomizer filled with distilled water to spray on my face before I put on my moisturizer. What I find especially effective is to work out or jog with a moisturizer-sunscreen on my face and neck. The exercise causes me to sweat. The cream keeps the water in my skin and prevents the elements from "pulling out" the moisture. My skin feels noticeably softer afterwards.

What about nighttime? What you put on your face at night depends on who you're with, what's on the agenda, and the state of your skin. For instance, if the mood is romantic and my skin seems normal, I will simply apply a little daytime moisturizer around my eyes, since that's the area that is the most dry and sensitive. If my husband, Tom, is away, I use an oil-based cream, like Caswell-Massey's Cucumber Night Cream or one of my vegetable oils. I think it's also good every once in a while, though I have no scientific proof, to let my skin breathe and rest for eight hours with nothing on it.

I tend to have puffy eyes in the morning, a real challenge to the ingenuity of cinematographers. The "puffs" are considerably worse if I ate within three hours of retiring the night before, consumed more than a minimal amount of fat, or had more than a glass of wine or beer. What a bore! These things make me retain fluid, always a problem for me. The fluid tends to collect in the connective tissue under the skin below the eye. Circulation and gravity, of course, will disperse this pooling during the day, and in the normal course of events I'm not too concerned about it. Filming, however, imposes greater discipline, so here's what I do to shrink the early-morning swelling. The night before, I soak two tea bags in water and put them in the refrigerator. First thing in the morning I place a cold tea bag on each eye for five minutes. Then I put on my cream and go for a run or workout. The sweating and exercise together with the cold poultices seem to reduce the swelling quite effectively. This will help if the puffiness around your eyes comes from edema, as mine does. It may not help if yours comes from other causes of swelling like allergy, sinus infection, and hayfever.

Repeated swelling—for whatever reason—that stretches the thin skin under the eyes can cause older skin to sag as it loses its elasticity. In addition, if the network of connective tissues under the skin below the eyes has relaxed, subcutaneous fat will move into pouches in the loose skin. There is nothing to be done about this unless one is prepared to undergo surgery. More about that later.

Let's not neglect the rest of your body. A good habit to get into, one that will make your skin tingle and glow all over, is to rub yourself down with a *dry* loofa brush before bathing, or with a natural

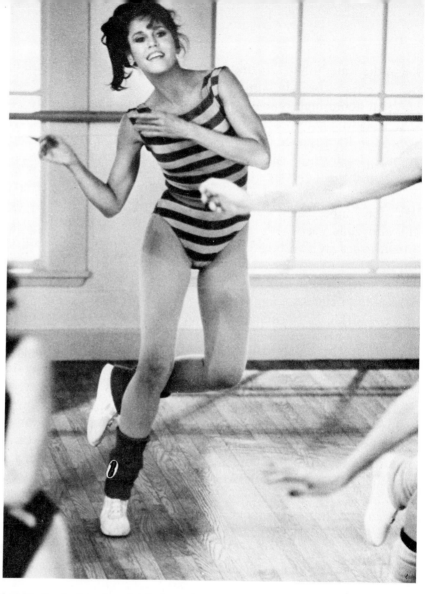

bristle body brush, which I prefer. Rub your skin all over, including your breasts, in circular motions. Your skin will redden as it's stimulated and as blood rushes to the surface (though don't rub so hard that you irritate the skin). In addition to stimulating the circulation, such a body rub will loosen your body's dead skin cells as well. Bathing afterwards will wash them away. Be sure to wash your loofa or body brush too in order to keep it free of bacteria, and allow to dry out for use the next day. This is a special treat after a workout.

Long baths in hot water and saunas are relaxing and they open the pores, but also be aware that they are very drying to the skin. If you bathe or sauna frequently, I suggest using a cream on your face to retain moisture. Afterwards rub a moisturizer into your body. If I have time to allow them to be absorbed, I like the natural avocado, almond, or sesame oils. Otherwise, I use Keri Lotion, especially effective in wintertime when the body skin dries out even more and tends to itch.

COSMETIC SURGERY

Before we conclude the subject of skin, let's talk more about wrinkles. There are three ways to go with wrinkles. We can do nothing. We can choose to take a radical approach like plastic surgery. Or there's a middle way to go, the course I prefer: making peace with the growing numbers of fine (and some not so fine) lines you see on your face and doing your best through nutrition, exercise, proper cleansing, moisturizing, sleep, and healthy living habits to avoid aggravated and premature wrinkles.

Wrinkles are part of who we are, of where we've been. Not to have wrinkles means never having laughed or cried or expressed passion, never having squinted into the sun or felt the bite of winter's wind—never having fully lived!

I'm in no position as a successful actress and happily married woman to castigate those who turn to cosmetic surgery in the hope it will enhance their ability to compete in the youth-oriented job market or as a way to attract or keep a partner—a hedge against loneliness, if you will. But I've seen many a "perfect" woman, nipped and tucked to within a taut and shiny inch of her life, who's still lonely. Perhaps these women think that how they look is who they are. Certainly our culture does everything it can to affirm that myth. But, ultimately, what matters is your *gestalt*, the many elements that combine to make you unique—your attitude, your energy, your humor, your ability to think straight, to listen and be listened to, and your depth of character.

However, if your personal or professional situation or a disliked facial feature militates in favor of cosmetic surgery, here is a word of caution. Once you have gone as far as interviewing a plastic surgeon, you have probably pretty much made up your mind to go ahead with the surgery. The tendency at that point is to hear only what you want to. Too many women simply dismiss the warnings and cautions. It's not difficult to ignore the risks of cosmetic surgery. The language used to describe the procedures—"nose bobs," "mini-lifts," and "nips and tucks," for instance—make it seem no more consequential than going to a dressmaker.

But consider the fact that, although facial surgery is rarely life-threatening, there can be serious physical and aesthetic complications. Unpublicized but not uncommon occurrences include blood clotting, temporary or permanent injury to sensory or motor nerves, infection, permanent deformities such as the inability to close the mouth or eyes (when too much skin has been removed or scarring has caused skin to contract), excessive scar tissue, and facial paralysis. Not to mention the face that no longer matches the body.

I don't mean to imply that there are not highly successful operations performed by serious, skillful surgeons, but I want you to realize that plastic surgery is not to be taken lightly and has many potential risks. If you decide to go ahead with cosmetic surgery, select your doctor with care.

Choosing a Cosmetic Surgeon

- Interview two or three licensed surgeons who are members of the AMA (American Medical Association) and the American College of Surgeons. This will assure you of their medical credentials. Choose those you visit from your own physician's referral and/or from the recommendations of friends whose results you've seen.
- The physician should be *Board Certified* in her or his plastic surgery specialty. *This is probably the most important determination you need to make and I suggest you do so before your first visit.* You can find out about board certification by calling the surgeon's office or by contacting the two plastic surgery associations I list in the Resource Guide.

  Board certification means the surgeon has had advanced training and passed an exam given by the Board of Specialists of the AMA. ("Board eligibility" means the training has been done but the exam not yet passed.) The two specialties certified to perform all facial plastic procedures are the American Board of Otolaryngology–Head and Neck Surgery and the American Board of Plastic Surgery. Board Certified ophthalmologists may perform eyelid surgery only, and dermatologists who are Board Certified can remove skin lesions. Surgeons or surgeon groups who advertise have not necessarily met these criteria.

- The surgeon should currently be on the staff of a major accredited hospital. If you call the surgeon's office to inquire about board certification, you can inquire about hospital affiliation at the same time. (Make sure the hospital privileges include those for the specific surgical procedure you need.)

  The following are two possible, cost-effective alternatives to hospitals: operating facilities in a surgeon's office approved by the Society for Office-Based Surgery, and Freestanding Ambulatory Surgicenters accredited by the AAAHC (Accreditation Association for Ambulatory Health Care).

- After confirming all of the above, select the surgeon with whom you have the best rapport and who examines your face the most carefully rather than giving you assembly-line treatment. It may be that your particular face, eyes, or chin require one type of procedure over another, or that surgery is actually contraindicated for you. You want a surgeon who informs you adequately of the risks rather than promising magic results. A cut-rate surgeon's fee should not enter into your final choice of a plastic surgeon.

A final word about face lifts—acupuncture face lifts. I've been treated successfully with acupuncture from time to time for fluid retention, fever, and various injuries, and I have even tried it on my face before filming because some claim acupuncture can bring temporary improvement to wrinkles. It was not true for me; in fact, while the fine acupuncture needles used in the body are not painful, for me the facial acupuncture hurt too much and caused temporary bruising.

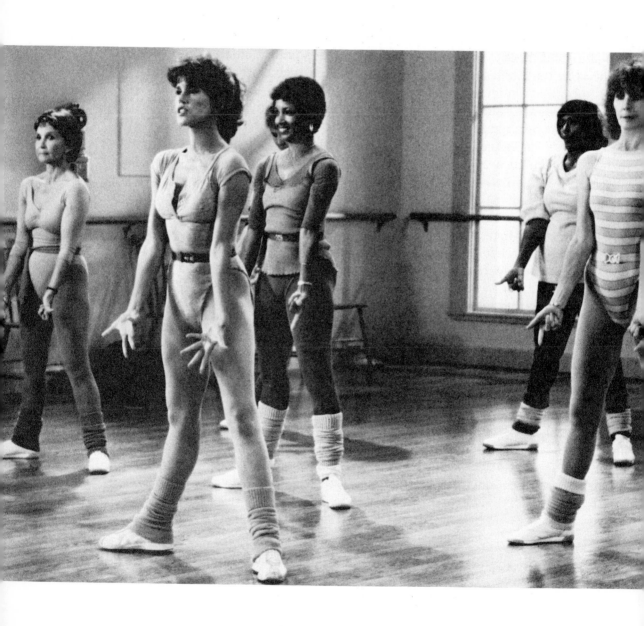

CHAPTER 5

MIDDLE-AGE SPREAD

SOME OF YOU WHO BOUGHT THIS BOOK have probably turned directly here. "What's she have to say about getting rid of this?" you're asking—perhaps even grabbing a handful of the flesh that's getting harder to dismiss affectionately as "love handles."

We've all noticed how much more difficult it is to lose those extra pounds now than it was five or ten years ago. Some of you have almost given up. Some of you may still be diet-hopping, consumed by the endless struggle against fat, trapped on the binge-and-starve seesaw. As one who's always had to fight her weight, I have a lot to say on the subject and I know there are thousands of you with the same problem.

Julie Jordan, now forty-five, and one of our Workout regulars, was seriously overweight by age thirty-eight. She was also smoking secretly. She'd raised two boys and had been immersed for fifteen years in her church community, a self-effacing, dedicated volunteer who spent a great deal of her time running bake sales and rummage sales. Alarmed by her lack of energy and ever-increasing weight, Julie finally made a life-altering decision to change all this. And change she did. From that moment, she began a slow weight-loss diet and the gradual elimination of cigarettes—forever. She also began running. A few blocks was all she could do at the start. Several years later when the doors of the Workout opened for the first time, Julie was right there to sign up. By that time she'd begun her own business and was down to a size 14½. Now, still a Workout regular, Julie is a size 8, just right for her frame. "I've lost fifty inches in my hips since I first came here," she told me during the recent videotaping of our Prime Time class. "Fifteen?" I asked,

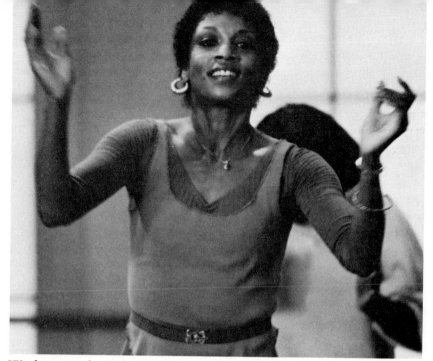

Workout regular, Julie Jordan, 45.

thinking I'd misheard her. "No," she said with a radiant smile. "*Fifty!* Never again will I weigh more than I do now. It's taken me six years to get here. One step at a time. I've come this far, into my mid-forties like many others, feeling good and looking good. What could be better?"

The Fire Inside

I have been exercising for twenty-five years and I've long known that exercise burns off fat faster than dieting alone without exercise. But it was while researching my first Workout Book that I learned why. It all comes down to metabolism and the key to metabolism—our muscles. If you're like me, you'll find this information the best incentive of all to get those muscles working—and burning.

Metabolism refers to the internal combustion that takes place in our body cells when already digested fats, proteins, and carbohydrates (in the form of glucose) are "burned" to create energy—with the help of oxygen. The energy released is measured in calories.

Why is it, you might ask, that some women seem to be better at this burning of calories than others? Do they have an inherently better metabolism? Is the slender person who eats heartily without gaining an ounce magically blessed with a good metabolism? Is the overweight person who eats modestly by comparison, barely holding the weight line, somehow cursed with a sluggish one—with nothing to be done about it? No. There's no mystery or luck involved. Your metabolism is what you make it and you can improve it at any time. But you have to work at it—by building and maintaining the active tissue of your muscles.

The muscles make up the largest part of the body and, together with the bones, constitute your *lean body mass*. Think of the muscles as your furnace, burning 90 percent of all the body's calories. They are *always* at work burning glucose and fat whether you are resting, exercising, or just going about your daily activities. The more of this lean tissue you have, the more calories you use up. A muscular 120-pound woman of forty, for example, will require more food to maintain her weight than a woman of the same age and weight who has relatively little muscle. She will be able to eat more without gaining weight.

Each of us arrives at midlife in various stages of muscular, hence metabolic, fitness. Years of crash dieting, unbalanced nutrition and, most of all, too little exercise will have cost us muscle while tuning *down* our metabolism. If we're not already putting on pounds, we will begin to do so now because there are certain age-related changes in our muscle that, however gentle, pull us in that direction.

All of us will experience a small loss of lean muscle tissue as a result of the aging process. With each decade after thirty, we can lose three to five percent on the average. If on top of this natural change we become less active, a "middle-aged" tendency in the past, we'll lose muscle even faster. Unused, muscles will atrophy, shorten and lose many of the enzymes that are crucial to their being able to burn calories. When you have less muscle—whether from age, lack of physical activity, or both—you will burn fewer calories. If you continue to consume the same number of calories, those not burned will turn to fat. For instance, if you eat just 100 calories more than you use up every day, you can expect to gain more than fifty pounds in five years. If the normal age change in muscle is allowed to get out of hand, calorie-burning tissue gives way to calorie-*storing* tissue—at an escalating pace.

This happens quietly at first. As lean muscle retreats, fat advances, penetrating first the muscle itself, altering its firm long contours. In the beginning, none of this will be evident on the scale since fat simply replaces muscle and even weighs less. We become *overfat* before we become overweight. Once the muscle is completely saturated, fat is next deposited outside the muscle, subcutaneously, under the skin. We all know its favorite pockets—the thighs, hips, waist, stomach, upper arms, and back. At this point, surplus fat does become excess poundage. Soft and shapeless, it also takes up more space than muscle.

As the body's percentage of fat rises, the metabolism slows down further and further. For unlike active muscle which earns its keep, fat is *inert*. Fat stored in the body doesn't burn calories. No energy is required for its upkeep. Fat *is* calories—3,500 of them contained in each fat pound—the body's densest fuel. Of course, a certain amount of body fat is essential—as an energy resource and for other specialized functions. For instance, fat plays an important role during a woman's fertile years in ensuring a healthy menstrual cycle, and after menopause in the production of estrogen. But while a little fat is necessary, not having enough body fat is rarely a problem, unless we tend to be anorexic.

The human body's ability to store fat is *unlimited*. The same is not true for the other major nutrients. The body can store only so much carbohydrate and use so much protein. When we surpass these limits by eating more than we need, the excess carbohydrate and protein turn to fat. When we eat too much fat, of course, it too converts to body fat. And, once there, *the only way to lose unwanted stored fat is to burn it away as energy.*

How often do we try fruitlessly to starve it away instead on unrealistic diets we can't possibly stick to? Eventually, after prolonged periods of dieting, the body will fight back, holding onto its fat stores when it thinks it must. This is one of the survival mechanisms of our species, a way of stocking up for times of famine and emergency. Some scientists speculate there may exist in each of us an internal set-point that regulates the amount of fat we carry—a kind of fat-o-stat that differs from person to person. This will kick into action, *conserving* fat when fat stores are too low or threaten to become so.

Understanding how this works is an important element in learning to drop excess fat pounds wisely and forever. The way most people choose to lose weight is counterproductive and tends to trigger the set-point mechanism. If the body perceives that it is starving, as it does if you are *always* on a diet or if you suddenly *crash* diet, its response is to keep a tenacious grip on fat stores. The body will first cause you to *crave* food in order to replenish itself—and the cravings will tend toward the fuel-dense high-caloried sugars and fats. If this ravenous pressure to eat is successfully resisted by the most determined dieter, the body's next line of defense is to slow down its metabolism in order to conserve calories and the fat tissue that remains. In other words, it adapts by burning up food less rapidly because you are supplying it with less—one of the reasons that losing those last few pounds on a diet can get harder and harder. Remember, if we're overfat our metabolism is already slower because there is relatively little muscle to burn ever greater amounts of fat.

Chronic dieting is known to lower the metabolism by as much as 10 to 14 percent! The set-point mechanism is believed by many to be a major reason. Another is that by trying to lose excess fat too quickly, we lose fat, yes, but we also *lose muscle.* This happens when a weight-loss diet is so low in complex carbohydrates that the body has to turn instead to burning protein in order to satisfy certain energy needs, specialized requirements for energy that can't be adequately met by fat. The body will have to use both the protein we eat that otherwise could have gone to the building and repair of muscle and the protein that already makes up muscle tissue itself. The fact is you can't run on empty for long without your muscles, as well as other parts of you, having to pay the price.

I'd like to tell you the story of my friend Hazel Washburn, sixty-two, who has tried every crash diet imaginable and who, finally, has given them up. In Hazel's words,

I was always on a diet. I'd start every Monday morning. By Monday night I'd be off it again. I craved sugar, ate too much fat, and ate on the run. I shunned vegetables and fruit and relished croissants and candy. Eventually, I became a closet eater and the excess pounds became a crisis. I went to talk to the Workout nutritionist. Now, one year later, the weight is gone. I lost slowly, never more than two or three pounds a week. I look forward to my fresh vegetables and fruits, previously scorned, and have no temptation to go back to sweets. I never thought I'd see the day.

I've known Hazel for ten years, since the days when she was working with the United Farm Workers. Now she directs fund-raising for the California Campaign for Economic Democracy. Over the last

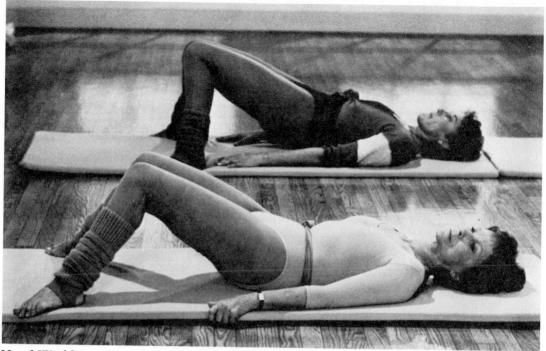

Hazel Washburn, 62, with Femmy DeLyser in the background.

year, I've watched Hazel embody the very things about diet and exercise that I was busy putting into words. She was among the first to join the Prime Time class at our Los Angeles studio. She lost twenty-five pounds. She walks regularly, wouldn't miss an exercise class, and eats well. She's an inspiration to those around her, women and men alike. "This is the first time in sixty years I've felt completely satisfied," Hazel told me. "I never thought I'd be able to exercise—now I'm planning to add the Beginner's Workout to my exercise schedule. I never thought I'd be able to stop thinking about losing weight—now I think about how good I feel. It began as a secret. I did it on my own, for myself, without telling anybody. But then my kids began to notice a change in me. I was more positive. I was less defeated. And, of course, I looked different. I feel that I've gotten my life back."

TUNING UP YOUR METABOLISM

When we need to drop weight, the goal is to lose almost exclusively from fat—not from muscle, or from water for that matter.

The *only* way to lose fat and *not* lose muscle is through exercise—combined with a balanced diet high in complex carbohydrates which will spare the protein you need for your muscles. Exercise, in fact, acts as a *muscle preservative* while unwanted pounds are shed safely. (It may also lower the set-point that regulates the amount of fat our bodies like to store.)

- *The only way to build muscle is through exercise.*
- *The only way to create more of the enzymes needed to metabolize fat in muscle is through exercise.*
- *The only way to slow the age-related loss of muscle mass is through exercise.*

If you're not already at your optimum, the ability to *increase* your lean body mass through exercise is lifelong.

For all these reasons, regular exercise is the best way to raise your body's metabolic rate—permanently—for the long term. Regular exercise also speeds up your metabolism in the short term. Calories are burned faster *while* exercising and, what's more, for hours *afterward*. More food energy is channeled into the working tissues of your muscles than is put into fat storage. And as your muscles heat up, your appetite is also cooled, especially if you exercise an hour or so before a meal. Lastly, regular exercise reduces fat tissue itself, especially so when the exercise is aerobic.

Aerobic exercise is unique in its ability to mobilize subcutaneous fat from *all over* the body as fuel for the large muscles in the legs and buttocks. Aerobic exercise also gets to the marbled fat deep inside the muscle—one of the things dieting, short of starvation, *can't* do. In fact, you can lose twenty pounds by dieting and still look "out of shape" because the fat inside the muscle hasn't been touched. In addition to aerobics, exercises that focus on specific muscle groups reach intramuscular fat too—like those in the Prime Time Workout and my first Workout program. If you combine a balanced *moderate* weight-loss diet with an exercise program like these that include aerobics, you won't just become thinner faster, you'll also have a new, toned, smoothly contoured shape. And as long as you continue to exercise, your body's higher metabolic rate will keep it that way.

Aerobic exercises work so well in all this because they actually favor burning fat as fuel. In the first minutes of aerobic exercise, the ready energy supply of glucose is used. As the activity continues though, the body turns to its fat supply, a more plentiful and denser fuel which needs a lot of oxygen in order to be burned. Aerobics, by definition, means exercising "with oxygen."

This brings me to the final aspect of a tuned-up metabolism—a healthy cardiorespiratory system. The heart, lungs, and blood-vessel network that compose it are responsible for delivering both oxygen and fuel to muscle cells. This system is affected by age, as we already discussed in "The Process of Aging." But like other muscles, your heart, as well as your lungs and your circulation, can be strenthened at any age—through a regular and sufficiently vigorous aerobic exercise program, combined with the kind of low-fat, low-salt diet I'll talk about later.

EXERCISING TO LOSE WEIGHT

- Exercise aerobically at least three times a week, preferably four or five times, but no more than six times a week.
- Exercise for at least 30 minutes—45 to 60 minutes is ideal if your schedule permits.
- Each session should burn between 300 to 500 calories (see page 245 of "Hitting Our Stride" for guidelines on very brisk and mildly brisk exercises).
- Reduce your caloric intake by *no more* than 500 calories a day. (Please see "A Word to Chronic Dieters" on page 220 for my dieting guidelines for losing weight.)
- If you combine burning 500 calories more with eating 500 less, you will have a deficit at your day's end of 1,000 calories—most of them in fat!

As women, we've always been taught, regrettably, that the body's bottom line is the number on the scale—not the composition of that weight, how lean we are inside, or how energetic we feel. But we're learning now that how much we weigh is only part of the picture. A relatively thin person can still be overfat inside, slow-burning, and low on energy. She may be in a constant battle to ward off the fat that shows. But if we build up our metabolic machines, the muscles will largely carry this battle for us. If you're overweight or out of shape now, it will take time to turn fat to lean because it's taken years to lay the foundation for unwanted "middle-age spread." Developing muscles always requires a greater effort than maintaining them. But it can be done—and the sooner we begin the easier it will be. Muscles that have been worked before will respond faster, because muscles seem to have a memory. No matter what our past and present levels of fitness, however, we *all* have to work a little harder if we want to burn rather than store fat, if we want to be fiery furnaces rather than cold storage.

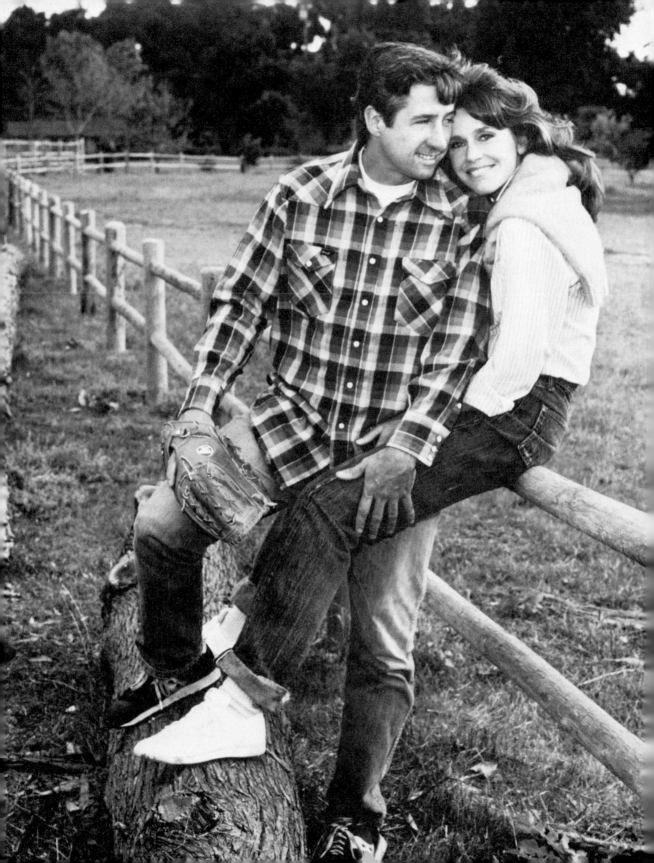

CHAPTER 6

BODY MECHANICS

AS WE REACH THE MIDDLE YEARS, even as early as our thirties, we begin to notice ourselves becoming more prone to aches and pains. We start to feel our muscles, joints, backs, and even bones in ways we hadn't before. Perhaps we suddenly become more conscious of our knees as we walk up stairs. A partner's arm under our back during lovemaking might bring on the wrong kind of spasm. Or a long-forgotten injury, like a personal weathervane, will begin to ache with oncoming rain.

Like every part of the body, the musculoskeletal system is subject to change as we age. Over time, the springy cushions between the joints and in the spine become more dry. Similarly, other supporting connective tissues become less elastic. And the bones become thinner. But as with other age-related changes, none of these need escalate into arthritis, chronic neck and back pain, or the "dowager's hump" of osteoporosis.

Faced with new kinks, stiffness, and pain, many of us tend to slow down—and some doctors still recommend this. But such passivity is the opposite of what's really needed. If we limit our activity in response to normal changes in our joints, back, and bones, their vulnerabilities will actually get worse. Joints will stiffen up even more, not so much wearing out as rusting out. Supporting muscles will atrophy and weaken, no longer able to provide stability to our skeletal structure or stimulation to the bones. If, on the other hand, we continue to use our bodies—wisely—the *strengths* of the musculoskeletal system will be emphasized.

We have to be viligant engineers of this dynamic, internal machinery, learning the basic tools with which to better manage this vital aspect of our midlife fitness. If we know how to prevent unnec-

om and me at Laurel Springs Ranch.

essary damage, to find the optimal balance between activity and rest, and to read the body's messages to us, our joints, back, and bones will last us.

THE JOINTS

Your joints consist of rubberlike connectors, dense shock absorbers, and natural lubricants—many times more powerful than any automotive oil you can buy. The drawings below show the basic structure of all the movable joints in the body, such as the knees, hips, shoulders, elbows, fingers, and toes.

- Tough, slightly flexible *ligaments* hold the joint together, attaching bone to bone and enclosing each joint in a protective sleevelike capsule.
- More flexible but equally tough *tendons* attach muscle to bone on either side of the joint. These are actually the narrowed extensions of muscle.
- Gristly, spongy *cartilage* covers the end of the adjoining bones, permitting friction-free, smooth motion between them.

The Structure of a Joint

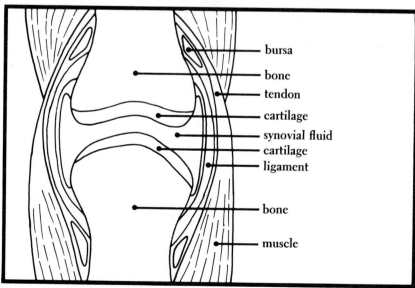

bursa
bone
tendon
cartilage
synovial fluid
cartilage
ligament
bone
muscle

The Nourishment of Cartilage

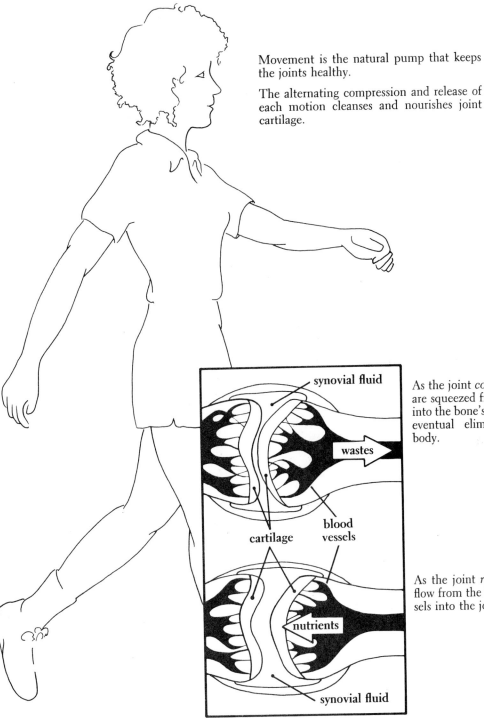

Movement is the natural pump that keeps the joints healthy.

The alternating compression and release of each motion cleanses and nourishes joint cartilage.

synovial fluid

wastes

cartilage

blood vessels

nutrients

synovial fluid

As the joint *compresses*, wastes are squeezed from the cartilage into the bone's blood vessels for eventual elimination by the body.

As the joint *releases*, nutrients flow from the bone's blood vessels into the joint cartilage.

- A thick slippery *synovial fluid* bathes and lubricates the cartilage as the joint moves.
- Near each joint, cushioning sacs called *bursas,* which also contain protective fluids, allow soft muscle tissue to glide easily over hard bone and across other muscle tissue.

The key to keeping your joints healthy is to take good care of the cartilage. It has no circulation of its own and depends on movement of the joint to receive its nutrients and to remove its wastes. When the joint moves, the bones on either side squeeze the pliant cartilage in between. The pumping action forces wastes out, to be taken up by the bone's own blood vessel network. When this pressure is released, rich nutrients from the ends of the bones and from joint fluids wash through the expanding cartilage sponge. Thus you will have healthy, nourished cartilage only if you *use* your joints.

With time, all parts of the joint alter—including the bone and synovia that keep it healthy and the ligaments and tendons that hold it stable. But it's the cartilage that feels most the effects of all this. In addition, as early as our twenties and thirties, the cartilage very slowly begins to lose water. By the time we're in our seventies, most of us will, if X-rayed, show signs of cartilage that's been worn away. Technically, this is arthritis, the most common form called osteoarthritis.

Arthritis

Arthritis is not just one disease. It refers to many different conditions that share common characteristics. The most serious is rheumatoid arthritis, a chronic inflammation which can damage joints and other tissues all over the body but which occurs in less than one percent of the population and is *not* age-related. The most well-known type of arthritis and the one frequently experienced with age is the cartilage degeneration of osteoarthritis just mentioned, as well as the soft tissue inflammations of tendinitis, bursitis and fibrositis.

Tendinitis is pain in a tendon that sneaks up on you over a period of weeks. It is usually caused by the overuse of a joint or by straining a muscle beyond the strength and flexibility of its tendons. Such an inflammation is a major cause of tennis elbow, a common joint affliction.

Bursitis, another local inflammation caused largely by overuse, is pain in one of the bursas near the joint, most frequently occurring in the shoulder, one of the most hard-working joints in the body.

Fibrositis, often described as an all-over body ache and a seemingly middle-years phenomenon, is less clearly understood. There is growing agreement that chronically contracted muscles are the cause. Tense muscles, without any counterbalancing relaxation, can produce premature fatigue and chronic soreness in muscles, as well as in ligaments and tendons of the joints.

These three essentially benign but painful conditions often trigger one another, and hence frequently occur in clusters. If we strain a tendon, for example, the bursas will work doubly hard to protect the hurt tendon and bursitis may result at the same time as tendinitis.

Osteoarthritis, which happens to virtually everyone in time, is caused by the gradual wearing away of cartilage tissue between the joints and in the discs of the spine. Localized and usually mild, osteoarthritis seldom cripples. In fact, only a few people experience symptoms which interfere with their normal activities.

Changes in cartilage progress very slowly over the years. They can, however, be accelerated by the underuse, misuse, or overuse of the joint. An inactive joint will leave cartilage inadequately nourished. A joint that is unstable due to weak supporting ligaments, tendons, or muscles will cause cartilage to wear unevenly, the way a tire tread does when your car is out of alignment. And an injury or repeated stress to a joint without giving it adequate rest can cause adverse effects as well. It is inevitable that we will have some cartilage deterioration as it loses some of its buffering and rebounding capacity, but we can keep that loss to a minimum.

As cartilage is worn away, the joint space between the bones becomes smaller. Instead of generating new cartilage, the body produces non-elastic scar tissue. And in advanced stages, bony tissues tend to grow around worn-out cartilage. These bony "spurs," as they're called, can result in stiffness, pain, and decreased mobility. The symptoms are usually worse in the morning, and tend to come and go in stages. Osteoarthritis can progress for a time and then plateau. For example, without adequate cushioning of the joint, bone may grate against bone. But with continued use, the ends of the

Cartilage Degeneration

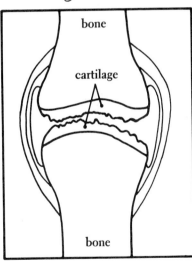

With increasing age, there is a tendency for cartilage to dry out, fray, split, and gradually wear away to some degree. Sensible joint movement is the best way to keep these changes to a minimum.

bones may polish each other to the extent that smooth joint movement is eventually possible again.*

Osteoarthritis occurs in three principal sites. The mildest and the earliest form to show symptoms occurs in the last joints of the *fingers*. This arthritis is largely hereditary, experienced primarily by women in their middle years whose aunts, mothers, or grandmothers may have had it. After a period of swelling and tenderness, this kind of arthritis subsides on its own, leaving behind bony enlargements in the finger joints it affected, with some possible stiffness but little pain.

The *weight-bearing joints* that work so strenuously, particularly the *knees* and *hips*, are the second most common location for osteoarthritis. These joints will be even more subject to arthritis if you are markedly overweight. Lastly, the cartilagelike discs in the spaces between the vertebrae of the *spine* are susceptible to osteoarthritis, and bony growths or spurs can appear in the lower back or in the neck.

Taking Care of Your Joints

The kinds of arthritis we've just talked about are easier to *prevent* than to treat, so it's important to start *now*. The following three remedies will help prevent arthritis and will be effective in treating it as well.

1. Maintain your normal weight.

Extra pounds will place stress on the weight-bearing joints as well as the lower back. Too much weight will also pull joint-supporting ligaments and tendons out of line.

2. Minimize joint stress.

Here are a few key rules of thumb:

- Use the strongest or largest joint possible to accomplish a task.

* Up until now, cartilage repair and regeneration was not thought to be possible. But ongoing research is finding promising evidence that it might well be after all. One major study at the University of Toronto, for instance, has been successful in regenerating cartilage in damaged joints through "continuous passive motion." When moved passively by machine day and night over a period of three weeks, damaged joints seem to build new cartilage rather than outgrowths of bony tissue in the joint.

- Distribute the load over several joints.
- Avoid prolonged periods of holding a joint in the same position.
- Avoid grasping objects tightly and keep your hands open and relaxed whenever possible.

3. Keep fit.

Regular exercise that uses the joints in their full range of motion is essential. It will prime the natural pump that keeps the cartilage nourished. It will also tighten, thicken, and enhance the resilience of supporting ligaments and tendons, while strengthening nearby muscle as well.

The Prime Time Workout has been specifically designed with joint health in mind. If you already have arthritis, you'll find Prime Time also well suited to your special problems. Whatever type of physical activity you choose to do, make sure you pay particular attention to these guidelines:

- Be sure to put your joints through their full range of motion *daily*, with or without aerobics.
- Never increase more than ten percent over your previous day's workout. This gives the ligaments and tendons a chance to catch up with strengthened muscles.
- Always warm up and stretch before you exercise and cool down and stretch after you exercise to avoid exercise-induced injury or reinjury. Warmed up, flexible joints and muscles are much more resistant to injury.
- Pay special attention to form when you exercise and to posture in your everyday activities of sitting, standing, walking, and sleeping. Keeping the joints in proper alignment will reduce abnormal pulls.
- Use protective equipment such as a cushioned mat if you do floor exercises, or stable shock-absorbing shoes if you walk, run, or do studio aerobics for exercise.
- When you're tired, or if something hurts, listen to your body's messages. If you're new at this, you won't always be sure when to exercise through discomfort and when to stop and rest. But this is something you'll get better and better at. The following suggestions may help. If pain is relieved with exercise, continue. If

pain lasts longer than two hours following exercise, that's a clue to cut back next time and pay close attention to whether you need to change the sport or specific exercise that may be causing or aggravating the problem.

- The only case in which you should *never* exercise is when a muscle or a joint is swollen or inflamed.
- If you presently have arthritis, try to select activities such as swimming, brisk walking, or slow stretching that allow smooth movement. Avoid high-tension exercises like weight-lifting that put stress across the joints.

A Word on Injuries

If you do have an injury such as tendinitis, a sprained ligament, a pulled muscle, or "runner's knee," the first order of business is to reduce the inflammation. The Rx for this is RICE—rest, ice, compression, and elevation.

Rest the suffering tissues for however long it takes for the pain and swelling to go away.

Ice the injured area for twenty to thirty minutes at a time, no longer, as soon as possible after the injury. Do this several times during the day. The cold constricts the blood vessels, preventing blood or fluid from entering, thereby reducing the swelling. After icing, the blood vessels return to normal, permitting an onrush of fresh blood which helps to heal the injury. I always keep several ice packs in my freezer. They are designed for this purpose and are available at most pharmacies. You can also wrap ice in a towel or Baggie then place or strap that onto the injured area. After two to three days, the application of heat will help relax the muscles and promote further healing.

Compress the area after icing by wrapping an elastic bandage around it, though not so tight as to be uncomfortable or to restrict circulation. This helps to contain the swelling and generally may be needed for two or three days following the injury.

Elevate the injured part in order to let gravity drain any fluid from the area, short-circuiting the tendency toward swelling.

Aspirin is also anti-inflammatory when taken in large doses, such as two tablets four times a day. It's a painkiller too, so be careful not to use it to "mask" the pain while you keep on moving the injured part. This is the time to rest it, not to work it. (Aspirin shouldn't be used if the area is bleeding.)

Once the inflammation is gone, resume gentle exercise in order to restore or maintain the full range of motion. Eventually, add strengthening exercises to prevent a recurrence of the injury.

Patience is essential for all joint injuries. Most problems involving the musculoskeletal system require the "tincture of time" for healing—usually anywhere from two to six weeks.

THE BACK

- Next to headache, backache is the most common painful condition in our society. Four out of five Americans will experience back pain in their lifetimes.
- For half of those who do, back pain will be a recurring affliction.
- Currently, we spend $14 billion a year on back problems, rivaling the cost of heart disease.
- Back pain results in as much long-term disability and as many lost work days as does any other illness or injury.

These are today's facts about our backs—those indispensable carriers of babies and bundles which we take for granted until the first episode of back pain brings us up short. Those who have already had back trouble, on the other hand, can be *so* sensitized that they start walking on eggshells, afraid that any vigorous movement will retrigger the pain.

But the return of back pain, as well as its first appearance, is *preventable*—and not by shying away from energetic activity, but by building safely up to it. An estimated 80 to 85 percent of all back trouble originates in weak, tense, or imbalanced muscles—the result of too little exercise and our generally tension-filled way of life. Exercise is the best known preventive for back trouble, and it is also the superior alternative to the treatment treadmill and to surgery in almost every case. My own story bears this out.

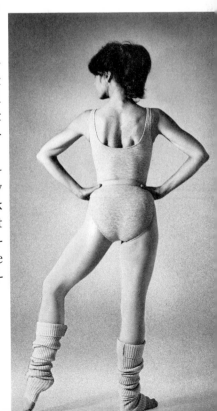

For a woman who likes to feel she can carry her own weight—and bags if necessary—having a strong healthy back she can depend on is of prime importance. How to achieve this starts with knowing how the back works, and also what can go wrong. You'll want to refer to the drawing on the opposite page as we go along.

The *spine* is the primary structure of the back. It's held erect by three stabilizing cables of muscle and tendon— in the abdominals, in the hips, and in the back itself. A column of twenty-four bones called *vertebrae*, linked together by ligaments, make up this firm yet flexible backbone. Cartilagelike *discs* with gelatinous centers cushion the spaces in between the intricately shaped vertebrae. A hollow canal running through the spine houses and protects the body's long *spinal cord* that extends downward from the brain. Pairs of *nerve roots* branch out through openings in the vertebrae and extend to areas all over the body.

Back Pain

The relatively mobile upper back and lower back—the neck and the lumbar region—are the sites of most back pain. And trouble in one often means trouble in the other. One third of low back pain sufferers, for example, will also experience neck pain eventually. There are many kinds of back pain that affect these areas with varying intensities. The three most common are the result of sudden or chronic back strain, injured discs, and arthritis, in that order and sometimes concurrently.

An acute spasm of back pain usually results from an immediate injury like mine, or the trauma of an awkward motion, or abnormal stress that exceeds the strength and flexibility of the back. But many people do not recall any particular incident as the cause. *Constant throbbing pain* usually indicates back strain that has resulted from repeated stress on the back over time, such as consistently slumped shoulders, swayback, sleeping on a poor mattress, or a poorly designed work station.

If you feel *pain shooting down your leg or arm*, it could be a sign that one of the discs of the neck or lower back has "slipped" and is pressing on one of the nerve roots, such as that of the large sciatic nerve extending to the lower limbs. Weakened ligaments allow the disc to bulge or even rupture through the fibrous capsule that nor-

The Structure of the Spine

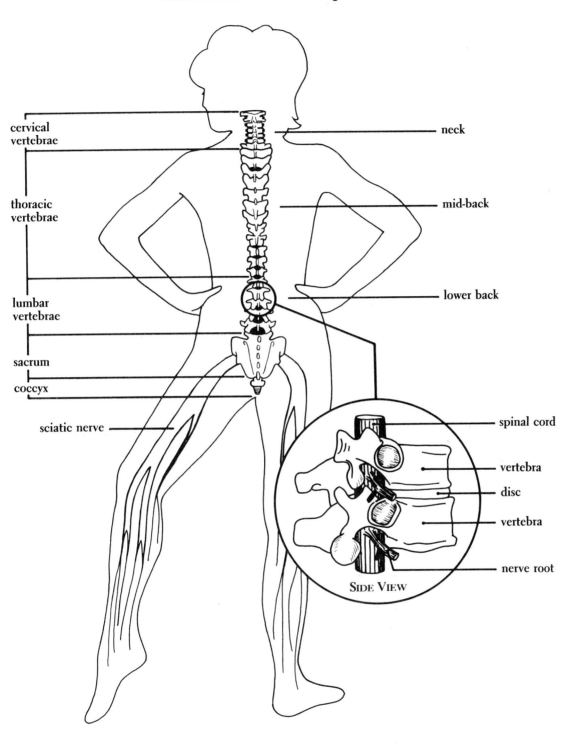

cervical vertebrae

neck

thoracic vertebrae

mid-back

lumbar vertebrae

lower back

sacrum

coccyx

sciatic nerve

spinal cord

vertebra

disc

vertebra

nerve root

SIDE VIEW

mally holds it in place. Such a protruding or herniated disc will heal, but will not return to its former placement between the vertebrae. It remains a weak area of the back that requires special strengthening and lifelong care.

Possibly related to this kind of disc problem are misalignments in the spinal column called "subluxations" which, according to chiropractic medicine, are very common in adults as well as in children, occurring simply from the everyday stresses and strains of normal living. Such misplaced vertebrae can also cause irritation to spinal nerve roots, which can in turn cause pain and malfunctioning not only in the back, but in other areas of the body. Unnatural pressure on these nerves can reduce their effective communication to the cells, tissues, and the organs they regulate.

If you have *backaches, pain, or stiffness that is worse in the morning,* you may have osteoarthritis resulting from an accumulation of back stresses and from normal changes to the disc structure over time. Beginning in our mid-twenties, the discs, like the joint cartilage, slowly start to lose some of their water content—30 percent by our seventies. Disc spaces correspondingly narrow very gradually. By late life it's common to have lost one to one-and-a-half inches in height due to this shrinkage in the discs, which normally constitute one quarter of the spine's length.

Taking Care of Your Back

Any kind of back pain is a sign that you need to start protecting your back more. When you have an involuntary muscle spasm, for example, it means that the muscles are closing ranks around damaged tissue in order to force you to rest it. In fact, in the acute stage of any back pain complete bed rest is usually the first course of action.

Less than five percent of people who suffer back pain will ever require surgical intervention. If you're one of the few who may need surgery as the result of chronic pain from a herniated disc, there's now an excellent alternative to cutting out the disc surgically. An enzyme called chymopapain derived from the papaya and injected into the nucleus of the damaged disc will dissolve the disc's center, taking pressure off the nerve and eliminating pain in almost all cases. Approved several years ago, this new procedure is less expensive than traditional surgery and requires a briefer hospitalization, if any. Many people have relief within hours. If you need to contemplate such a step, make sure the physician you select is experienced in this new and very precise procedure. Also, be sure you are allergy-tested for the enzyme first, because allergic reaction is the principal risk factor with chymopapain.

Back pain of any kind is Nature's way of telling you that you're developing a weakness in your back and that it's time to take the necessary steps to compensate. You can prevent almost all back pain by reducing swayed lower backs, protruding necks, and sagging stomachs; by relaxing tense muscles and strengthening weak ones; and by learning a few basics of back mechanics.

Here's my recipe for a healthy back.

1. Think tall, straight, relaxed.

Poor posture is the principal cause of back trouble. The tendency to slouch pulls the head and neck forward, placing stress on the lower back. The tendency to allow stomach muscles to neglect their job does the same to an already arch-prone lower back. This kind of exaggerated curvature puts tremendous stress on the inside curves of the neck and lower back, and is the cause of almost all chronic pain in those areas. The vertebrae and the discs in between take the brunt of this excessive force. The body is thrown out of line. Muscles have to work overtime to try to correct the imbalances.

Aligned properly, the body is balanced. Stresses are evenly distributed across the back and along the spine. Movement is more efficient and easier. Muscle energy is conserved, so you are less fatigued. The very slight natural curve of the back is restored.

Becoming aware of your posture is the first step—eventually it becomes second nature. Just sitting or standing in a way that requires the muscles to support the back properly will strengthen them, as will the practice of flattening your neck and lower back.

Here are the principles of good posture, the biomechanics of body alignment that we use for every exercise class at the Workout.

- Pull up tall, lengthening from the waist, stretching and straightening the spine. (Think of curling the pubic bone upward toward your navel.)
- Head is held high.
- Chest is lifted.

The Strength of the Spine

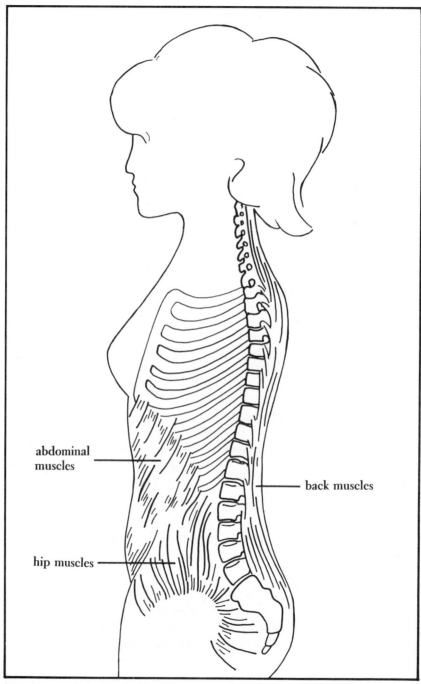

Strong supporting muscles hold the spine erect and in ideal alignment. A healthy spine, as illustrated here, has a slight natural curve.

- Shoulders are pressed down and back.
- Stomach is pulled in.
- Weight rests slightly forward, not back on the heels.

2. Exercise regularly.

Keeping good posture is a matter of developing and maintaining the muscles that hold you erect. To start with, you have to *strengthen the back, stomach, and hip muscles* that support the back. The abdominals tend to be the weakest of these three groups of muscles. When they abdicate their responsibility for holding the spine in place, more stress is placed on the others. Back muscles will tire easily when they have to fight the unnatural pull of a sagging stomach on the lower back. Strengthened stomach muscles, on the other hand, hold the intestines in, pressing them backward and providing support for the spine. When all the muscles are balanced and fully functioning, the back is much more able to withstand the force of a sudden stress or awkward movement.

Regular exercise together with good posture will also *relax tense muscles*—stretching out tightness and breaking a cycle of chronic unreleased tension which can wreak havoc on muscles already stiff or weakened. Tension can pull the body out of line as easily as an imbalance of muscle strength—in fact, the two usually go together. Common reactions to tension are, for example, tight and lifted shoulders, a stiff neck, a rigid spine, the head thrust forward, and clenched jaws and fists. On the other hand, a slouching or collapsed posture may also be your body's way of trying to ease the pain of excess tension. The goal is to build firm yet supple muscles, strength with fluidity, the basis of good posture.

The Prime Time Workout is designed to stretch and also to strengthen all skeletal muscles, especially those of the neck and lower back. Both preventive and therapeutic, these exercises will also help you to release any tension you may have stored deep in your muscles. Swimming is also excellent for the back, as are cycling and brisk walking—up and down hills is ideal. (Going downhill uses more of the back muscles, so build up slowly.) If you already have a back problem, build up gradually in these sports; be sure to cycle upright, avoid the breast stroke in swimming, and be especially careful if you run.

Many of the guidelines for protecting the joints while exercising apply to the back too. Always warm up and cool down. Watch your form. Use whatever protective equipment may be necessary, if any. And respect your body's warning signals. *Don't* try to exercise if your back is in pain. Use rest and ice instead. Only when the pain is completely gone should you begin to build with gentle exercise.

3. Minimize back stress and everyday activities.

Standing and walking: If you have to stand for a long time, rest one foot on a low stool or similar support in order to rest and flatten the lower spine. Wear medium or low heels, which encourage a flatter back. Walk with weight slightly forward, pushing off with your back toes.

Sitting: Sitting places more stress on the back than standing, so observe the first rule of thumb: don't sit for long. A firm chair is infinitely preferable to a soft seat you can sink into. Rest the small of your back against the back of the chair with your feet flat on the floor. If you could obtain the ideal chair, it would tilt, swivel, curve into your lower back, have arm rests and an adjustable height so your knees are slightly higher than your hips when your feet touch the floor. When driving, follow this same principle: keep your knees at hip level or higher by sitting close enough to the steering wheel. Enter the car by sitting first, then bringing your legs in. Pillows specifically designed to support the lower back in a chair or driver's seat are available.

Lifting: Always use the longest, strongest muscles of the arms and legs to help provide power for strenuous activities, such as lifting, pushing, and pulling. Make it a habit to *think* before you attempt a lift, whether it's a baby, bulky box, or stuck window. If the object must be lifted from the floor, no matter how light or heavy it may be, always bend from the knees, not from the back or waist. Keep the back straight and the object as close to the body as possible. Never bend or lift from a twisted position. Always face the object squarely. The more work you can pass on to the legs the better. Let your powerful thigh muscles do as much of the lifting as possible. Also avoid lifting extremely heavy objects above the level of your elbow.

If an object is too heavy to lift, slide it, roll, push, or pull it first. Broaden your base of support by placing the feet wide apart, keeping the knees slightly bent. This lowers your center of gravity, giving you more stability and allowing you to apply the strength of your powerful leg muscles. You actually transfer the force produced by your legs through your upper body muscles to the object you're trying to move.

Carry shopping bags or other bundles close to the body and, if possible, evenly on both sides. Watch the weight of shoulder bags and shoulder luggage that rest on one shoulder, and try to alternate sides.

Sleeping: Sleep on a firm mattress with either a thin pillow or no pillow. If your bed is soft, put a three-quarter-inch plywood board under the mattress. A thinner board won't be solid enough. Your spine will rest better if you sleep on your back or on your side with one or both knees drawn up. Sleeping on your stomach is discouraged because it exaggerates the curve of the lower back and arches the neck upward and out to the side. If you have neck problems, there are specifically designed neck pillows available, or you might want to try a rolled-up towel placed under your neck. If you have a lower back problem, you might want to sleep on your back with a pillow placed under your knees to help flatten the lower back while you sleep.

Back Doctors

Five principal kinds of practitioners specialize in problems of the back. Their different designations and approaches are easily confused, so the following is a brief description.

An *orthopedist* is an M.D. (Doctor of Medicine) with a specialty in treating the entire musculoskeletal system, who is also licensed to perform surgery, including back surgery.

A *rheumatologist* specializes in musculoskeletal disorders and a *physiatrist* specializes in physical therapy and rehabilitation. Both are also M.D.s who take care of back diseases, but neither performs surgery.

A *chiropractor* is a D.C. (Doctor of Chiropractic) who works primarily with the back, usually through the manual manipulation of the spine, on the theory that many back problems as well as other conditions are due to misaligned vertebrae. Chiropractic care may also include other treatments such as ultrasound, acupuncture, kinesiology, and electrical and nerve stimulation. This is a robust but small profession of 22,000 which currently has sixteen four-year colleges of chiropractic.

An *osteopath* is a D.O. (Doctor of Osteopathy) who works similarly to the chiropractor but is considered somewhat higher in the treatment hierarchy. Both practice spinal adjustment, but the older discipline of osteopathy is broader and closer to established medicine. Its schools are largely indistinguishable from medical schools except that osteopathic students are encouraged to go into general practice. Twenty thousand D.O.s are licensed to practice medicine in all fifty states on the same basis as an M.D. They can prescribe drugs and perform surgery. Recently, the American Medical Association (AMA) invited D.O.s to join their organization and to receive M.D. degrees, but the American Osteopathic Association (AOA) has not accepted their offer.

THE BONES

The masterly detective writer Agatha Christie weaves a brief bone lesson into *The Mirror Crack'd* when supersleuth Miss Jane Marple suddenly falls after losing her balance at an afternoon lawn party. Miss Marple's longtime physician and friend runs to her assistance.

"I assure you, Dr. Haydock, I'm perfectly all right," says the vigorous, gray-haired Miss Marple.

"You had a nasty fall," says the concerned doctor.

"Nonsense, I'm not even shaken."

"Yes, I am amazed there's nothing broken, and you got away with just a sprain. I never did discover the secret of your bone structure!"

"Hm," she reflects. "Long, brisk walks as a young woman, I expect." And she goes on to solve another murder mystery.

Christie's two colorful characters reflect the good and the bad news about our bone health as we age. Miss Marple models the possibility for an older woman to have strong resilient bones—if she has exercised. The doctor, however, still holds the familiar but not necessarily correct notion that an older woman will automatically have brittle, easily broken bones.

Bones which thin to the breaking point remain one of the *most common* and *greatest* health threats to our later years. Once considered inevitable for women, however, severe bone loss is now known to be preventable and potentially treatable.

We don't often think of the bones as being alive, but they are as dynamic as any other living tissue in the body. Their network of blood vessels even helps to nourish joint cartilage. Fibrous collagen gives bone the elasticity of wood; calcium, phosphorus and other minerals its amazing strength. Bone cells are in a constant state of breakdown and repair. In the average active body, every bone is completely replaced over a period of seven years. In fact, except for your skin, no other tissue in your body has such excellent regenerative powers. Like all tissues, however, there is a decline in the rate of cell replacement over time. Bones begin to thin when new bone formation no longer keeps up with bone loss. A gradual decrease in bone mass is therefore to be expected. As we've seen with many age-related changes, however, this normal condition can accelerate into a destructive one.

Osteoporosis

Osteoporosis is the end result of severe, prolonged bone loss. If you're new to this medical term, your tongue will probably trip over it as mine did just months ago. You'll forget the word and confuse it with others the first few times you try to recall it. But "osteoporosis" is finding its way slowly into our everyday vocabulary. The increasing numbers of midlife and older women, the most vulnerable to osteoporosis, are making it a public issue of enormous magnitude.

Osteoporosis now affects one in four women after menopause, one in ten severely. More women over fifty-five have osteoporosis than diabetes. The bones don't become smaller, but rather so thin and porous they are easily susceptible to fracture, which can lead to a loss of height or, worse, disability. *One billion dollars* a year is spent on hip fractures alone, one of the most common indirect causes of death for older women.

We reach our peak bone mass at thirty-five. After this time, women begin to lose bone at an *average* rate of about ½ percent a year. This rate can double to one percent in the five years following menopause. Women are eight times more likely to develop osteoporosis than men, who, having larger muscles, larger bones and a

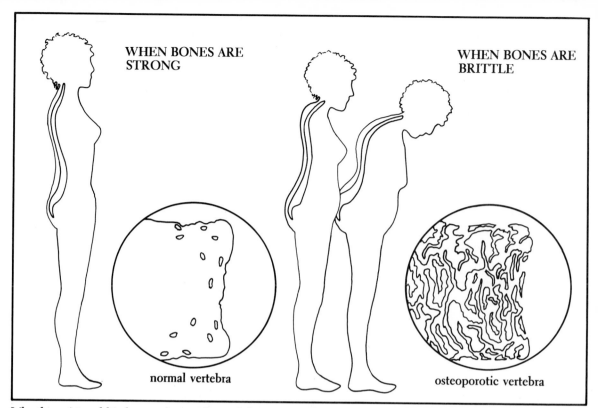

normal vertebra

osteoporotic vertebra

Like the wrist and hip bones, the vertebrae of the spine tend to thin faster than other bones in the body and are, therefore, more vulnerable to osteoporosis. If vertebrae become too porous, they eventually break and collapse. By a woman's seventies, the outward signs of this may be extreme—as shown in illustration—loss of height from the upper body, inward curvature of the lower back, outward curvature of the neck, and a significantly protruding stomach.

higher calcium intake (due to greater consumption of food), start to lose bone about ten years later and at a somewhat slower rate. By age seventy-five, a woman may have lost 30 to 40 percent of the bone in her spine and 20 to 30 percent in the long bones of her arms and legs.

There are three principal areas most vulnerable to thinning and ultimately to fractures, which tend to occur between the ages of fifty and seventy: the spine, hips, and wrists. Bone in these areas can become so weak that it spontaneously collapses just from the weight of the body. More commonly, a break will happen as a result of a fall or an abnormal stress. Fractures of the vertebrae usually bring abrupt, severe back pain, a loss of height, and in advanced states can cause the upper back to round into a classic "dowager's hump." Hip fractures are the most disabling and life-threatening—a woman's life expectancy is reduced by 12 percent if she has had a hip fracture. More women die as a result of osteoporotic fractures each year than are killed by breast cancer, hence the importance of learning about it. Death is not caused directly by the fracture itself, but by a secondary condition, like pneumonia, which may arise during the rehabilitation period.

Bone loss happens to all vertebrates. But our knowledge of it and why it escalates into osteoporosis is limited. There may be no *one* cause, but rather a constellation of interacting factors.

We know that bone formation slows down with age. Bone loss also results from a drain on the large calcium reserves in the skeleton. One of the reasons this occurs is thought to be due to age changes in the special hormones that directly regulate our calcium balance, as well as in the estrogen that appears to play an indirect but protective role in preserving bone during our fertile years. After natural *and* surgical menopause (the removal of the ovaries), when estrogen levels decrease, the risk of developing osteoporosis seems to increase dramatically.

But the most important reason for the loss of bone calcium may be nutritional. Most of our body's calcium, 98 percent of it, is stored in our bones; one percent is in our teeth; and the remaining one percent circulates throughout the rest of the body assisting in many vital functions such as the transmission of nerve messages and the contraction and relaxation of muscles. If this last small percentage of calcium falls too low, the body will automatically draw calcium out of its stores in the bones—even if it has to be at the expense of the bones' health. A diet low in calcium can cause such a negative calcium balance to occur.

It is well established that *most women have a chronically inadequate consumption of calcium.* The recommended daily allowance (RDA) for calcium is 800 mg a day, but the average woman of any age consumes less than 500 mg a day—a level associated with a 1.5 percent loss of bone per year. And now there is evidence that the RDA itself is considerably less than the optimal level of calcium women need in order to maintain strong bones. Habitual dieting also means taking in less calcium. In addition, quick weight loss means bone loss as well. The calcium demands of childbearing and breastfeeding can further deplete our calcium reserves unless mothers have been careful to consume enough for both their own and their baby's needs.

How well the body absorbs and uses calcium is another key factor. Normally, we only absorb about 10 to 30 percent of the calcium we consume. With age, this *absorptive capacity decreases* even more. In addition, *excessive alcohol* consumption and *too much fiber* can interfere with calcium absorption—though we don't have to worry so much about fiber since, regrettably, the average American diet is fiber-poor. A *high protein diet* can add to calcium loss, although protein intake has to be fairly high before you begin to lose calcium—over 95 grams a day. After menopause, vegetarian women have been shown to have stronger, denser bones than women whose diets include a significant amount of protein-rich red meat. Red meat is also high in *phosphorus*, which, if consumed in excess of calcium, may negatively affect the body's calcium balance. Other potential "bone robbers" are believed to be *caffeine, salt, smoking* and *stress*.

Along with nutritional factors, *lack of exercise* may be one of the most important causes of accelerated bone loss. Bone mass decreases when physical activity decreases. Regular exercise, on the other hand, builds bone as it builds muscle. When muscle pulls on bones to work, they respond to this stress by becoming bigger and stronger. The increased circulation brings more oxygen and bone-building nutrients to skeletal cells as well. And the hormonal balance shifts in favor of new bone formation. But chronic lack of exercise will cause the same kind of serious calcium depletion that has shown up in astronauts after their relatively short periods of enforced inactivity and weightlessness during space missions.

Certain *genetic factors* in bone loss seem to be outside our control. Small-framed, fair-skinned, blond or red-haired, very thin women, especially of Northwestern European ancestry, as well as Asians, are at a higher risk of developing osteoporosis than other women. (Blacks are spared this disease for the most part.) A family history of osteoporosis, as well as never having had children or having had an early menopause are additional risk factors. This is all compounded if a woman has never exercised much and has a history of poor calcium intake.

The excellent book *Stand Tall: The Informed Woman's Guide*

to Preventing Osteoporosis emphasizes the point that one of the greatest problems with osteoporosis is that it produces absolutely no symptoms until a fracture occurs. It is a silent disease, difficult to detect early. Backache, a gradual loss of height, and periodontal or gum disease may be warning signs. But one third of your bone can be lost before the condition shows up on a conventional X ray—and once bone is lost, it may be impossible to rebuild. If a vertebra fractures, there's no going back. So *prevention* is the key—maximizing the bone you have at skeletal maturity (age thirty-five), slowing the rate at which you subsequently lose bone, and maintaining a positive calcium balance. The longer we live, the longer our bones have to last us.

Taking Care of Your Bones

There is no established treatment that can *restore* lost bone once osteoporosis develops. But there are definite steps you can take to strengthen your bones whether or not you show signs of accelerated bone loss. If you are under thirty-five, you want to work at maximizing your bone mass. If you are over thirty-five, you want to work at slowing its decrease.

1. **Maintain a positive calcium balance.**

An adequate intake of calcium won't cause new bone formation, but it can slow its loss and arrest the development of osteoporosis. The USDA Human Nutrition Research Center at Tufts University and many others now recommend that women consume 1,000 mg of calcium a day in the years before menopause and 1,500 mg after—as both prevention and treatment.

All dairy products are calcium-rich—yogurt, cheeses (hard more than soft) and, of course, milk. Skim and low-fat milk have the same amount of calcium as whole milk, so try to stick with using these, as well as low-fat cheeses. Sardines, collard, turnip and mustard greens, kale, broccoli, and tofu are also good sources. If you make soups or stews with meat bones, put a small amount of vinegar into the water for the stock; this will draw the calcium out of the bones. (The vinegar is neutralized so there is no acid taste.) When you make sauces, spoon in some nonfat dry milk.

The Best Calcium Foodstuffs
High in Calcium, Low in Fat, Low in Calories

Plain nonfat yogurt, 1 cup, 125 calories, 452 mg calcium
Plain low-fat yogurt, 1 cup, 145 calories, 415 mg
Sardines*, with bones, canned, 3 oz., 175 calories, 372 mg
Collard greens, cooked, 1 cup, 65 calories, 357 mg
Nonfat milk, 1 cup, 85 calories, 302 mg
Low-fat milk, 1%, 1 cup, 100 calories, 300 mg
Low-fat milk, 2%, 1 cup, 120 calories, 297 mg
Buttermilk, 1 cup, 100 calories, 285 mg
Turnip greens, cooked, 1 cup, 30 calories, 252 mg
Nonfat dry milk, ¼ cup, 61 calories, 209 mg
Mozzarella cheese, part-skim, 1 oz., 80 calories, 207 mg
Kale, cooked, 1 cup, 45 calories, 206 mg
Mustard greens, cooked, 1 cup, 30 calories, 193 mg
Broccoli, cooked, 1 stalk, 45 calories, 158 mg
Low-fat cottage cheese, 2%, 1 cup, 205 calories, 155 mg
Low-fat cottage cheese, 1%, 1 cup, 165 calories, 138 mg
Molasses, blackstrap, 1 tablespoon, 50 calories, 137 mg
Tofu, 3.5 oz., 72 calories, 128 mg
Corn tortillas, 2, 126 calories, 120 mg

* Sardines are relatively high in cholesterol and also usually canned in oil, so eat in moderation. Salmon with its bones and oysters are also excellent, low-calorie sources of calcium, though medium-fat.

For many it will be difficult to obtain enough calcium from meals alone. We have to watch calories more as we age; some women develop a lactase deficiency which makes it hard to digest milk or milk products; and knowing just how nutrient-rich our foods are these days can be a problem. It can also be difficult to obtain your optimal calcium intake through a multivitamin and mineral supplement. A special calcium supplement is an excellent way to be sure you're getting the 1,000 to 1,500 mg of calcium a day that you need.

There are a variety of calcium supplements with different advantages and disadvantages, so always *read the label* carefully before buying yours to check both the source of the calcium and how much is in each tablet. The FDA warns against the use of bone meal and dolomite. These have high, potentially toxic levels of lead, which seeks out bone as a storage site. Calcium lactate and calcium gluconate are absorbed well but supply little calcium per tablet, requiring you to take many. Calcium carbonate is often recommended because it is the most concentrated form, though not as easily absorbed as the others. To maximize absorption divide your intake into several doses during the day, on an empty stomach if possible or with a little yogurt or milk. Try not to take your calcium along with a fiber product, such as bran, which can decrease the amount of calcium, as well as other minerals, that is absorbed through the intestine. Taking a half or third of the daily consumption at bedtime is a good idea because we tend to lose more calcium at night during the inactivity of sleep (and also because calcium is a good natural tranquilizer).

If you have a history of kidney stones, be sure to discuss the dosage of your calcium supplementation with your physician. (Your dosage should probably remain below 250 mg a day.) For most of us, a daily intake of up to 2,500 mg is considered a safe calcium consumption, though exceeding 1,500 mg is unnecessary. It's always a good idea during routine physical exams to ask for a measurement of calcium in the urine or blood. Remember, though, a deficiency of calcium rather than an excess is the more likely danger.

There are two minerals whose intake should be in balance with calcium. According to nutritionists, your intake of *magnesium* should be half that of your calcium (calcium supplements like mine often come already combined with this proportion of magnesium). Your intake of *phosphorus* should never exceed and preferably be less than your calcium intake.

VITAMIN D stimulates our absorption of calcium. In fact, it's essential for it. We usually get all the vitamin D we need from our cumulative exposure to the sun during the day. But if you don't consistently get from fifteen minutes to an hour of total sunshine a day, be sure you obtain 400 I.U. of vitamin D through food or supplementation. Cod liver oil, butter, and fish are excellent food sources; especially so is milk fortified with vitamin D, which gives you calcium at the same time. If you do take a supplement be sure not to exceed 1,000 I.U. a day because too much vitamin D can have the opposite effect on calcium absorption. In addition, because vitamin D is fat-soluble it's stored in the body, and therefore it is potentially toxic if you take doses of 25,000 I.U. or more a day over a prolonged period of time. Supplements like "Os-Cal" are available, which conveniently combine calcium and vitamin D, though these tend to be more expensive than other forms of calcium supplementation.

VITAMIN K is another fat-soluble vitamin now thought to be vital to the calcium absorption in bone. Very small amounts are essential, and rarely is supplementation needed. Vitamin K is found in yogurt, green leafy vegetables, alfalfa, cabbage, cauliflower, and potatoes.

Avoid extremely high amounts of protein in your diet, phosphorus-rich soft drinks, and red meat, as well as excessive alcohol, caffeine, salt, and smoking. (You'll find more on calcium later in the nutrition chapter on pages 211–17.)

If physicians were to prescribe calcium for women over thirty, we could reduce the number of osteoporotic patients by at least 60 percent. . . .

Women who run regularly are going to increase their bone mass by 30 percent more than women who lead a completely sedentary life.

Joseph Lane, M.D.
Chief, Metabolic Bone Disease Services
Hospital for Special Surgery, New York

---

2. Exercise regularly.

Exercise is the only known and currently recommended practice that actually *enhances bone formation.* Combined with enough calcium in the diet, exercise can make the crucial difference in building or preserving strong bones. Calcium is deposited in the bones in proportion to the load they have to carry or the work they must do. We can see evidence of this in the longest-lived peoples in the world. No sign of osteoporosis has been found in certain remote communities tucked away in Russia, Pakistan, and Ecuador, where the people routinely live well into their eighties and nineties, some into the hundreds. The key? They are physically active, out-of-doors, far into their old age.

Exercise is already fundamental at bone treatment centers like the Hospital for Special Surgery in New York, where patients have succeeded in *increasing* bone mass by three percent a year. A study at the University of Wisconsin Medical School showed similar bone growth. Women who were in their eighties had an almost *two-percent gain* in bone after thirty minutes of continuous exercise three times a week over a three-year period. Another study of women in their fifties reported an almost *three-percent gain* in just one year after an hour of regular exercise three days a week; the control group of women who didn't exercise *lost* close to an equivalent amount of bone in the same year. "Age doesn't seem to be a major limiting factor in the bone's response to stress," reports Dr. Everett Smith, Director of the Wisconsin study's biogerontology laboratory.

Movement seems to be Nature's way of enabling us to maintain erect, strong, supple bodies throughout our entire life span. As Miss Marple knew, activity is good for the bones. We're still learning exactly what kind and how much is *best*, particularly for *building* bone. Properly performed studio aerobics, walking, running, cycling and other aerobic sports, as well as weight-training, are thought to be especially good. If you already have osteoporosis, you need to take special safety precautions when exercising—finding a balance between an activity which places positive stress on the skeletal structure and one that could cause a fracture. For you, swimming is especially recommended, and long walks twice a day.

3. Keep informed of other options.

ESTROGEN THERAPY is often recommended for women who are known to be at especially high risk for osteoporosis due to their genetics or because an early surgical menopause means many more years without the bone-protective effects of high estrogen levels. If you are thinking of taking estrogen, please read carefully pages 169–79 in "Is There Life After Menopause?" This type of treatment should not be taken lightly. Estrogen therapy for osteoporosis is always long-term—lasting until about age sixty-five for the naturally postmenopausal woman (after that age bone loss tends to slow down on its own) and most likely for the surgically postmenopausal woman as well.

Estrogen therapy will *not* stimulate the formation of new bone, but it will slow bone loss—if combined with the recommended amounts of calcium and vitamin D. No one knows how long estrogen therapy can protect against bone loss. Some say six years, others eight. But it is generally agreed that its efficacy in protecting bone wears off after ten years.

Because of the long-term nature of the treatment, you should take extraordinary care to weigh the benefits of estrogen therapy against the risks, the most serious of which is the increased possibility of developing uterine cancer. There are women whose likelihood of developing osteoporosis is considerably greater than that of developing uterine cancer. In these cases, because osteoporosis is potentially more life-threatening, estrogen therapy will be the best course of action.

EARLY DETECTION of osteoporosis could make a tremendous difference. At the present time, however, the technology is either too expensive or available only to the few who live near research centers with the highly specialized and sensitive X-ray equipment needed to measure bone thickness. Less expensive, more accessible equipment is expected to be available in the next five years or so—hopefully

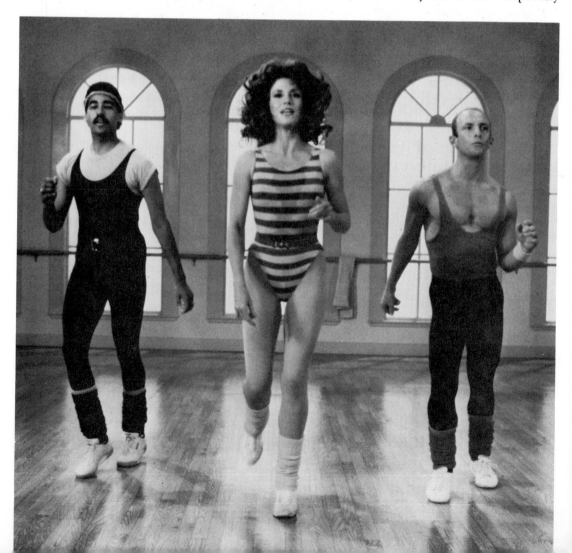

sooner if we create a consumer demand for it. If you have access now to such technology, it's a good idea to get a basic bone assessment, ideally while in your thirties or forties, another at menopause, and then annually for several years following in order to determine your rate of bone loss. (Dental X rays can sometimes pick up bone loss in the jaw, which can be an early indicator of osteoporosis.)

4. Pass the word.
Tell your friends and family about this silent disease and how to prevent it—especially your daughters and women under age thirty-five who can still take steps to maximize their peak bone mass.

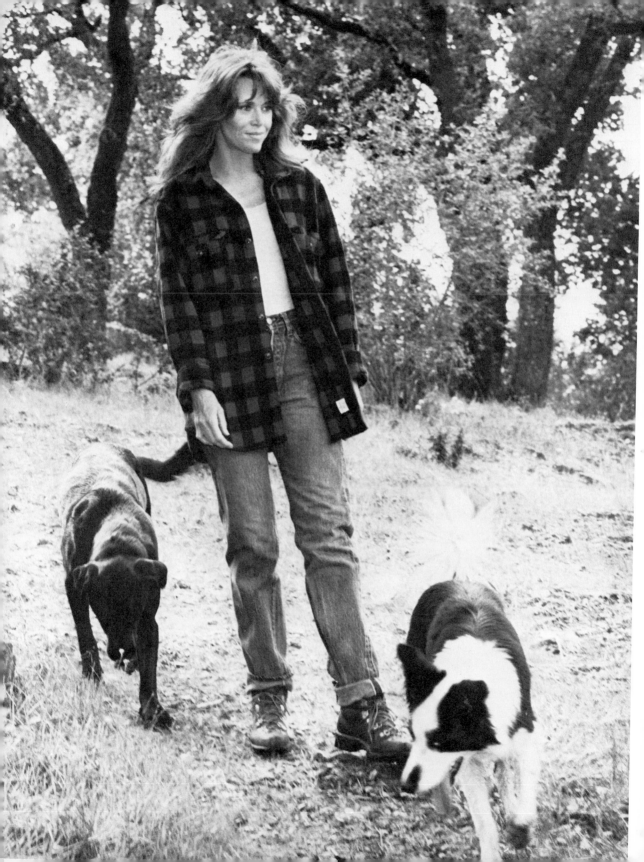

PART THREE

Is There Life After Menopause?

To me, this generation of women, first awakening, coming into the power of middle age, now knowing how to move from sexual symbol into symbol of wisdom, how to have a period of menopause or what I call "a pause without men," frightened of that limbo, thinking we may become wise but are no longer sexual, or thinking if we are sexual we are not supposed to be wise, that one has to be at the expense of the other—just poppycock! Rubbish!

Randi Gunther, Ph.D.
Therapist

CHAPTER 7

NATURAL
RITE OF PASSAGE

IN THE COURSE OF WRITING THIS BOOK there have been times when I've actually hoped I'd have a hot flash. I know my editor secretly wishes I'd have an early menopause so this chapter would be more "personal." But no such luck. I've been a late starter in every other arena and I'm sure this one will prove to be no exception. But bear with me anyway. I'm sure that no matter where you are along the road into or out of fertility, you'll find this chapter as fascinating to read as I did to research it.

The more I learn about menopause the more I'm reminded of how closely women's bodies are linked to Nature, how closely we reflect the symmetry of the natural world around us. During the fertile years, our menstrual patterns revolve with the lunar calendar— the moon's twelve monthly cycles mirrored in ours. At the end of these years, in midlife, there is one final revolution and Nature finishes its turning of the human reproductive wheel. The full circle from menarche to menopause, from the first to the last menstruation, closes with the precision of a fine timepiece. Our fertility's end is as natural and inevitable as was its preordained beginning. Arriving at menopause is actually a sign of physical health—a sign that our body's inner clock is humming along.

But what this event is actually like for women depends on many things and, to a large degree, on how menopause is culturally perceived. Historically, it has been shrouded in superstition. Myths about menopause, woven into the stereotypes of aging in general, have cast an aura of apprehension around this aspect of our growing older—even though for most women the transition away from fertility is a smooth and gradual one, with nothing to fear. Until now, the cultural cloud surrounding menopause has darkened the whole experience and discouraged women from acknowledging with pride this natural rite of passage.

In other cultures, for many religions, such times of letting go and moving forward are celebrated with ritual. Bat and bar mitzvah celebrations, for example, mark the exit from childhood and the entry into adulthood of the Jewish girl and boy at puberty. Rabbi Laura Geller, one of the first women in the country to be so ordained, spoke with us about the need for ritual at menopause. "Such a ritual will not come from the top down—positions usually occupied by

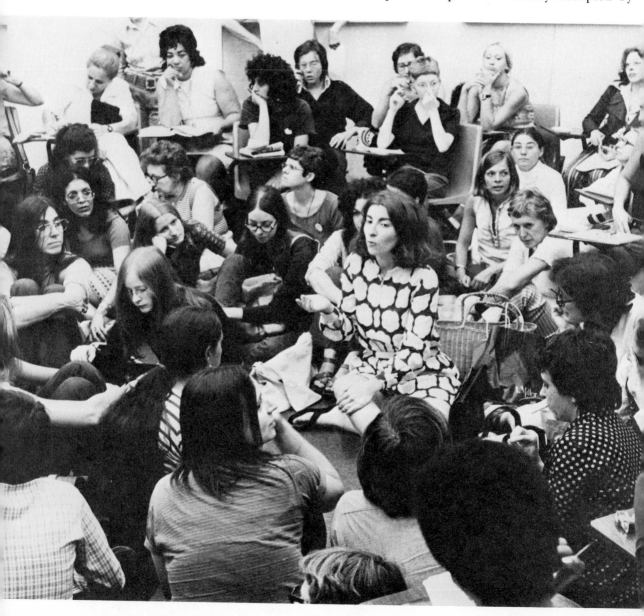

men," she said. "It will come from women themselves. Menopause cuts across racial and socioeconomic lines, bringing all women together. There is a certain collective power in that." The special value of ritual, she explained, is that it provides for us a time of preparation for whatever transition lies ahead, gives permission to talk about it, and, finally, helps us actively to accept and consciously to celebrate the change.

While there may never be a formal "bat mitzvah" for menopause, and in fact we know of no menopausal ceremony anywhere in the world, perhaps our generation of midlife women can begin to create informal, but equally significant equivalents. Educating ourselves about the facts of menopause will better prepare us. Talking about menopause to each other will break the silent taboos. And making menopause an acknowledged part of our culture can transform this part of Nature's design for us into a potentially positive moment in our lives.

Changing "The Change"

Most women and men today have learned about menopause through a hazy folklore of old wives' and old docs' tales. Like myself, you may not recall this dubious education. You may not remember your mother or anyone ever talking about menopause directly. Rather, you may have absorbed many shadowy impressions now difficult to piece together, vague outlines which portrayed menopause as catastrophic—physically, psychologically, or both. Most of my friends say that menopause was an unmentionable subject, such a dark area that their mothers and grandmothers were reluctant to admit to their doctors and even to themselves that they were going through it.

In the recent past, to read about menopause was to cut your way through a plethora of frightening and misleading information of what a woman was supposed to be at this time of life. *Everything You Always Wanted to Know About Sex* told its readers in the early 1970s that "having outlived their ovaries, they [women] may have outlived their usefulness as human beings. The remaining years may be just marking time until they follow their glands into oblivion." This was the literary offspring of the earlier eminent best seller *Feminine Forever*, which sold off the shelves in the mid-1960s to millions and millions of women the idea that menopause meant a loss of womanhood, a loss of good health, and "the transformation . . . of a formerly pleasant energetic woman into a dull-minded but sharp-tongued caricature of her former self . . . one of the saddest of human spectacles." In addition, along with many women's magazines at the time, these books popularized the notion that without estrogen treatment after menopause, we were doomed to become the passive victims of raging hormones and mental aberrations.

Suppose that we had a menopausal woman president who had to make a decision on the Bay of Pigs. . . .

Edgar Berman, M.D.
Personal physician to Hubert Humphrey
Washington, D.C., 1970
Appointee to the Democratic Party's
Committee on National Priorities

Today, these tragic exaggerations have become ludicrous, even comic. Women are striding away from the obsolete caricatures of the "menopausal woman," leaving only their empty shells. And it is these cultural remnants, not ourselves, that are in the process of falling into ruin. If menopause has been a crisis, it has been more a crisis of perception than of biology.

And we can help to change the perception of menopause only if we understand fully the biology. We need to learn as much as we can about what to expect and why. By asking the questions, we are lifting the taboo against discussing menopause openly. The effects of this are already reflected in the new visibility and viability of menopausal research in many different fields. Women are playing pivotal roles as scientists and scholars, as well as healthy subjects in increasing our understanding of menopause. And because of all this, our generation has the opportunity to know much more than our mothers did at that juncture of their lives, when the experience of menopause was largely in the closet and still considered, mistakenly, to be a disease.

I guess I don't like being defined by the tense of my ovarian functions [as a "menopausal woman"]; I would not have liked to have been called a "reproductive woman" in my early years, though I really loved the facts and the acts of reproducing.

Grace Paley
Author

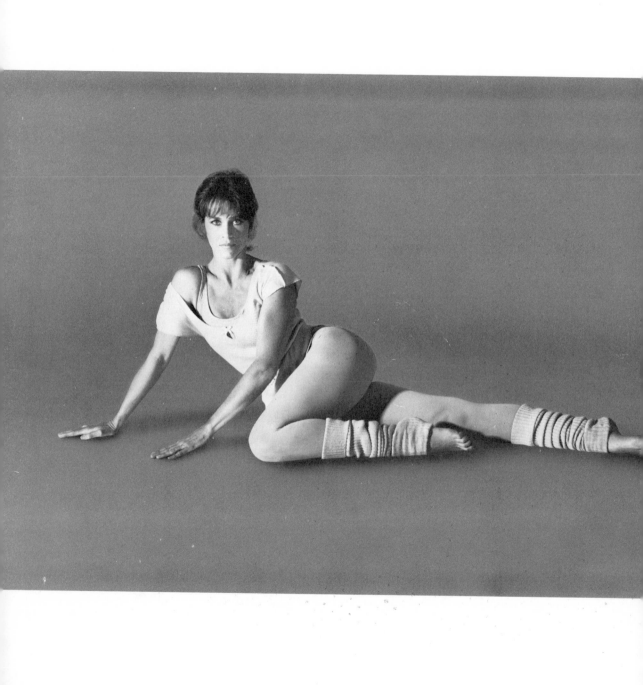

CHAPTER 8

WHAT IS MENOPAUSE?

LET'S START by taking a laywoman's trip through the reproductive system—that part of our anatomy that has already brought us so much pleasure and so much pain. Getting to know its inner workings and its hormonal underpinnings is essential to understanding what occurs before, during and after menopause.

At birth, women already contain the seeds of new life. We are born with nearly *one-half million ova* or eggs held in saclike follicles in our ovaries—a generous gift since only about five hundred of these will be needed throughout the three or four decades of our reproductive life span. Each month during the menstrual cycle, an egg will ripen and be released by the ovary. Unlike the male sperm cells and other cells of the body, these original ova are never replaced by new cells. Rather, there is a gradual attrition of female eggs until menopause. By a woman's late thirties and early forties she has fewer eggs and may occasionally skip ovulation, making it more difficult to become pregnant in those years. Eventually, at an average age of fifty, no eggs remain, or only a relative few that are no longer sensitive to the chemical messages that previously would have caused an egg's release. Ovulation ceases, menstruation stops, and the cycle of fertility has completed itself.

Strictly defined, menopause occurs at the *final menstruation*. It is generally agreed, however, that one full calendar year without menstruating at all must pass before we can be certain we are no longer ovulating, no longer fertile.

Some women experience an abrupt end to menstruation, although that is uncommon. Most go through a period of gradual transition that includes a winding down of the cycle in *premenopause*; its closure in *perimenopause*, the time closest to the last menstruation; and the body's final adjustment in *postmenopause.* Medically referred to as the *climacteric,* these three stages take place over a matter of years and embrace the entire changeover from the reproductive to the nonreproductive phase in women. During this transition subtle changes in our remarkable internal reproductive system begin to occur, five or even ten years before menopause.

Endocrine Ecology

If we view the ova as having a leading role in the great reproductive drama, then the endocrine system can be seen as providing the supporting cast and the technical talent to ensure a smooth and successful production every month.

The endocrine crew is a group of small organs called glands that secrete minute but very powerful chemical substances called *hormones.* These hormones travel from the glands through the bloodstream carrying messages to specific organs in the body. The hormones "urge on" virtually every cell in the body to do its proper work, influencing all the activities of daily life. In Eastern practices, such as yoga, the endocrine glands are considered the *chakras* or energy centers of the body. Each of these glands with their particular hormones and specialized functions works in a team with all the others. Any alteration in the balanced pattern of chemical relations, any change to one part, can cause a shift in the whole system.

Four hormone producers are especially significant to us at menopause: the hypothalamus, the pituitary, the ovaries, and the adrenals. The hypothalamus and the pituitary gland—the producer and the director of the whole endocrine system—are located in the head. About the size of a walnut, the *hypothalamus* is part of the lower brain. It serves as a link between the endocrine system and the brain and nervous system, keeping both systems sensitive to the environment of the other. Through the hypothalamus, for example, our thoughts and emotions can affect the functioning of the glands and their hormones; likewise, the glands can influence our state of mind—a reciprocal relationship that science is just beginning to understand and which may be crucially important for understanding the experience of menopause. The hypothalamus controls all hormone release in the body and is directly involved in regulating the reproductive cycle as well as the body temperature. It directs the

The Key Glands

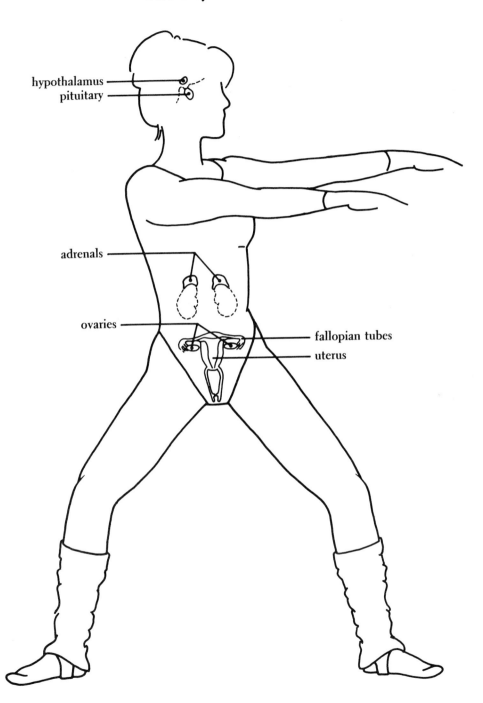

hypothalamus
pituitary

adrenals

ovaries

fallopian tubes
uterus

entire endocrine system by secreting specialized hormones that release the pituitary, the "master gland," to do its work.

The *pituitary*, resting just beneath the brain, controls each individual gland of the endocrine system and through them all body activities. After being triggered by the hypothalamus to start the reproductive cycle going, the pituitary produces its own specialized hormones which in turn activate the ovaries.

Located in the pelvic area, the *ovaries*—about the size of two almonds—are situated at the fingerlike ends of the fallopian tubes which lead to the uterus. These glands are the principal producers of women's *sex hormones* (or sex steroids as they are sometimes called), the most important of which are *estrogen* and *progesterone*. These are the hormonal focal points of menopause. Both hormones have dominated the fertile phase of our lives and are, accordingly, significantly altered at menopause.

The Changing Cycle

Now let's put all these glandular pieces together to see what happens at menopause.

During the menstrual cycle, the hypothalamus-pituitary-ovarian glands form an information exchange loop between them. Through hormone messengers, a feedback system from gland to gland ensures that a regular sequence of events makes conception possible each month, providing a welcome environment for an embryo in case fertilization occurs, and shedding the prepared uterine cells if it doesn't.

In the first half of the cycle, hormones from the pituitary stimulate an egg to ripen in the ovary. The ripening egg then stimulates the production of increasing amounts of estrogen which begins to prepare the uterus for an embryo. At midcycle, estrogen is at its peak and the now mature egg is released into the fallopian tubes where it may or may not be fertilized. In the cycle's second half, progesterone is secreted in increasing amounts which further builds the uterine lining and, if fertilization doesn't take place, eventually causes this lining to be shed in menstruation. At that point the levels of estrogen and progesterone both drop dramatically. The cycle immediately begins anew and the hypothalamus again tells the pituitary to signal the ovaries to release an ovum. This self-cycling system will repeat itself month after month, year after year, until premenopause, when irregularities may begin, and menopause, when it ceases completely.

What happens to change all this? Probably several factors. But one, a profound, programmed alteration in part of the system, ultimately rings down the curtain on the whole reproductive cycle. The ovaries reach their zero sum of ova. The rare few which may remain can no longer respond to the stimulation of the hypothalamic-pituitary messengers. The ovary ceases its cyclic production of estrogen, mature eggs, and progesterone.

The reproductive endocrine network enters a time of disequilibrium and readjustment that manifests itself with great variation among women. Lower levels of estrogen may appear even before the final menstruation. The pituitary hormones, on the other hand, usually increase dramatically as though working overtime to try to stimulate unresponsive ovaries; these remain at high levels for two to three years after menopause. In spite of these ups and downs, however, the hormonal system is not runaway, out of control. It is simply realigning itself, bringing with it a new state of balance.

A New Equilibrium

Contrary to popular belief, our bodies *do not* cease producing sex hormones after menopause. They are merely produced in smaller amounts. There's a rise and fall of estrogen production over the span of our lives just as there is each month during the period of our fertile years. Until first menstruation, our bodies produce estrogen at a steady and relatively low level. At puberty, the level of estrogen begins to increase because one of its key roles is to develop and maintain the tissues of our sexual organs—the breasts, uterus, vagina and urethral area. The production of estrogen reaches a peak for most women in our twenties and thirties. Later, when the task of reproduction is completed, we return to our originally lower, more stable levels.

But in this last phase, we begin to produce estrogen in several new ways. First, half will now come from the *conversion of the male hormones* testosterone and androstenedione into estrogen. Second, the major responsibility for all estrogen production now shifts from the ovaries to the *adrenals*, the small crescent-shaped glands that sit atop the kidneys. The ovaries continue to secrete small amounts of estrogen and testosterone. But the adrenals now take over more responsibility for all sex hormones, a role much less well known than the part they play in secreting the hormone adrenaline during times of danger or stress.

Healthy adrenals, as well as healthy ovaries, can mean a relatively stable production of estrogen for many years following menopause, though we will never need as much estrogen as we once did for reproduction. They may make a tremendous difference in how we experience menopause and the years afterward. How well we produce the sex hormones is partly up to our individual genetics. But it is also influenced a great deal by how fit we are, a subject to which we'll return shortly.

Another factor in estrogen production is possessing an *essential* store of body fat—something few of us fall short on. The fat cells play a unique role after menopause in providing the site for the conversion of male hormones into estrogen. Hence, we don't want to have less than 15 percent of our body weight in fat—a guideline true for any age. Of course, neither do we want to exceed 22 to 25 percent fat. Few of us have access to the kind of equipment that measures body fat, nor is it essential that we do. These figures are just to give you an idea of the range that's optimal for health as well as appearance. Dropping below the minimum is *very* difficult to accomplish, generally only at the cost of extraordinarily compulsive exercise and a near-starvation diet. The vast majority of us have our worries on the opposite end of the body composition scale.

WHAT YOU CAN EXPECT

Ultimately, as our cycles wind down, all of us will stop menstruating. Almost one-third of us will have our last period by the age of forty-eight, half by fifty, and three-fourths by fifty-two. As far as we know the latest a woman has ever menstruated was at age fifty-eight. We have no sure way of foretelling when our own menopause will happen. Some have thought the age a woman begins to menstruate contains a clue to the age she'll stop; so far, however, no clearcut evidence of such a connection has been found. Our mother's age at menopause *may* help to predict our own, though that too is uncertain. Smoking, as several studies have shown, appears to cause an earlier menopause, as might poor nutrition. Beyond these bits of information, all we can know with confidence is that optimal health is the best way to maximize our reproductive life span and to remain healthy, vital, and happy through menopause and beyond.

Changes Large and Small

So long a part of life's routine events, the monthly period begins to lose its regularity for most women some time in the premenopausal years. What is "normal" becomes hard to define at this time, but there are several patterns that might be expected before the final menstruation. First and least common, a woman's periods may continue as they always have, with no observable changes, until at some point they simply stop. More often, periods gradually taper off, their duration shortening each month until finally no menstruation occurs at all. Last but most common, we may have irregular or missed periods that happen only occasionally at first but then increasingly often until the periods cease altogether. We may also experience a heavier or lighter flow, longer or shorter times in between periods, and a more noticeable cramping or breast tenderness.*

During this period, variation and flux are as much the rule for ovulation as for menstruation. Ovulation can be sporadic and come at unusual times of the month. You may have periods without ovulation. Though much more rare, you may also ovulate without an accompanying period and this can occur even following your final menstruation for a time. All of this means that in some cases becoming pregnant can become more difficult, as I mentioned earlier. In others it may happen when you least expect it.

If you do not want to become pregnant in these years, you should use a safe and effective method of contraception until *at least a year has passed after your last period.* Do *not* take birth control pills,

---

* Prolonged, profuse bleeding with clotting *may* be abnormal, as may spotting between periods or after you've already stopped menstruating for a year. If abnormal bleeding does occur, you should always check with your physician, who may prescribe an endometrial biopsy or, more likely, a dilation and curettage (D&C) of the uterus, which is the best course for diagnosing the cause. A D&C will thoroughly scrape the inner lining or endometrium of your uterus; endometrial tissue can then be examined for any abnormality. This is minor surgery that usually itself solves the problem in 80 to 90 percent of the cases. (A Pap smear should always be done before a D&C to help rule out the possibility of cervical cancer.)

which are unquestionably unsafe for women in midlife. After age forty, there is a decidedly greater risk of death from blood clotting, heart attack, and stroke—especially but not exclusively for women who smoke. Even after thirty-five, the pill is less safe.

Condoms and diaphragms are effective methods of contraception when used properly; they are also the *safest.* Voluntary surgical sterilization is the *most effective* and also now the most widely used method of birth control in the country, the favored choice of women over age thirty-five. Most choose to be sterilized by a process called tubal ligation. Others rely on the sterilization of their partners through the process of vasectomy. Both methods make it impossible for sperm to contact the mature egg. Tubal ligation is relatively minor surgery, though it still requires anesthesia, with the attendant risk of complications.*

The IUD is less safe than either the condom or the diaphragm and less effective than sterilization, but it is nevertheless a viable choice if you can accept the risk of infection that is higher for IUD-users. (The fewer partners a woman has, the less risk.) If you have an IUD, be sure to have it replaced every three years to lessen the probability of an infection.

Although it is unreliable as an aid to birth control because of uncertain fertility patterns, I keep a personal record of my menstrual cycle as a preparation for menopause. Even before their middle years, many women keep such a cycle diary. On a very simple chart, like the one included here, you can note the day your period starts, how many days it lasts, the kind of flow, and anything else you may want to keep track of. You'll learn your own body's pattern and when to expect your next period. It can be reassuring to know you're on top of things when and if irregularities begin to appear, and you'll be well prepared for any visit to the doctor. You may also want to use this self-tracking system for the other signs of menopause—especially the hot flashes experienced by so many women.

---

* For more information on sterilization, contact the Association for Voluntary Sterilization whose address is given in the Resource Guide. If you become pregnant after age thirty-five, your chances of having a baby with Down's Syndrome are relatively low (only 4 percent), but they do continue to increase as we get older. You should therefore consider having an amniocentesis, a procedure which permits the examination of amniotic fluid surrounding the fetus. This test makes it possible to detect Down's Syndrome and other genetic defects early in your pregnancy.

X = day of menstruation
/ = day of spotting
● = breast self-exam

PERSONAL CHART

	1	2	3	4	5	6	7	8	9	10	11	12	13	14	15	16	17	18	19	20	21	22	23	24	25	26	27	28	29	30	31
JAN																															
FEB																															
MAR																															
APR																															
MAY																															
JUN																															
JUL																															
AUG																															
SEP																															
OCT																															
NOV																															
DEC																															

X = day of menstruation
/ = day of spotting
● = breast self-exam

PERSONAL CHART

	1	2	3	4	5	6	7	8	9	10	11	12	13	14	15	16	17	18	19	20	21	22	23	24	25	26	27	28	29	30	31
JAN	X	X	X	/										●																	
FEB			X	X	X	/									●																
MAR								X	X	X								●													
APR								X	X	X	/								●												
MAY											X	X	X							●											
JUN											X	X	/							●											
JUL												X	X	X							●										
AUG												X	X	/							●										
SEP													X	X	X						●										
OCT													X	X	/								●								
NOV													X	X	X	X							●								
DEC														X	X	X							●								

131

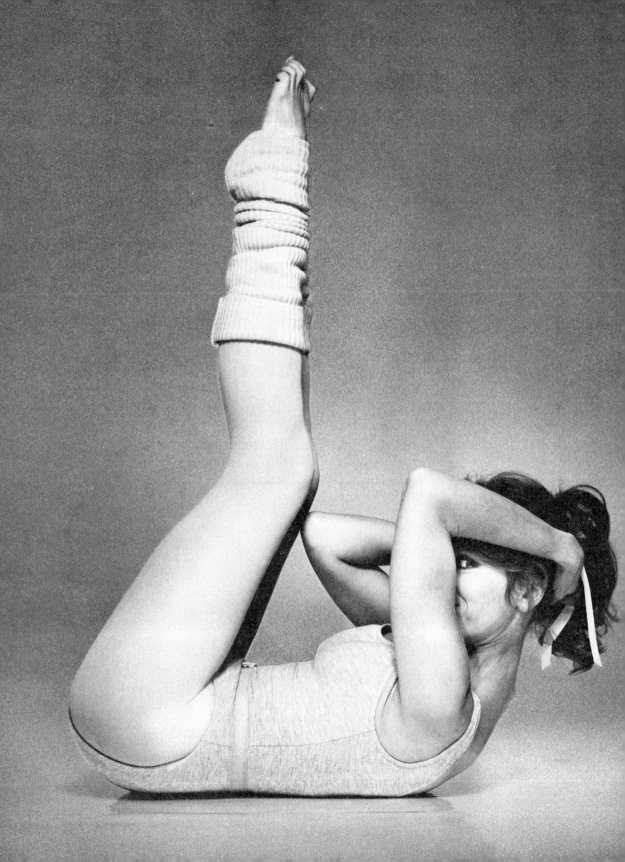

CHAPTER 9

SWEATS
AND FLASHES

WHAT WE HAVE come to know as *hot flashes* are sudden, intense sensations of body heat with no immediately apparent cause. They are the feverish, "common cold" of menopause that usually produce sweating and are sometimes followed by chills. They are often, but not always, accompanied by a *flush* or reddening of the skin. They may occur less abruptly, coming on more like the allover warmth of a general *sweat.*

As far as we know today, 75 percent of all women who go through menopause will experience hot flashes in some form. Fortunately for most of us these sensations will be mild. Usually a feeling of heat will begin in the upper body and travel further upward to the neck and head—perhaps to the scalp, the ears, the cheeks, or maybe even the entire face. But a hot flash can begin at any point in the body. It may spread down rather than up, or in both directions, or it may not spread at all.

What exactly causes hot flashes to occur is still imperfectly understood, nor do we know why some women seem immune. Until recently, hot flashes were virtually ignored and not considered worthy of serious investigation by the medical community, even though they were treated for years with oral estrogens. Now, fortunately, a number of researchers are focusing on the phenomenon of hot flashes and, hopefully, will soon be able to provide answers to the questions remaining. What mechanism sets off a hot flash? How does it take place inside the body? When will hot flashes stop naturally for most women, without drug therapy?

At this point, the hypothalamus is thought to be the internal switch for the hot flash mechanism. Remember, among the many functions of this key part of the brain is the regulation of our body temperature. When the body is too warm, the hypothalamus will send chemical messages to the heart prompting it to pump more blood and to dilate the blood vessels, especially the tiny capillaries in the upper layers of the skin. This relieves the excess body heat and causes us to sweat, which cools the body even more.

Around the time of menopause, for reasons yet unknown, the hypothalamus may adjust the body's thermostat *downward* in response to the significant hormonal changes that are occurring. At such a lowered set point, temperatures that before would have felt comfortable now become too warm. The body proceeds to do all the things it normally might to cool itself—dilating the blood vessels in a flush and perspiring in a sweat to release the unwanted body heat. What is 70 degrees may suddenly feel like 100 degrees to a woman about to have a hot flash.

The experience of hot flashes and how they occur are different for each of us. Most hot flashes last a matter of two or three minutes—although some are less than a minute. For some women, they happen mostly at night during sleep; these women often awaken in a sweat. For others, hot flashes occur mostly during the day. They can also be completely unpredictable. There may be as few as one a week or as many as one an hour or more. Whatever the pattern, only about ten percent of women report their hot flashes as severe—inordinately frequent, lengthy, or chronically exhausting if sleep is continually disrupted. For the large majority of women, hot flashes are mild or moderate and not a significant problem. Some women even find them a sensual, pleasurable experience. In fact, hot flashes are considered signs of health in some cultures—the more the better, I'm told, as far as Welsh women in South Wales are concerned, for example.

The majority of women begin experiencing hot flashes a year or so before menstruation stops, though for some hot flashes can begin earlier or later. Continuing to have hot flashes for at least a year is common. Having them for five years or more, usually in our fifties, is likely for the majority of us. And some women report experiencing hot flashes as late as the age of sixty and beyond.

WHAT IS TO BE DONE?

When you begin to experience hot flashes, it can be tremendously useful to document them in the interest of uncovering their unique pattern for you—if one exists. The best calendar is a daily one, with enough room to record the *time of day*, the *duration* of each hot flash, how it *spread* if at all, and *what may have precipitated it.* In a short time, this not only helps you to understand what is happening, but also to establish a greater feeling of control over your hot flashes and, as you know your body better, over the menopause experience in general. Some women are able to isolate what triggers their hot flashes, giving them even more information to work with. For a few women, paying too much attention to hot flashes seems to make them worse. If that is the case for you, I recommend trying to devise another method for monitoring your own susceptibility to hot flashes.

So far, there doesn't appear to be a common trigger among women who experience hot flashes. But we do have a few clues. Negative stresses, both emotional and physical, seem to be involved in setting them off. Everyday normal stresses to our bodies can become even more stressful at this time when the body is getting its internal bearings, seeking a new hormonal balance. You should watch the following possible triggers carefully. (You'll find these stress-producers resurfacing throughout the book, so note them well.)

Alcohol—which dilates the blood vessels.

Smoking and *caffeine* in teas, coffees, colas, and chocolate—which both influence the central nervous system and constrict the blood vessels.

Swings of blood sugar that come from consuming too many simple carbohydrates and simple sugars, including alcohol.

Spicy, highly seasoned foods, including *salt*—which not only is involved in high blood pressure, but which also contributes to *water retention*, itself a potential problem during this time of hormonal readjustment and a possible catalyst for hot flashes.

The *loss of potassium* that can occur through profuse sweating from frequent hot flashes, though probably not a trigger in itself, should be offset by eating foods rich in this important mineral, such as bananas, oranges, apricots, and raisins.

We know that hot flashes can happen to any woman, active or sedentary, homemaker or paid working woman. But we also know that we can, to a degree, control whatever may trigger hot flashes, and there is a lot of room to lessen their impact. I'm convinced that proper diet and exercise are critical for every woman. They can make a huge difference in alleviating or even stopping hot flashes. There's no question we'll be better able to cope if we're fit.

Later, in Part IV, "Making It Last," you'll find the basics of my complete midlife program of diet and exercise. Here, I want to identify some of the specifics that apply especially to hot flashes.

The Diet Factor

First, nutrition. You already know about eliminating smoking, alcohol, salt, sugar and caffeine. Here are some things you can add.

VITAMIN E: There has been no scientific research about vitamin E that can either affirm or refute the claims of its effectiveness in alleviating hot flashes. But there is enough testimony in its favor from physicians as well as from women who've taken vitamin E to include it here as a possible help for hot flashes. According to the medical newsletter *Women's Health '82*, vitamin E lessens the intensity of hot flashes in 50 percent of women who experience them. We know that this major midlife vitamin is essential for the production of all sex hormones and for the health of strong, flexible capillary walls.

It's difficult to find vitamin E naturally because a great deal of it is lost in the milling and refining of processed foods. Its greatest concentrations are found in whole grains, nuts, and in *unprocessed* vegetable oils, such as corn, safflower and soybean oil. The best natural sources are raw wheat germ and wheat germ oil. You will find information about the dosage physicians sometimes recommend for hot flashes on page 214 in the chapter on nutrition. If you decide to take a supplement be sure to build up gradually. Whether you increase your vitamin E intake through food or supplementation, it may take a month or longer to see results, so give it a good try for at least several months.

SELENIUM AND VITAMIN C: Some women take a combination supplement that includes both vitamin E and the vital trace mineral *selenium*, which enhances the action of vitamin E. Selenium is also found naturally with E in wheat germ and wheat germ oil. You can also take vitamin E with a *vitamin C* supplement because C protects E from destruction and enhances its activity.

HERBAL REMEDIES: Herbs and herb teas are our original medications, and some have been used for hot flashes. Like any medicine, however, they should be used carefully. The best rule of thumb is to use them always in moderation.

Used for thousands of years in the Far East as tonics for general wellness, the traditional female root *Dong Quai* and its male counterpart *Ginseng* may each help to alleviate hot flashes. These herbs may contain estrogenlike substances and are reported to be especially effective if taken in addition to vitamin E.

Other herbs that may also be helpful are black cohosh, red raspberry, life root, squaw vine, sarsaparilla, blue vervain and fo-ti-tieng. You might want to try these as teas, alone or in combinations.

The Exercise Angle

As a kind of "home-brew estrogen" and stress-reducer, exercise done regularly can profoundly influence our experience of hot flashes, as well as the other signs of menopause. Exercise tunes up the entire endocrine system, producing positive hormonal changes.

At the time of menopause and in the years following, two hormonal elements are particularly important. First, how much estrogen we continue to produce. Second, how well this estrogen is received and utilized by the tissues. The belief is that exercise can enhance *both* of these processes—before, during, and after menopause.

Consistent vigorous exercise increases the levels of estrogen circulating in the blood, as well as adrenaline, testosterone, and other hormones. Exactly why this happens remains unclear. It may be that exercise causes more hormones to be produced. Or it may also be that exercise alters how our hormones enter the cells of the body. In other words, the higher levels of hormones may be the result of an increased production, a reduced uptake by tissues, or even a reduced excretion of hormones through the urine. But for whatever

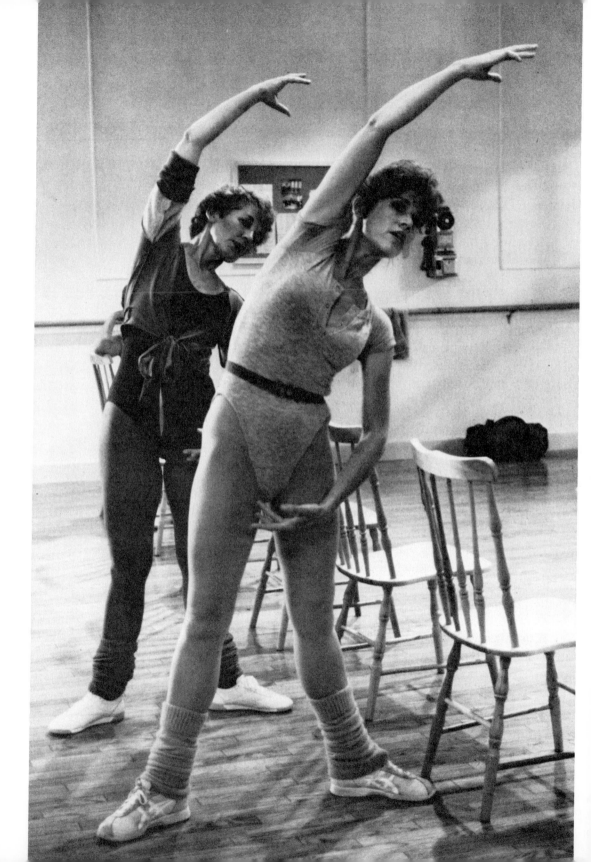

reason we do have more estrogen circulating in the blood after exercise. We're just beginning to learn the effects of strenuous exercise on the endocrine system. But the good news thus far indicates that regular workouts keep the sex-hormone glands—the ovaries and the remarkably hardy adrenals—in top form.

Our systems also have to be effective in putting the hormones to work in the body after they are produced. "To be effective, the hormones you make have to find their appropriate locks," Dr. Estelle Ramey, an endocrinologist at Georgetown University Medical School, explained to us. Hormones must be able to "key" into specific receptors or doors found on cell walls in order to enter the tissue these body chemicals are designed to influence. If the tissues themselves are kept healthy through exercise, they are better able to receive and to utilize the estrogen and other hormones that our bodies do produce. All of this can mean the alleviation, and in some cases even the prevention, of hot flashes and other signs of menopause.

Done vigorously, exercise may offer an *added* benefit for the specific experience of the hot flash. Physically active women are now known to have a much greater tolerance for heat stress. Physiologist Dr. Barbara Drinkwater of the University of Washington is in the forefront of exercise research that includes midlife and older women. According to her well-documented studies, "Active women begin sweating sooner and have a higher sweat rate [than inactive women]. The body is able to cool itself faster and more efficiently. Physical activity enhances the responsiveness of our sweating mechanism, and this capacity, it has also been discovered, does *not* diminish with age."

When we visited The Menopause Clinic in San Diego, one of the first among a growing number of such clinics across the country, we found that women there attributed a similar importance to sweating. They had observed that women who weren't "great sweaters," chilled easily, and had poor circulation, seemed to have the greatest problems with hot flashes. Those of us who exercise regularly know how our improved circulation makes us less apt to feel chilly, especially in the hands and feet. Extremes of temperature become easier to tolerate, especially heat, since our ability to sweat improves with exercise. It may be too that the more accustomed we are to working

orking out with Femmy DeLyser, the Director of
Pregnancy, Birth and Recovery Program at the
orkout studios.

up a good sweat with exercise—which can feel great and which cleanses the body—the less bothered we are by the experience of a hot flash.

Common-Sense Cool-Downs

1. **Don't fight it.** You can't argue with sweat. Hot flashes are natural and safe. They are a sign that your body is doing its work, adjusting to a new internal environment. Don't panic, just let the flash pass. Accepting it can be an important part of making the hot flash a non-problem.
2. **Rethink your wardrobe.** For a time your changing body may require a changing wardrobe. Wear fabrics like cotton that allow your skin to breathe, and avoid non-breathing polyesters and snuggly, but roasting, woolens. Don't wear long sleeves and high necks. Rule of thumb for a hot-flash wardrobe: less, looser, and layered.
3. **Create night strategies.** If you get hot flashes during your sleep, the layers here should be in blankets that keep you perfectly warm but can, when necessary, be peeled off one by one to keep you perfectly cool. You might want to sleep on a large towel. If you have a partner, try an electric blanket with separate controls in the fall and winter months. With good covers, you can wear the lightest or least bedclothing any time of year. Always be sure to have a fresh, warm change of sleepwear ready, within easy reach, in case of a night sweat and the usual chill that follows.
4. **Drink water.** A cold glass of water can help and is always good for you. You may want to get in the habit of carrying your own thermos of ice water. When available, cool showers and swims can give a cool splash to a hot flash.
5. **Talk hot.** Being a "closet flasher" may hurt. Talking about hot flashes spontaneously or when you think it's appropriate can be a positive step.
6. **Relax and think cool.** Find a place where you can sit or lie quietly. Concentrate on deep breathing, inhaling and exhaling slowly, relaxing your entire body. Feel all the tension drain from

you. Once you are relaxed, think of a cold, snowy landscape, a cool forest glen, or whatever your favorite cool image might be.

7. **Watch the temperature.** Unless it will get you in trouble with other members of your household, try to keep room temperatures low at home, perhaps at 65 degrees. Indulge in fresh air whenever you can. Always take advantage of windows, fans, and air conditioners. Avoid hot environments, if at all possible. (Be sure, on the other hand, not to become over-chilled.)

8. **Ignore it.**

9. **... and remember,** the flush of the hot flash that feels so scarlet is barely visible to anyone else.

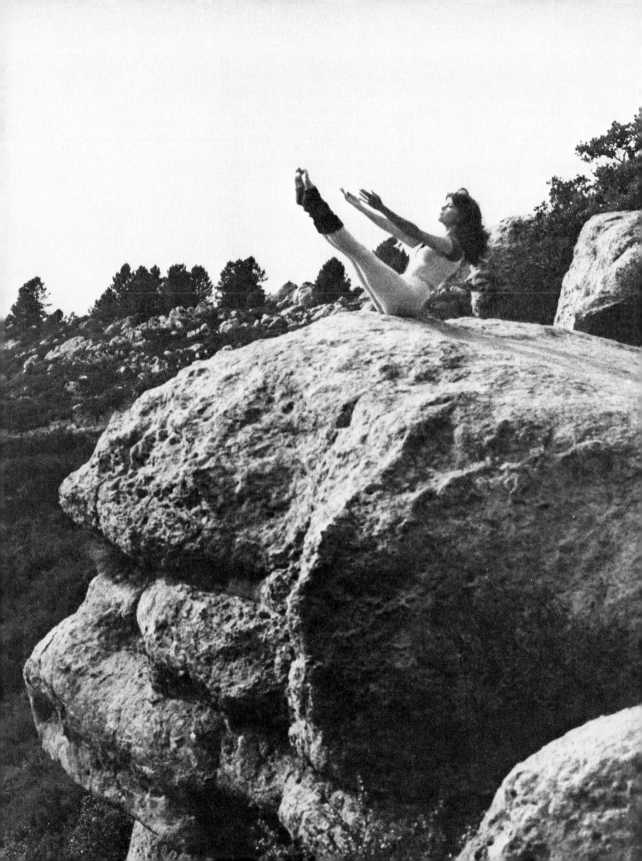

SEXUAL PASSAGES

FOLLOWING MENOPAUSE, a number of physical changes in our sexual organs begin to occur as a result of our bodies' new hormonal environment, as well as the aging process in general. None of these changes, however, need alter our status as sexual beings. We do not cross some natural Rubicon in midlife that somehow separates women and men from their own sexuality, or from each other. Sexual problems of any significance that do arise in these years are less frequently physical in origin than they are the result of restricting social attitudes, the absence of a sexual partner, or lack of knowledge about our changing bodies.

In the postmenopausal years, our lowered production of estrogen means subtle alterations in the reproductive tissues—how subtle depends largely on genetics, good health, and the general state of our physical and sexual fitness. The changes come about gradually and differently for each woman. Overall, there is a small decrease in the size of both the internal and external sexual organs—the vagina, uterus, and the ovaries, as well as the inner and outer vaginal lips and the clitoral hood—though there is no loss of sensation in the clitoris. The color of the external vaginal tissues gradually lightens from maroon to rose to pink by the later years, and there may be a lessening of pubic hair. Lubrication during sexual activity may take longer. And the membranous walls of the vagina may generally become smoother, thinner, less moist, and less elastic.

When these vaginal changes do occur, they sometimes go unnoticed unless there is itching or burning, or until intercourse becomes uncomfortable or even painful, especially if you and your partner haven't taken the time necessary for complete lubrication. You may also have a little bleeding if the vaginal walls have become too thin.

Before such outward signs manifest themselves, however, it is possible to recognize any internal vaginal changes by sight and touch through your own or your physician's regular gynecological exam.

After menopause, there is also a tendency toward more vaginal and urethral infections. The change in the outer vaginal lips provides less protection for the vagina, as well as for the urethra, which leads to the bladder. Further, there can be a disturbance in the vagina's acid balance. Maintaining a slightly acidic environment prevents bothersome bacteria and other microorganisms from flourishing. A sugary, alkaline environment, on the other hand, is a breeding ground for infection. The cells of the vaginal wall normally store sugar in the form of glycogen, but the average diet rich in sugar and refined carbohydrates will tilt us toward an alkaline imbalance.

Lastly, the pelvic muscles which contain and support the vagina and its surrounding organs may slacken. These muscles are hormone-sensitive, as well as inactivity-sensitive. This muscular relaxation is also a result of having given birth. One of the most common results of a loss of pelvic muscle tone is the occasional, uncontrolled loss of a little urine. Referred to as urinary or stress incontinence, this is caused by a relaxation of the muscles around the neck of the bladder. Some women may have already encountered this during or after pregnancy. As many as half of all midlife and older women now experience urinary incontinence, most frequently while coughing, sneezing, lifting, or laughing, and it is twice as common in women as in men. But such urinary leakage is not inevitable, even though the urinary tract thins with age as does the vagina. Proper exercise, discussed later in this section, is a strong preventive. Another less common but far less correctable problem occurs when the pelvic muscle weakens to the extent that the urethra, the bladder, or the rectum prolapse, that is, fall out of place into the vaginal space. The uterus can also drop. Strong, exercised muscles can likewise help to prevent this from happening.

All of these changes are possibilities. How probable they are and when they occur is less well known than information about hot flashes. Women may have a reluctance to talk about these physical changes and may be unaware of their connection to menopause— partly accounting for our relative lack of information. We do know that these pelvic changes can begin anytime in the ten years following the last menstruation, and as early as the first year. It appears that about 25 to 30 percent of women experience discomfort as a result of thinning vaginal walls. We need to know more about what variability exists between sexually active and sexually inactive women. The strong belief among authorities now is that sexual activity, defined in its broadest sense, can make a difference in significantly slowing or even postponing the normal, but modifiable, sexual aging process.

Male Menopause?

What about men? Are there corresponding changes in their bodies? Is there a "male menopause"?

"Menopause" is a literal misnomer when applied to men, who have nothing comparable to our menstrual cycle and who have no abrupt hormonal punctuation mark in their midlife. But rhetorically it fits. Like midlife women, midlife men have a new sense of strength but also of vulnerability in many areas of their lives, including the physical. They encounter a sexual aging process similar to ours, sometimes referred to as "andropause."

The pelvic muscles in midlife and older men can lose their tone. Like the ovaries, the testes decrease in size, become more flaccid, and the tubes that transport sperm from the testes become more narrow. Until recently, it was believed that after a man's twenties, production of testosterone in the testes slowly and very gradually begins to decrease. Men have reported urinary irregularities, fluid retention, and even hot flashes (though quite rarely)—all of which could be the result of such hormonal change. But the largest aging research project in the country, sponsored by the NIA, has found no changes in the sex hormone levels of men who've been consistently studied for nearly three decades—even up into their later years. This could mean that a testosterone decline is not inevitable for men, so more research will have to be done in order to answer this newly reopened question. Men do have rising levels of the pituitary hormones, as we do, though these reach their maximum a decade later—in their sixties.

In sexual activity, men experience a gradual slowing of the arousal process. It takes longer to reach orgasm and orgasms are spaced more widely apart, unlike the process for women, whose ability to experience multiple orgasms seems to increase with age (!). If men don't understand or expect these changes of pace, they can develop a tremendous anxiety over "performance" and a fear of impotence. But actually this slowing down contains the wonderful possibility of a more neatly matched sexual relationship with women. More time is usually needed by both men and women for sex in each of its phases, which means more time for tender and imaginative love-making. As it may take a woman longer to lubricate, it may take a man longer to become erect. Also, arousal may require more stimulation and varied touch. The erection can be held longer and there is less of a need to reach orgasm with every sexual experience. The *process* of lovemaking itself can become more important than the *outcome*, and there is more room for emotional closeness to grow as well. When orgasm does occur, there is a faster loss of erection, a smaller volume and less force to the ejaculation, and over time there are fewer sperm and still fewer that are capable of fertilizing an egg—though most men remain fertile throughout their lifetimes. None of these changes need mean a lessening of sensual pleasure or sexual satisfaction.

There are two potential health problems for men in these years that are important for us to know about. The most common is an enlargement of the prostate gland that surrounds the urethra and that supplies about one third of the fluid portion of the ejaculate. This can interfere with the ease or force of both ejaculation and the urinary function. Eighty to 85 percent of men *over age fifty* will experience this, and for now this is considered a normal part of the aging process. Far into the later years, ten percent may require surgery. (Prostate cancer is less common but the risk does increase over the age of fifty. It is the third-ranking cause of cancer death among men.)

Impotence, the inability to achieve or sustain an erection, is the other potential difficulty, but far more a fear than a reality. While a common complaint among half of all men, impotence is one of the most treatable of sexual problems, according to many physicians and sex therapists. Impotence of an organic origin occurs in only a small percentage of men, possibly caused by some underlying disease like diabetes, for example. The vast majority of cases in midlife men are psychological in origin, the result of not understanding or not being prepared for the body's changes, or the result of more long-standing performance anxieties.

A WOMAN FOR ALL SEASONS

I am sixty years old and they say you never get too old to enjoy sex. I know because once I asked my Grandma when you stop liking it and she was eighty. She said, "Child, you'll have to ask someone older than me."

Hilda D.

What is the fate of the female libido in the midst of these possible physiological changes? Does the decrease in our primary sex hormone mean a lessening of desire as well?

From a purely physical perspective, a woman's sexual desire should *increase* at menopause. The hormone most directly associated with sexual desire is not estrogen, but rather *testosterone.* The production of testosterone by our adrenal glands is virtually unaffected by menopause. In the postmenopausal woman it achieves a new, more dominant position alongside the now lower levels of estrogen. And, indeed, there is increasing evidence to support the fact that for most women there *is* more sexual interest, pleasure, and capacity for orgasm. In fact, for many the desire for and enjoyment of sex appear to rise continuously into our middle years and remain stable from that time on. This, of course, overthrows the old conception that sexuality somehow disappears for the mature woman. People of all ages are awakening to the reality that sex is not just the private preserve of the young—"a myth perpetuated by our adult children, who have an immaculate conception of their own creation," says Maggie Kuhn, founder of the Gray Panthers.

A whole constellation of factors contributes to a mature woman's capacity for heightened sexual response. Sexual conflicts may be resolved, or nearly so, releasing the hold that old inhibitions may have had on our sensuality. Energies previously tied to child-rearing are more available for opening, renewing, or deepening intimacies with a partner. A mature woman is likely to give more priority to lovemaking in all its dimensions.

But desire isn't static. It varies from day to day. It can come and go in different periods in your life. Many women also choose celibacy at some times during their lives. More often, though, we become sexually inactive because other problems have intervened and need to be addressed—we may be bored by our sexual routine and have lowered expectations or we may be troubled about our self-image, especially in regard to aging. The stress of money worries, the time demands of work, chronic psychological depression, the fear of not measuring up in the new "sexual Olympics," and too much food or drink can also affect our sexual desire. Alcohol, as well as certain other psychoactive drugs, has an ambiguous effect on sexual response—it can excite or sedate—but over time its effect is more negative. Some common depressive medications also suppress sexual desire and performance, such as tranquilizers, antihypertensives for high blood pressure, and antihistamines for allergies.

The most important factor in sustaining sexual desire is regular sexual activity. The more sex a woman has, the more she'll maintain her sexual fitness as well. Of course the availability of partners *is* an important issue for women in midlife, and even more so in the later years when there are still fewer men than women. In midlife, men may become less available for a number of complex reasons. For example, according to researchers Masters and Johnson, the problems men tend to have in this period, especially the fear of aging and of losing sexual vitality, may often be projected negatively onto their female peers. They may pursue younger women as a way out, and the cultural images around us have tended to support this pattern. Women who want a sexual partner need to make this decision consciously, let their friends know, and in general do their best to meet new people.

The pleasure that sexual activity brings to us contributes to a total sense of well-being. The physical stimulation keeps us in the best possible shape for however full a sex life we want—as will the right kind of regular exercise.

Sex Fitness

Most of us are unaware of the muscle deep in our pelvic area, much less the need to exercise it.

The pubococcygeus (pew-bo-cox-uh-geé-us) or PC muscle is a broad band of tissue that stretches like a taut hammock from the

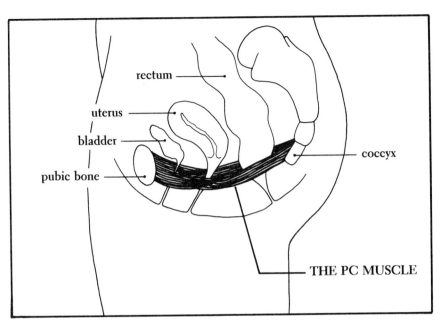

rectum

uterus

bladder

pubic bone

coccyx

THE PC MUSCLE

pubic bone in front to the tailbone or coccyx in back. Sometimes called "the love muscle," it supports all of the internal pelvic organs and includes the muscles of the vagina. And like any muscle group, this one needs to be kept strong.

If this muscle is not exercised, in both women and men, it will, like any muscle, weaken and eventually atrophy. A lack of PC muscle tone may cause urinary incontinence. It can also mean the lessening of sensitivity in the vagina and hence the lessening of sexual pleasure. Decreased sensation can also be caused if the PC muscle is held in a chronically tense state. *Weak* muscles and *tense* muscles both can inhibit strong active pelvic movement and block the flow of physical and even emotional feelings that are part of healthy sexual release and activity.

Regular exercise of the PC muscle is a way to reverse all of this. With conditioning the entire pelvic area will become stronger, more limber, and less tense. It will allow a greater flow of blood to the genitals, which is so important for orgasm. The muscles themselves become healthy and toned so you will have a healthy vagina, more pleasure in sex, firm placement of the pelvic organs, and an end to urinary troubles. It also means better posture and a stronger lower back.

Sexual intercourse exercises the PC muscle naturally. There are also specific exercises that similarly work this muscle. In the 1940s, the physician Arnold Kegel developed a series of exercises as a non-surgical alternative for urinary incontinence. These have proven a success in slowing the unwanted flow of urine—and, in addition, some women have reported experiencing orgasm for the first time after doing the exercises!

The Kegel exercises, as they are called today, involve the concentrated contraction and release of the PC muscle, which you can activate when you squeeze your vagina as though trying to interrupt a flow of urine. With good muscle tone and good muscle control, you will be able to start and stop your flow of urine at will. If you place your finger inside your vagina to test yourself, you will be able to feel the muscles tighten.

The PC Exercise

To *improve* your PC muscle tone, squeeze and release the PC muscle 200 times a day in slow movements and in rapid movements.

1. **The Slow Squeeze**
    Squeeze for ten seconds, relax for ten seconds. Do ten times.
    (Begin, if you can, with three seconds and gradually build to ten seconds. Always be sure the duration of your release equals the duration of your contraction.)
2. **The Quick Squeeze**
    Squeeze and relax the PC muscle as rapidly as you can. Do for two minutes.
    (Begin with as many seconds as you can and gradually build up to two minutes.)
3. **Make Your Personal Plan.**
    Design whatever plan will work best for you that ensures you will have done a total of 200 contractions by the end of the day.
4. **Breathe Normally** during the exercises.

The PC exercise can be done spontaneously anytime—driving the car, watching TV, sitting at your desk, or relaxing in bed. Some women like to do their Kegels five times a day when they urinate (except first thing in the morning when the bladder is most full). The regularity of urination serves as a good reminder to exercise and you can really see the muscle at work as you start and stop the flow; whether you use this method or not, the image of it is a good one when first trying to identify and work with the muscle. You might also think of folding up this sling of muscle as you squeeze it, drawing the anus closer toward the urethra, or imagine sucking air up into the vagina.*

It's important to begin gradually, but to do the exercises regularly. In a short time, you'll notice how much better you've become at identifying and controlling the muscle during the exercises. Overall, they take very little time, and you'll get faster at the quick flutters.

The new Prime Time Workout includes the Kegels. Prime Time is also an *all-over body workout*, equally important to a healthy sexuality. The stronger your general musculature, the more limber your joints, and the more aerobic stamina you have, the better your sexual experiences are going to be.

Other Helps

The isometrics of the Kegels will bring blood to the vagina tissues, helping to make the walls thicker and more moist, in addition to improving lubrication. During lovemaking, if you need to add to your body's own ability to lubricate, there are a variety of appealing, good products to use. *Vegetable and fruit oils* are among the best. Try coconut, apricot kernel, safflower, and even baby oil. A whole range of *body and massage oils*, flavored and unflavored, pleasant to the touch, fragrant and unscented, can also double as vaginal lubricants. Avoid oils containing alcohol, which can irritate the vaginal mucous membranes, lotions or creams too readily absorbed by the skin, and non-water-soluble Vaseline or petroleum jelly, which can be irritating and cause infection. Some women use Ortho Personal Lubricant, cocoa butter, A&D ointment, or KY-jelly, though the jelly tends to dry too quickly. *Vitamin E* oil, which you can take from a vitamin E capsule, is a good healer in between times of sexual activity for fragile vaginal tissues that may have torn, and it also relieves dryness. And make sure you get enough vitamin A, vitamin

---

* Ask your doctor about the use of a resistive device as an aid to exercising the PC muscle.

E, and the mineral zinc in your diet—all three are important for healthy vaginal tissues.

Taking external estrogens can significantly improve the health of the vagina as well. I will discuss the pros and cons of estrogen therapy later, but for now I want to mention several things about *estrogen cream*, the form most commonly used for vaginal problems. First, estrogen cream is *not* a lubricant for lovemaking. It's taken up by the bloodstream through the skin and shouldn't be used during sexual intercourse when it can be absorbed by your partner as well as by yourself. This is a therapeutic cream to be used as your physician prescribes. It needs to be left undisturbed in the vagina for several hours in order to be effective. Also, the most minute amounts are frequently all that are necessary to promote improvement of vaginal dryness. "There is reason to believe that the manufacturer's suggested dose is too big," writes Dr. Barbara Edelstein in *The Woman Doctor's Medical Guide for Women.* "Doctors may prescribe 1/5 to 1/10 the recommended amount with excellent results." Women who do use estrogen cream should therefore be sure to work out with their physicians the lowest possible dose that will bring results.

In the case of urinary or vaginal infections, there are several natural solutions. For a urinary infection, drinking lots of *water* will flush bacteria out of the urinary tract. Drinking lots of *cranberry juice* can also help to restore its acidity. For a vaginal infection many women report success treating the vagina with *yogurt.* The plain lactobacillus acidophilus kind is best. You can use one to two tablespoons in warm douche water, or several teaspoons of yogurt inserted with a vaginal-medication applicator, foam applicator, or tampon container, allowing it to remain in the vagina for a few minutes. You may want to use a mini-sanitary napkin for a few hours afterwards because you will probably have some leakage.

These steps often are sufficient to solve problems of infection. If not, you need to consult your physician. *Antibiotics* may be prescribed which, unfortunately, have both good and bad effects. In the process of wiping out the bad guys, antibiotics simultaneously kill off good bacteria in the vagina, the lactobacilli that keep the vaginal wall acidic. Yeast infections are often the result. If you're particularly prone to yeast outbreaks when taking antibiotics, insert yogurt vaginally while you're on the drug. Eating yogurt is also a good idea.

As a preventive against urinary infections, it's a good idea to empty your bladder immediately before and after sex to keep bacteria from entering the urethra. To protect against both urinary and vaginal infections, wearing the right clothes is also important. A hot, moist environment encourages infections, so the idea is to keep yourself as cool and dry as possible. Always wear clean cotton underwear or panties with a cotton crotch. Look for pantyhose with a cotton crotch too. Make sure your panties, hose, and trousers are all loose enough to permit the vaginal and urethral tissues to breathe.

From all I've said about the benefits of sexual activity, exercise, and the other suggestions just discussed, I hope you can see there's plenty we can do to ensure our lasting sexual health and vitality.

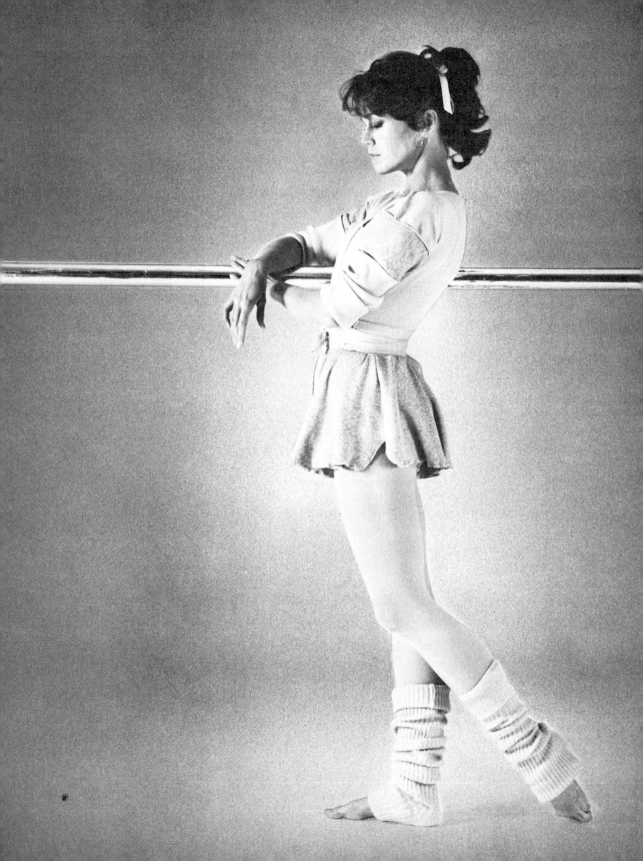

CHAPTER 11

DEPRESSION

Somewhere in my middle years, I began to feel unexpectedly different—volatile moods, feeling up one minute and down to the depths the next. I felt irritable, had trouble sleeping, and seemed to be losing my ability to think (one day I could not remember how to measure my windows for new curtains). This deepening depression was a new experience for me and for almost a year I kept pushing it away, feeling I could handle it, as I had all other crisis periods of my life. My gynecologist patted me on the head like a little girl and said, "This too will pass. It's just menopause." He prescribed 1.25 milligrams of estrogen daily. One morning I just didn't want to get out of bed. I could see no reason for my being alive. I felt that there was no meaning in my life and was sure that the world and my family had no further use for me. There were a number of social reasons for this depression. I had seven children (three of whom had already left home) and it was apparent that in a few short years they would all be gone, leaving me with no clear role. My husband and I had just left the church which had been the foundation of our lives for some forty-five years. But more than all of these life events, I believe that I was among the approximately twenty percent of all women who suffer a sharp and abrupt drop in estrogen. At that time, it was difficult for me to understand why this was happening to me. I was a modern, liberated, active woman, with never a thought about menopause being a difficult time. All of the scant literature on the subject, and my doctor, suggested that menopausal problems only occurred to neurotic, unfulfilled women and that my symptoms were purely psychosomatic. Now I know that most of the stress of that period, which was the worst time in my life, could have been avoided if I had been more knowledgeable about menopause and had received some support from other women. I thought I was alone in experiencing these traumatic symptoms.

> Claudia, Age 56
> *Growing Older, Getting Better*

PROBABLY the least understood aspect of menopause is its psychological dimension. The hormones estrogen and progesterone are known to affect our moods and to be related indirectly to our nervous systems. The brain, for example, is known to have cells that are receptive to estrogen. When this body chemical decreases dramatically at menopause, it's not surprising that for some women certain psychological effects emerge alongside hot flashes and changing sexual tissues. Remember, since puberty our bodies have been accustomed to the regular cycling of *high* levels of estrogen and progesterone.

But this is not to say menopause means "woman mizry" after all, a point that must be clarified before we go on. So many in our generation grew up with the frightening expectation that with menopause comes severe depression or serious mental instability. Until recently, this was commonly believed, even among the medical profession. *Any* emotional distress of whatever kind in a woman in her late forties or early fifties would summon up the "aha-she-must-be-menopausal" response. Suffering was labeled and dismissed as neurosis. Now, the idea that menopause and emotional illness go hand-in-glove is considered nonsense. No evidence has been found to support the view that a mysterious surge of psychic breakdowns occurs during these years. This scary myth has to be separated from the *real* psychological side of menopause, infinitely less dire.

The *majority* of us will be aware of little or no psychological reaction due to menopause. In fact, many women in their fifties and sixties report reaching an *improved* sense of emotional well-being—what the late anthropologist Margaret Mead called *PMZ* or *postmenopausal zest.* But some women—like Claudia, whom I quoted above—describe experiencing a whole list of seemingly unexplained but related neurological symptoms—depression, insomnia, fatigue, irritability, nervousness, weepiness, and lack of concentration, as well as water retention, rapid and strong heart beats, and numbness in the hands and feet. A number of us who think of ourselves as being on top of it as women, who feel we manage our own lives and our families well, may suddenly feel that things are falling apart. What we coped with easily before suddenly becomes too much.

None of this is particularly new to women. We've taken these roller-coaster rides long before menopause, at other times of extreme

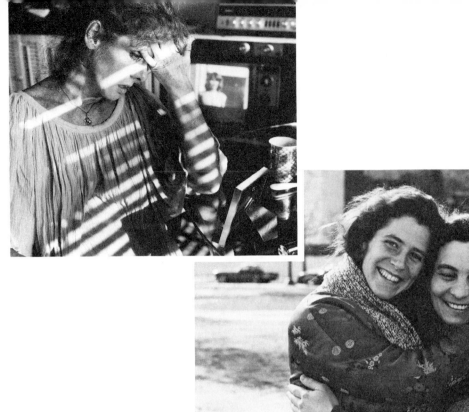

hormonal change. Anxiety, crying spells, and migraines before monthly menstruation have sent some of us to seek psychological counseling. And how many mothers have experienced postnatal blues, as I did after the birth of my first child? I felt I'd hit bottom with no idea why. For weeks I cried and cried. Everyday problems took on enormous significance. I thought my life had fallen to pieces, and had no idea this depression was the result of the enormous chemical upheaval taking place inside my body after giving birth. Like Claudia, I think now how different the experience would have been had I understood what was happening to me and had I known what to do.

Because of experiences like these, most of us arrive at menopause no strangers to hormonally triggered mood changes. But we may be strangers to understanding what steps might be taken to move more easily through such periods of disequilibrium. And added to the changes within our bodies are others that make this an especially emotionally charged time. We are faced with a host of new questions that have no ready answers. What does the future hold? Is my life going to get better? Will anyone love me? Any period of transition brings with it moments of fear and moments of sadness at what is passing, even if we are looking forward to an exciting future. I see this in both my daughter, now sixteen, and myself, like two bookends on either side of the menstrual arc. She is entering her phase of fertile womanhood as I prepare to leave mine. Here we are, the two of us, trying to figure out who we are and how to handle all the tumultuous changes as we each enter a new phase. I'm hoping she adapts to her hormonal changes before I begin menopause. Otherwise I'm not sure how our household would handle all the excitement.

It's important to know as much as we can about how our physical states affect our moods, and equally important, how our emotional states affect our bodies. This is one of the least understood areas of health. And menopause is no exception. But we have useful information with which to work. Clearly, not every factor that tilts us toward depression or nervousness at menopause is within our control, but there are positive steps we can take to minimize them if we begin to feel down.

Water Retention

Excess water in the body, even a modest amount, can have an emotional as well as a physical impact on us. Many women report experiencing some degree of water retention at menopause, especially during pre- and perimenopause. In fact, for some, water retention may be as much a sign of shifting hormones as are hot flashes. The good news is that we can control fluid retention with relative ease.

One of estrogen's little-known roles is its regulation of the fluid balance in the body. Unusual fluctuations of estrogen can cause the body's sodium or salt levels to rise. This in turn causes the cells of the body to retain water. In the menopausal years, only a few extra ounces of water can cause breast tenderness and bloating, just as they can in the menstrual years during the two weeks before the monthly period when estrogen levels shift the most. (In fact, water retention is one of the principal symptoms of premenstrual syndrome or PMS, an imperfectly understood group of physical and emotional symptoms occurring most frequently in women in their mid- to late thirties and sometimes called the "mini-menopause.")

There are several other effects of water retention at menopause. A surplus of water in the body can trigger, accompany, or intensify the experience of hot flashes. And it can also mean more water in the brain tissues which can cause feelings of depression, anxiety, and nervousness.

When we have more sodium in the body, another related reaction takes place. We begin to excrete potassium automatically if our salt levels go up. This only compounds the effects of water retention because the mineral potassium, like the hormone estrogen, helps to regulate the body's water balance. In addition, potassium and sodium working together have a profound effect on the nervous system. Both minerals are essential for the healthy transmission of nerve messages. If an excess of sodium causes a loss of potassium, we not only miss out on potassium's moderating influence on water retention, but irritability and other neurological symptoms can result.

Natural Diuretics

1. **Less salt.** Cut down, or preferably eliminate, all table salt and sodium products from your diet. (You'll read more on this in the chapter "Eating for the Long Run.")

2. **More water.** Increase your intake of water (remember, it's good for hot flashes as well). This is a case where more means less, because reducing your fluid intake can actually exacerbate water retention, while adding more water causes you to lose fluid. Water is a natural diuretic because it helps you to excrete excess sodium. As you lose the sodium, your body retains less and less of the water it doesn't need for optimal functioning. (Avoid water with meals, though. Liquids in the presence of the sodium in most foods encourage fluid retention.)

3. **Vitamin B$_6$ (pyridoxine).** A natural diuretic, vitamin B$_6$ helps directly to maintain the body's balance of sodium and potassium and so indirectly affects the body's fluid balance. (Amounts recommended by physicians are given on page 215. Be sure not to exceed the dosages given there.)

4. **Exercise.** All exercise helps to regulate water balance in the body. When vigorous, it also may induce sweating, which excretes water-retaining sodium.

5. **Foods and herbs.** Certain foods and herbs are also natural diuretics and will help you to excrete unwanted water.

   FRUITS: Strawberries, watermelon, grapes, pineapple, cantaloupe.
   VEGETABLES: Parsley, cucumber, watercress, artichokes, asparagus. Parsley juice is especially effective.
   HERB TEAS: Alfalfa leaf, raspberry leaf, hibiscus, or a combination of parsley, thyme, and chamomile. (Always use herbs in moderation.)

6. **Protect your potassium.** Natural diuretics cause you to excrete not only the water you are retaining and excess sodium, but also potassium. Less healthful diuretics such as caffeine and alcohol do the same. And too much sugar in the diet causes the loss of potassium as well. Be sure to have a good supply of potassium from the fruits and vegetables in your diet. (In fact, a high intake of potassium can promote sodium loss.)

Insomnia

The inner chaos of depression, waking episodes of hot flashes, and the slightly decreased need for sleep in some of us can cause insomnia to be a problem around the time of menopause. The lack of sound sleep, in turn, can unquestionably exacerbate depression. So making sure we have good rest is essential to our physical and emotional health.

How much sleep we need is very much an individual matter. Sleep researchers tell us that on the *average*, by the time we reach our sixties, most of us will need an hour less sleep each night than we needed forty years earlier in our twenties. Some experience this relatively small change as a positive gain of time, others as troubling insomnia. We may expect to "sleep like a baby" even though as we age it seems to take many of us somewhat longer to fall asleep and our sleep may be lighter. If you're used to falling asleep quickly and sleeping soundly through the night, a 15-minute delay can seem like an hour and a couple of awakenings can make it seem as though half the night has been spent tossing and turning.

The vast majority of cases which seem to be insomnia are benign and will yield to simple home remedies like the insomnia remedies following. You'll notice first the oldest remedy of all, milk, and

Insomnia Remedies

- Milk before bedtime, warm if you like. (Milk contains calming calcium, magnesium, and tryptophan.)
- A warm relaxing bath—followed with an all-over moisturizer.
- A soothing cup of chamomile herb tea—with a little honey.
- No caffeine after 12 noon.
- A good mattress.
- Don't go to bed too early. If you are one of the many people who need less sleep as you grow older, enjoy the extra time bonus.
- Exercise vigorously and regularly, but not close to bedtime.
- Don't go to bed angry.
- Learn to fall asleep without the radio or TV on. Research has shown a radio or TV running while we are asleep will cause us to be more wakeful.

listed with it the all-too-*un*familiar ingredient tryptophan. Trypto-phan is an amino acid found naturally in milk and other foods rich in protein. It's a precursor to the brain chemical serotonin, known for its calming, pain-killing, and sleep-inducing effects. Sleep experts now commonly recommend taking 1 to 2 grams of tryptophan in tablets or capsules before bedtime as an aid to insomnia. If I'm having trouble sleeping, I take two tablets at bedtime of just 100 mg each. (More often you'll find tryptophan in 500 mg doses.) If I don't fall asleep within 30 minutes, I take another. Though these are relatively expensive, no side effects have yet been discovered so trypto-phan is a natural and safe alternative to habit-forming sleeping pills, now the most frequently used medicine in the world.

Daily Stress-Producers

In times of distress we may unknowingly *add* to any depression by automatically reaching for certain foods or drugs that provide an initial sense of improved well-being, followed shortly thereafter by fatigue, anxiety or other such uncomfortable feelings. Not surprisingly, these are the same energy-robbers that can exaggerate a hot flash.

A *high-sugar diet* jolts the body into action. The pancreas over-produces insulin which then causes the blood sugar to drop too rapidly and you end up feeling the low "sugar blues." *Alcohol* may cause the adrenals to overproduce adrenaline, taxing you as well as your adrenal glands. Alcohol *in any quantity* can intensify depression, make insomnia worse, and interfere with our deepest dream sleep. *Caffeine* stimulates the whole central nervous system and can also cause insomnia, nervousness, irritability, heart palpitations, anxiety and even higher body temperatures. And *overeating* overworks our whole system, while simultaneously slowing it down and causing water retention. It adds the weight of both guilt and pounds to an already troubled spirit.

Any chronic negative stress like depression, the stress of too much sugar, alcohol, caffeine, food or some combination of these may mean the loss of essential nutrients. We can be left with a shortfall of certain nutrients just when we need them most. For example, vitamin C, whose largest concentration is in the adrenals, is thought to be especially called upon during times of stress, as are the B-complex vitamins—which potentially means running low on these nutrients. Emotional stress is also associated with a loss of protein and slight losses of certain minerals: calcium, magnesium, potassium, zinc, and copper.

We need to avoid the things that make hard times worse, while at the same time making sure to have a good, balanced diet. When the stress level is high, there is all the more reason to eat well. We need all the essential nutrients daily not only because stress can otherwise deplete them, but also because nutrition influences our moods in other ways. Certain nutrients are now known to have both a direct and an indirect effect on chemicals in the brain that influence behavior. The foods we eat provide the dietary building blocks for these "mood juices," hormonelike substances that transmit messages between nerves in the brain. Vitamins B_6, C, and niacin and the amino acid tryptophan, for example, are all essential for the production of the brain chemical serotonin, which I just mentioned in the discussion of insomnia. Serotonin, just one of several brain chemicals associated with mental health, is important in helping us to relax and to sleep. A deficiency in this key substance, as well as in others, is believed to produce irritability, insomnia, and depression itself. Our bodies may manufacture less of these essential brain chemicals as a normal process of aging, but nutrition and exercise are thought to play an important role in keeping the supply adequate.

Nature's Tranquilizer

Exercise is probably the strongest antidepressant we have—whether psychological symptoms have their origins in changing hormonal patterns, changing life patterns, or both. There isn't one of us who's done regular exercising who hasn't known its tonic effect. Physicians in private practice and stress researchers in the laboratory increasingly emphasize exercise as one of the best antidotes to mental distress of any kind. Many psychiatrists are regularly prescribing exercise as a powerful drug-free therapy for their depressed patients.

When your brain perceives a stressful situation, a cascade of reactions is triggered in the adrenal glands, so important because of their indirect role in producing estrogen after menopause. The adrenals can be chronically activated by depression, secreting in response abnormally large quantities of the hormones adrenaline, noradrena-

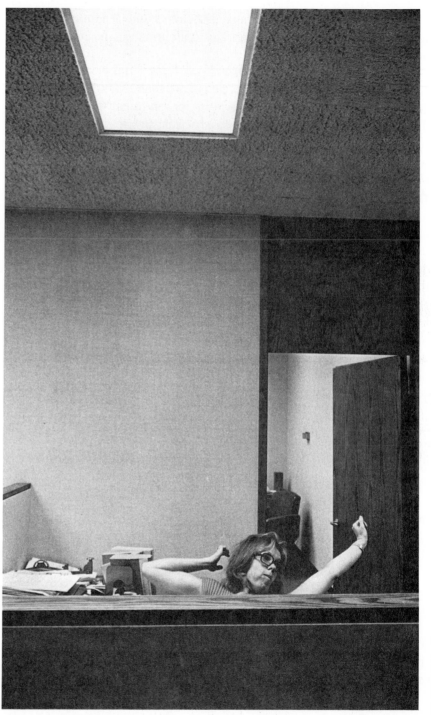

Either . . .

Or . .

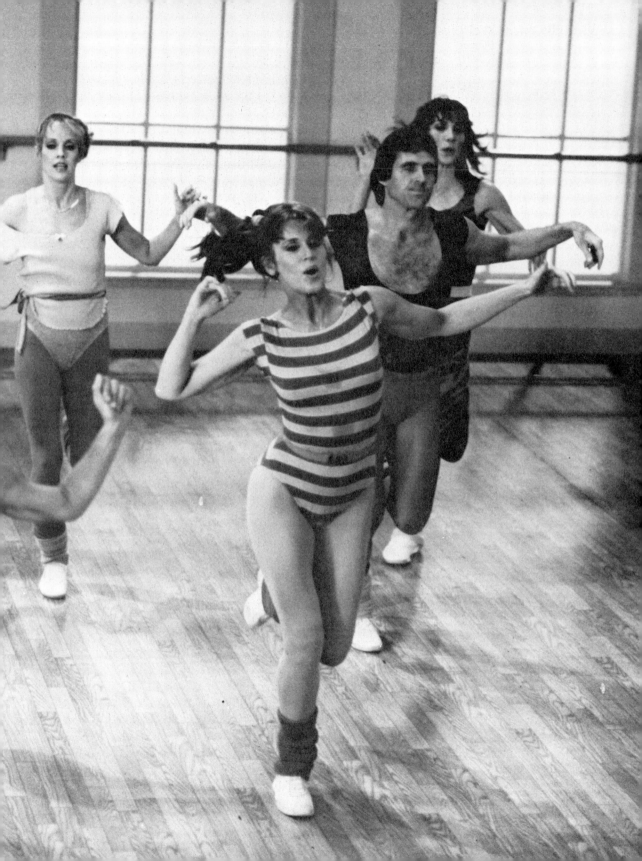

line, and cortisol. These increase our heart rate and blood pressure, and, if persistent, cause a state of perpetual alertness. Cortisol will tend to peak at 4:00 A.M., causing the early-morning wakefulness depressed people so often report. It remains elevated throughout the day. The body is frenzied, extra blood sugar is released, and the sodium/water balance is disturbed, as is our biological orderliness in general. The nervous system is put into a state of hyperarousal. But because its circuitry is overloaded, the system actually operates less efficiently. Thinking becomes clogged and tangled. Everything seems to slow down. Sexual desire may be extinguished. The adrenals also produce higher levels of the hormone aldosterone which causes us to retain water and sodium in the body—and I've already talked about the psychological effects of water retention.

When the adrenals work this hard (which they can also do in times of positive stress), the internal tension generated needs to be released. If not, long-term excess levels of adrenaline put harmful wear-and-tear on the central nervous system and its partner the endocrine system. "Each exposure to stress leaves an indelible chemical scar," explains Dr. Hans Selye, who first researched the concept of stress over forty years ago.

Exercise gives trapped energies somewhere to go, breaking up chronic stress patterns. It's a harmless way both to produce and to channel excess adrenaline. The great balancer, exercise tranquilizes at the same time that it energizes. Bound energy is released into action while energy is also conserved because the body develops an increased efficiency. We sleep better. We're less fatigued. We build up a physical as well as a psychological reserve that helps us to tolerate stress better overall. The increased blood supply carries more oxygen and more energy-rich nutrients to every cell, from those in the muscles to those in the brain.

There may be a direct relationship between exercise and the production of certain brain and pituitary compounds that give us a kind of natural "high." These natural painkillers, called the *endorphins* and the *enkephalins*, seem to be increased during rhythmic, aerobic exercise like walking, running, swimming, and cycling. Although researchers emphasize these findings are preliminary, both body chemicals appear to be released at the same time as the adrenal hormones in response to this kind of exercise. These substances not only have a calming effect, they also tend to have a moderating influence on the pituitary hormones, which are exceptionally high at menopause and may be related to hot flashes.

There are profound emotional benefits to exercise that go far beyond these physical explanations. Severe depression, a shaky identity, a battered or worn-out self-image—even a lack of humor—can turn around largely because a woman has turned to regular exercise. As exercise gets you moving, other things in your life begin to move too. Exercise can help you to develop a sense of self-reliance, power, and control that can be generalized to other areas of your life. You can learn so many things about yourself and about how to move forward and when to rest. You may discover the joy of setting your own goal, figuring out how you're going to get there, and then doing it. But the relationship to exercise is a very personal experience, different for everyone. Each woman, finally, will discover for herself and in her own way the fulfillment of physical expression and the psychological rewards that consistent physical activity is known to bring.

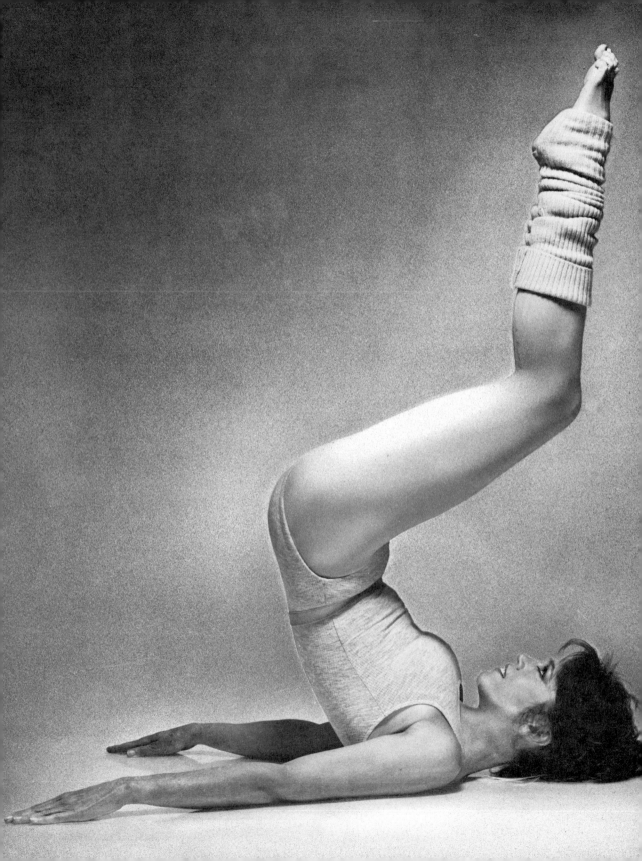

THE HORMONE THERAPY DECISION

We concede that no simple equation can be derived to demonstrate a positive or negative balance sheet for estrogen therapy. This is true because of gaps in our knowledge about the full effects of exogenous [external] estrogens, vagueness in the measures we use to value the risks and benefits, and widely different standards of practice which could affect the risks and benefits.

> P. A. Van Keep, M.D., W. H. Utian, M.D., and
> A. Vermeulen, M.D.
> *The Controversial Climacteric*

IT IS POSSIBLE to add to the body's own production of estrogen at menopause by taking manufactured estrogens. The decision to do so, however, is a hard choice when even the medical community differs in its opinion about the wisdom of estrogen replacement therapy (ERT), as it has been called. After exaggerated claims in the mid-1960s that estrogens could make you "feminine forever," their use quadrupled. But in the mid-1970s research revealed a significant increase in uterine cancer among women taking estrogens. As a result, the decade of initial enthusiasm was followed by another ten years of fearful concern over the cancer connection and a markedly reduced use of estrogen therapy. An emotional debate about its benefits, its risks, and the unknowns continues today.

While conflicting research results and perspectives keep the controversy alive, there are several points of general agreement about estrogen drugs:

- The promise of prolonging youth is a *false* promise.
- Estrogens should *not* be given to women as routine therapy at menopause.

- When estrogens *are* given, they should be accompanied by the separate administration, at a specified time each month, of a *progestin* or manufactured progesterone which significantly modifies the potentially harmful effects of estrogen.

No *conclusive* recommendation for the safe administration of estrogens for all women, however, has yet emerged from any source. Without such a definitive stop- or go-signal, a woman thinking about using estrogen drugs must learn what they are and what is known about the real benefits on the one hand, the real risks on the other, and the many shades of gray in between, before making her personal decision.

The Drugs

Estrogens are now available in pill, injection, cream and suppository form. The most frequently used are the pill taken orally and the cream applied vaginally. All of these are either synthetic estrogens produced from chemicals, or what are called "conjugated" estrogens manufactured from natural sources, usually the urine of pregnant horses. The most commonly known brands are Estrace and Premarin. Some estrogen drugs, such as different forms of Premarin, may contain tranquilizers, and women taking estrogens should be sure to know whether theirs do. (Occasionally, Bellergal may be prescribed as an alternative or supplement. This drug also contains phenobarbital, which has sedative and addictive effects, and belladonna ingredients, which give rise to other side effects). When a separate progestin is combined with estrogen therapy, the most commonly used is Provera, a derivative of progesterone in pill form.

The search for the safest methods of administration, for new routes and forms of the drugs continues. Time-released implants placed under the skin and creams applied directly onto the skin are being tested and have already been used successfully in France. In these ways, estrogen is absorbed into the body through the skin where it is then picked up by the bloodstream. Also, Estrace has been administered at half the oral dosage in pill form through the vagina, where it too is absorbed into the bloodstream and circulated throughout the body to target tissues. While still giving almost the full effect of the drug, these non-oral routes reduce the body's exposure to it by allowing the estrogens to bypass the gastrointestinal tract through which they otherwise would flow.

Benefits

Estrogen therapy has been proven to alleviate or prevent effectively the *hot flashes* and *vaginal-urethral changes* of menopause. In addition, there is increasing agreement that estrogen therapy can also help to retard the *bone loss* that tends to accelerate in women after menopause (or following the surgical removal of the ovaries), bone loss that can escalate into the brittle bones of osteoporosis. (Please see the chapter "Body Mechanics" for a complete discussion of osteoporosis and the role of diet and exercise in sustaining and even regaining good bone health.)

Whether other benefits exist for estrogen therapy is less clear. No firm evidence has shown estrogens effective in regard to *psychological symptoms* at menopause, for example. "The emotional problems which may occur during the time of life associated with menopause should not be treated with estrogen," concludes the *Harvard Medical School Health Letter*. The manufacturers of estrogen caution a similar prohibition, although some studies have reported a positive response in some women; hence, research is continuing.

There is also no real proof that estrogens can slow certain aspects of the *aging process*, even though the skin, for example, is one of estrogen's target tissues. "Estrogens do not appear to prevent age-related changes in skin, hair, and breasts," concluded the Consensus Development Conference on Estrogen Use sponsored by the National Institute on Aging in 1979. To assign the cause of these aging changes to lowered estrogen levels is "total hogwash," says Harvard's Dr. Johanna F. Perlmutter. The skin is the most exposed organ in the body and ages similarly in men, who don't experience the hormonal shifts women do. But research continues here too as estrogens have been shown to have some effects on these tissues.

Research also continues on the role of estrogens for cardiovascular health. A woman's risk of heart disease appears to increase after menopause. Because this risk also goes up after surgical menopause, when a woman's ovaries as well as her uterus have been removed, scientists have hypothesized that natural estrogen must normally protect women against cardiovascular illness. In fact, this has often been given as the reason why we live longer than men. The body's estrogen may raise the blood levels of HDL (high-density lipoproteins), the so-called "good cholesterol" that has been associated with a reduced risk of heart disease. Whether artificial estrogens can play a similarly protective role has not been conclusively shown. Research results have been contradictory, and have shown that external estrogens may even be detrimental. The NIA Conference on Estrogen concluded, "Although it was once hoped that estrogen would protect against heart disease in aging women, this effect has not yet been demonstrated." Sorting out the conflicting information is essential as cardiovascular disease is still the number one cause of death in our later years.

Risks

The most serious risk of estrogen therapy is cancer of the endometrial lining of the uterus. As you know, estrogen stimulates the buildup of this lining. Without sufficient progesterone to cause the regular shedding of the uterine lining as it did during the menstrual cycle, a woman taking estrogen will have excessive endometrial cells, making her very susceptible to cancer. The incidence of endometrial cancer in postmenopausal women who are not on estrogen therapy is normally one out of 1,000. This increases four- to eightfold in women who have been on estrogen therapy for two to four years, *without* the combined administration of a progestin, and fourteenfold if over seven years.

These are alarming statistics, but we must keep the issue in perspective. Most women do *not* get uterine cancer from external estrogens. In addition, the "cure rate" for women who have taken estrogens is higher (90 percent) than when uterine cancer is not drug-related (60 percent). Still, the increased risk *is* significant and climbs with the dose and duration of estrogen use. Research to date has been done primarily with women using the pill form orally, but we have to assume the same risks might apply to estrogen creams which are also absorbed systemically, even though they bypass some of the body's organs. (Fortunately, no cases of uterine cancer have been reported from using only the cream form.)

Those are the facts when estrogen is administered alone. If a progestin drug is given in addition to estrogen, the risk of endometrial cancer has been reported to decrease to a level *below* that which occurs in non-estrogen-using women. In fact, combining progestins and estrogens is now the most widely accepted method of administration. Progesterone's role is to balance the action of estrogen throughout the body. The monthly buildup of the uterine lining by estrogen, for example, was always opposed by progesterone's breakdown of it during the cycling years. The outcome was our menstrual period. Synthetic progesterone, mimicking this natural pattern, can stimulate the same sloughing off of the endometrial cells that are produced so abundantly during estrogen therapy. Women taking estrogen and progestin, in fact, usually begin to have light monthly periods again.

Unfortunately, while we know the protective benefits of adding progestin to estrogen therapy, we don't yet know its own long-range risks. "Currently, sufficient information is not available on the risk associated with simultaneous administration of estrogen and progesterone," reports Dr. Howard L. Judd of the UCLA School of Medicine. A higher incidence of cancer with progestins has shown up in animals. Before we know the real human risks, we need long-term studies. The use of progestins with estrogens at menopause is still quite new. Cancer, as is well known, can take many years to show up; it's a time bomb with as much as a twenty-year fuse. The initial good news about progestins may turn out to be only one side of the story.

If estrogen is given alone, there are other possible risks, although these are based on higher doses of estrogen than a woman would normally take after menopause:

- The chance of developing gall bladder disease may double.
- The incidence of blood clots, high blood pressure, stroke and heart attack may increase. Cardiovascular complications may also occur with the use of progestins.
- The deterioration of carbohydrate metabolism, which causes a blood sugar problem, may occur in as many as 40 percent of estrogen users. This effect and an impaired fat metabolism may also result from progestins.
- The growth of liver tumors may increase. These are usually benign but can cause internal bleeding.

There are several other possible risks that remain of concern:

- There is increasing evidence of a link between estrogens and breast cancer in animals, though there is no corresponding evidence among humans at this point.
- We don't really know what the cumulative exposure to external sex hormones will mean for women who use estrogen and progestin medication at menopause if they have also previously used the birth control pill, which contains considerably higher doses of both hormones.

Other Considerations

Women on ERT have also had other problems. These are probably not dangerous, but they are potentially bothersome: rashes, weight gain, water retention that may in turn cause breast tenderness and depression, an increase in the size of already existing benign tumors of the uterus, and the most common side effect, "breakthrough bleeding." Because bleeding is also a sign of endometrial cancer, if it occurs it must *always* be diagnosed immediately by your physician, who will usually do a D&C and/or an endometrial biopsy to examine the cells of the uterine lining. The addition of a progestin may help to control this breakthrough bleeding, but as I said earlier, will probably mean the resumption of a light monthly period as it stimulates the shedding of the endometrium. Progestins may also cause water retention. According to the Tufts Nutrition Research Center on Aging, estrogen users may be exposed to nutritional deficiencies similar to those that occur in women who use birth control pills: Vitamin C and the B vitamins, especially B_6 and folic acid, may become depleted.

The risks and side effects of estrogen therapy exist among other general concerns. Taking estrogens may mask natural menopause, merely postponing the body's gradual adjustment to its shifting internal hormonal environment. Hot flashes, for example, seem to return immediately after a woman ceases medication. Estrogen therapy may also alter our ability to adjust well on our own. We don't know exactly how estrogen drugs affect our body's own internal production of them. There's evidence, for example, that the ovaries and adrenals become indifferent or lulled into inactivity by the presence of external estrogens. Estrogen therapy may also have other broader effects on the endocrine system, effects we haven't yet discovered. Lastly, a practical concern. Estrogen therapy requires a woman to be diligent about taking medication, to make frequent and regular visits to the doctor and to have considerable testing done for side effects—there's also the expense of all of this.

Who Should NOT Take Estrogen or Progesterone?

If you can answer in the affirmative to any of the following questions, you should not take estrogens or progestins.

Do you have:

- A personal or family history of breast or uterine cancer?
- A history of blood clots, heart attack or stroke?
- A history of liver disease?
- A history of benign breast or uterine tumors?
- Undiagnosed vaginal bleeding?

Heavy smokers and women with diabetes, gall bladder disease, migraine headaches, high blood pressure, and varicose veins should be particularly careful.

Should I or Shouldn't I . . .

Some physicians to whom we've shown this section feel we're not as supportive as we should be of hormone therapy. Other physicians agree completely with the approach we've taken. My natural bias is to be extremely conservative when it comes to the administration of any drug or hormone.

Every drug entails a measure of risk, and for estrogens that measure has been a significant one. The addition of progestins to estrogen therapy has thus far reduced the risk of uterine cancer considerably, but we're still awaiting news on their long-term effects. Accordingly, we have to proceed with the utmost care and thoughtfulness in deciding whether or not to take hormones. Ultimately, the final decision must be made individually. Each of us should have an informed physician who will help us to weigh the known benefits and risks of hormone therapy in light of our own bodies and our own lives.

Let's recall for a moment that menopause is a *natural* event. With reproduction over, we no longer *need* the amount of estrogen we once did. We don't have a *deficiency* of estrogen. We simply have less. In fact, some consider the "replacement" in ERT a misnomer; the term implies we're putting back that which naturally should be present.

That *is* the case with surgical menopause, when the removal of both the uterus and the ovaries unnaturally causes premature menopause, a "menostop" to the production of estrogen. The conversion of androgens to estrogens that occurs naturally in an older woman is not so reliable in a younger woman who suddenly has no ovaries. She will probably experience all the signs of menopause. Estrogen replacement therapy may indeed be in order for her at least until age forty-five or fifty, when menopause normally would occur.

But this is *not* the case with natural menopause. The idea that estrogen needs to be replaced has in the past led to the overuse of estrogen therapy and the overtreatment of women at menopause. For *most* women, in view of the fact that menopause is actually a sign that the body is following its proper course and because of the still imperfectly understood effects of taking sex hormones, hormone therapy may be unnecessary and even unwise.

For *some* women, however, when the physical or psychological consequences of menopause are very serious, the balance may weigh in favor of taking hormones. For numerous individual reasons, the benefits may make such a huge difference in a woman's life that they do outweigh the risks. Perhaps you have tried dietary changes, vigorous exercise and the other alternatives suggested here, but are still experiencing intense and prolonged hot flashes that interfere with daily life, or severe vaginal dryness and thinning that cause pain during intercourse. You may be going through a particularly stressful time—a death in the family, a divorce, loss of a job—so it is more difficult to cope with menopausal symptoms at the same time. You may have had surgical menopause or ovarian failure before the age of forty. You may have determined that you are at high risk for developing osteoporosis. For any of these reasons, you may want to discuss the pros and cons of taking sex hormones with a physician who is fully familiar with hormone therapy and with your specific health status. If you do decide on hormone therapy, whether short- or long-term, the following guidelines will help you to do so as safely as possible.

Guidelines for Hormone Therapy

1. **Talk to a trusted physician.** This is the first and probably most important step. Discuss the benefits and risks of hormone therapy for your individual case and in light of your medical history and present health.
2. **Take the appropriate tests if recommended.** Two tests may be suggested before you begin taking any sex hormone drug, to make sure there are no existing contraindications you may not have known about: an endometrial biopsy for detection of uterine cancer, and a mammogram for detection of breast cancer.
3. **TAKE THE LOWEST DOSE THAT BRINGS RESULTS FOR THE SHORTEST PERIOD OF TIME.** The risks increase significantly with higher doses of estrogen over prolonged periods of time. Discuss the dose and duration carefully with your physician. Unless your case involves surgical menopause or osteoporosis, your physician may suggest you not exceed six months on estrogens.
4. **TAKE ESTROGEN CYCLICALLY.** The basic rule of thumb is always to have one week a month free of hormone therapy. This means your physician will usually prescribe taking estrogen for about three weeks (or 21 days) followed by one week off (7 days or a little less).

    If you are premenopausal, you will probably be advised to begin taking estrogen on day 5 after your period begins (day 5 of the menstrual cycle). If you are postmenopausal, starting on the first day of every month will make it easier.
5. **TAKE IT WITH A PROGESTIN.** A progestin should be prescribed during the last 10 days of estrogen administration each month. Stop at the same time you stop taking estrogen for your drug-free week.

    Progestins should be taken even if your uterus has been removed by hysterectomy, eliminating the possibility of endometrial cancer. Progestins act as buffers for *all* estrogen target-tissues and may play a protective role in the prevention of other cancers of the reproductive tract, as well as cancer of the breast.

    Occasionally, a physician may prescribe progestins intermittently, perhaps four times a year rather than monthly, to minimize the resumption of monthly periods. This may, however, weaken its protective effects.
6. **Remain under the close care of your physician.** A thorough examination should be done after six to twelve months, possibly including an

endometrial biopsy. If your estrogen therapy extends beyond this time, a schedule of regular visits to your physician must be set up, and testing, usually to include an endometrial biopsy, must be conducted annually or every two years. These regular tests may include an assessment of blood pressure, blood fats, and blood sugar as well.

7. **Remain alert.** Pay attention to your body for possible side effects and report any abnormal bleeding to your physician immediately. *Don't* wait until your next scheduled visit.

8. **Keep informed.** Be sure to work with a physician who makes it a point to keep up to date on the latest hormone therapy research. It's also a good idea to stay informed yourself through the kind of resources I recommend in The Resource Guide.

9. **Develop new health habits.** Try diet and exercise alternatives, if you haven't already, especially in preparation for the time when you stop taking hormones. Make sure you get adequate vitamin C and B-complex vitamins, especially B_6 and folic acid.

Needing Answers

In order for us to make the best decisions in managing our menopause, with or without hormone therapy, we need to know more. Research must be done to satisfy questions that are now only partially answered. Leaders in menopause and endocrine research are the first to point out that we have a long way to go before fully understanding the impact of our changing hormonal and reproductive status at menopause. Georgetown University's Dr. Ramey told us, "Less than two percent of the national health budget is used for research on women's reproductive system and this will have to change." The demand for better information is higher than ever because more and more women are now approaching menopause, and we all expect to have three potentially vital decades ahead of us.

Fortunately, there has been a dramatic increase of research interest in menopause, as there has been in midlife generally. And new channels of communication are opening up as well, providing a number of valuable resources to women: national newsletters and journals, and local menopause and midlife clinics with physicians and nonphysicians participating. These are fast becoming an inte-

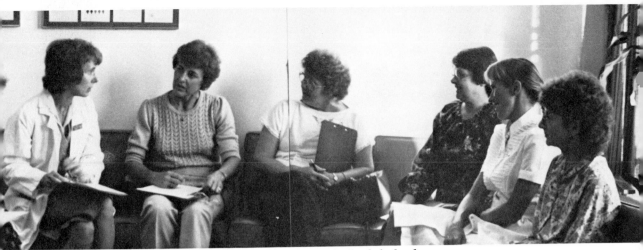

Co-coordinators Sonia Hamburger and Evelyn Anderson on the left, leading a discussion with women at the Menopause Clinic we visited at the University of California, San Diego.

gral part of women's health care at menopause. They go a long way toward transforming the old wives' tales about the end of reproduction into a real understanding of menopause. (In the Resource Guide, you'll find several of these resources that I especially recommend as a way of staying informed.) Our knowledge is growing largely because more of us are arriving at menopause eager for information, openly and unashamedly talking about it, much more aware of this unique natural rite of passage in midlife. The health community, accordingly, is responding. The preface to a current internationally known textbook on menopause alerts medical students and practicing doctors, "There are more women who will be spending a greater proportion of their lives in the postmenopausal years. . . . They will have questions and they will be looking for answers." We have, and we are.

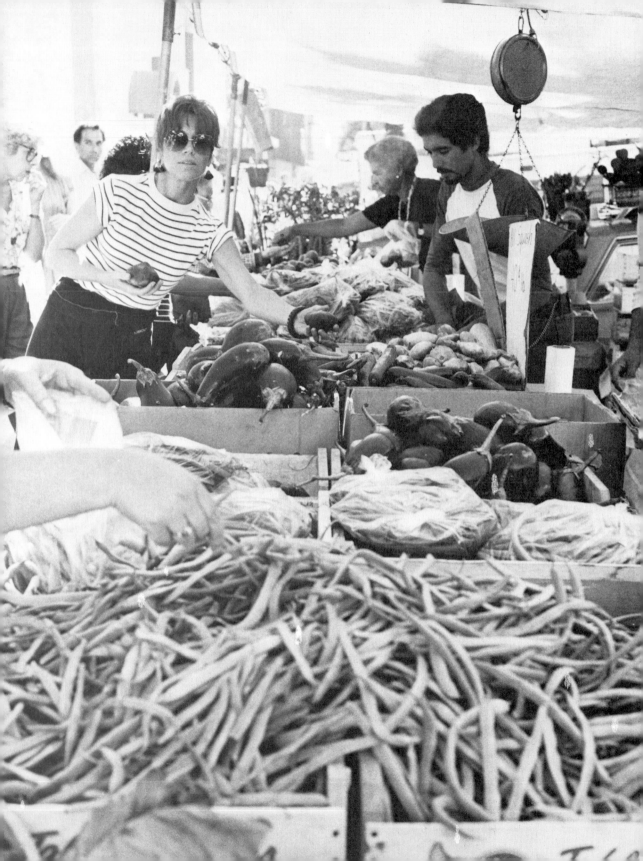

PART FOUR

Making It Last: My Program for Midlife Well-Being

CHAPTER *13*

EATING
FOR THE LONG RUN

IN THE LAST FIFTEEN YEARS I've learned a great deal about good nutrition. Food—so long a foe in my earlier years of starving and bingeing—has finally become my ally. Oh, there's an occasional skirmish now and then, but essentially we've made peace. And I'm more convinced than ever of how crucial a healthy diet is—to my mental and physical well-being, as well as to my family's. It can also help us all to put the brakes on fast aging, ease the menopause experience, prevent the onset of chronic illness, and give us the vitality we all want and need in midlife.

The food we eat affects every cell in the body—from the hormones to the bones, from the nerves to the skin, from the enzymes to the muscles. And whether we exercise regularly affects how well the food we eat is utilized by the cells for fuel, for building, and for repair. In midlife the quality and quantity of the nutrients we take in and use become increasingly important because of the normal changes that come with age.

In Chapter Three, "The Process of Aging," I described how the body's cells gradually slow down and are increasingly error-prone in regenerating and repairing themselves. Hence these miniature cellular factories require the *best raw materials* to reproduce the healthiest, strongest cells possible—otherwise they are starved of the nutrients needed for continual rebuilding, and damage accelerates. In addition, because the metabolism slows down a little as well, each of us needs fewer calories—all the more reason that the food we eat must be nutrition-packed. We can't afford empty calories. So, we have to master the dietary art of getting *more out of less*.

As we age we don't digest or absorb food as well as we once did. The enzymes that convert food into usable material may no longer perform at their maximum. Because of this, some foods begin to produce unexpected allergies or irritations to the digestive tract. It's not uncommon, for example, to develop an intolerance for milk because the intestinal enzyme lactase, necessary for the breakdown of lactose in milk, can diminish with age. The cells may lose some of their efficiency in absorbing as well as using nutrients over time. For example, there seems to be a decrease in the ability to handle glucose or sugar, which I'll talk more about later. How easily we eliminate the waste products of food may also change. Our kidneys, which filter waste from the blood, slow down to some extent. And we are more likely to be constipated if we reduce our fiber intake or drink less water. We can minimize all of these effects through exercise, but the results will only be significant if we combine exercise with healthy eating habits.

THE BASICS

A healthy diet remains healthy regardless of age. A good diet at twenty is a good diet at forty, sixty, and at eighty. In considering what foods we all need, let's start with the basics—the Big Three.

- CARBOHYDRATES give the broadest, most readily available energy to the body and those with fibrous residues keep the digestive tract clean and healthy.
- PROTEINS are the building blocks for every cell in the body.
- FATS lubricate each cell and provide the body's most concentrated form of energy.

Most foods contain all three of these nutrients, but with one predominating. For instance, potatoes contain a trace of fat, a few grams of protein, but ten times as much carbohydrate. One cup of low-fat cottage cheese contains 4 grams of fat, 8 of carbohydrate, but 31 of protein. Occasionally, there's more of a balance—spinach is half protein and half carbohydrate, with barely a trace of fat. Only a few foods provide only one of the Big Three, such as vegetable oils that are completely fat, or cod, which is virtually all protein. A fruit like watermelon is the closest we can come to a "pure carbohydrate."

There's no evidence that our nutritional needs decrease with age. Each of the major nutrients is essential to a healthy diet—with complex carbohydrates occupying center stage. But because of all the changes we go through as we age, some elements of our daily protein, carbohydrate, and fat requirements will alter as well. We will need more of some nutrients, less of others. In addition, because we don't absorb vitamins and minerals as well as we once did, our requirements for many of these tiny nutrients may indeed increase.

The Standard Aging Diet

Each of the three major nutrients has a downside. With proteins, it's an excess of animal protein. With fats, an excess of saturated fat. With simple carbohydrates, an excess of sugar—and the corresponding lack of fiber. Too many calories from all three add unwanted pounds.

Unfortunately, these negative sides of the Basics make up an all-too-familiar eating pattern—the Standard American Diet (SAD). This high-fat, high-sugar, high-calorie, low-fiber SAD regimen, bereft of vitamins and minerals, could just as easily be called the Standard Aging Diet!

The facts are quite shocking. Sixty-two percent of the calories we consume come from sugar, alcohol, and animal fats. This means *well over half* of the food we eat has no nutritive value, nor any fiber, and that only 38 percent of our food intake can be used to meet all of our nutritional needs. As a society, we couldn't be digging our graves faster with shovels than we do with our forks. The situation is critical and dangerous—for us, and for our children. We must change our eating habits. In the pages that follow, you'll learn, as I did, how to change to a life-saving low-fat, low-sugar, low-calorie, high-fiber, and high-nutrient diet. Keeping in mind the basics, the essential nutrients for a healthy diet, let's look at the most important elements to begin *subtracting* from your midlife diet. I call them "The Aging Eight."

THE BASICS: GOOD AT ANY AGE

PROTEINS

Protein builds, maintains, and repairs cells in virtually every body tissue. Protein is composed of twenty-two amino acids that replace old cells and build new ones in your skin, muscles, bone, cartilage, blood vessels, and each internal organ. The amino acids are also necessary for the formation of hormones and enzymes, which are necessary for every chemical process in the body.

Protein also serves as a back-up energy supply if carbohydrate and fat reserves become exhausted. Such a depletion is not desirable, however, since the protein you consume cannot be stored and must be replenished daily for the body's continuous maintenance needs. A diet balanced with carbohydrates and fats is the natural insurance against having to dip into your protein allowance.

*Daily need: 35–55 grams or 1–2 ounces of protein a day is ample—*protein should make up 15–20 percent of your total daily calories. Keeping within this range is important through midlife and beyond. A diet *too high* in protein, like the typical American diet, can be hard on the kidneys. It also accelerates the loss of calcium from the bones, which can lead to the development of osteoporosis.

Food sources: The body is able to manufacture most of the necessary amino acids. Nine of these, however, are available only through food and are best utilized by the body when consumed at the same time. The foods highest in protein that also contain all nine of these "essential" amino acids are called *complete proteins.* These are the animal products: fish, poultry, beef, eggs, milk, yogurt, and cheese. While not complete in themselves, *plant proteins in certain combinations provide an equally rich source of protein* and the essential amino acids. One of the most basic combinations is legumes (such dried beans, peas, lentils, and p nuts) served with seeds or wh grains (such as rice, wheat, corn, oa barley, and cereals).

CARBOHYDRATES

Carbohydrates are the chief sour of energy for all body functions. Th are readily digested and convert into the blood sugar glucose whi fuels the brain, the nervous syste and the muscles. Glucose works li kindling, helping the body to bu the denser fuel of fat more efficient A certain amount of glucose is stor in the muscles and liver as the reser fuel glycogen.

Carbohydrates are both simple a complex. Simple carbohydrates a sugars and are the most rapidly br ken down into glucose—giving us energy jolt followed by an equa sudden energy drop—with few or nutrients. Complex carbohydrate made up of starches and fibers, are duced to glucose more slowly, provi ing a more sustained energy relea over a greater length of time. Unle refined and depleted of nutrier through processing, the complex ca bohydrates are a treasure trove of tamins, minerals, and the indigestib

FATS

Fat provides the most concentrated form of energy to the body. This is true whether it is provided by the diet, or by the body's stored deposits of fat. Fat is the fuel you train your body to burn in long, endurance types of aerobic exercise. It also insulates you, lubricates the cells, protects the skin and other tissues from dryness, and assists the body in its absorption of the fat-soluble vitamins.

Fat is made up of fatty acids of two basic kinds: saturated fat, which is usually hard at room temperature and is derived primarily from animal fat, including butter and lard; and unsaturated fat, which is liquid at room temperature and comes largely from the oils of vegetables, nuts, and seeds. The hard saturated fats contain cholesterol, a waxy substance necessary for good health and a key component of your sex hormones but which in excess is associated with potentially fatal chronic artery and heart disease. The unsaturated fats, on the other hand, have no cholesterol and may actually, in moderation, reduce the cholesterol carried in the blood. Also, only the unsaturated fats contain linoleic acid, the "essential" fatty acid that we must get from food, and which we need for normal growth, metabolism, and healthy blood, arteries, and nerves.

Daily need: Just one tablespoon of a polyunsaturated liquid vegetable oil will supply the day's basic nutritional requirement for the essential linoleic acid. *Your intake of fats overall should be less than either of the other basics.* The calories per gram are twice those for protein and carbohydrates, hence your fat intake should not exceed 25 percent of your total daily calories. The average American diet is composed of more than 40 percent fat, most of it coming from saturated fat, and that largely from beef, poultry, and whole milk products.

Food sources: In moderation, the best sources of fat are vegetable oils, especially the polyunsaturated corn, sunflower, soybean, and safflow oils—safflower being the richest linoleic acid. Peanut, olive, and s ame oils are less liquid and should used sparingly. Coconut and pal oils, often added to processed foo are nearly solid and should avoided.

ITAMINS

*Absolutely essential to good health,
?amins are tiny chemical substances
? food that assist proteins, fats, and
?rbohydrates in fulfilling their differ-
?t functions in your body.* These mi-
?onutrients provide no calories or
?ergy themselves, but help as com-
?nents of enzymes to metabolize or
?nvert carbohydrates and fat into
energy, as well as protein into cells
and tissues. They also assist in the
formation of your hormones and the
chemicals of the nervous system such
as those in the brain, some of which
are known to influence mood.

Vitamins are often supplied in the
very foods that require them for their
own utilization in the body. Complex
carbohydrates, for example, are full of
B vitamins, which help to convert
carbohydrates to glucose. Polyunsaturated vegetable oils contain vitamin
E, which protects the oils from oxidation; the oils in turn ease the absorption of vitamin E throughout the
body.

There are two main types of vitamins: water-soluble and fat-soluble.
Those soluble in water are essentially
unable to be stored in the body and
must be continually replenished.
These are vitamin C and the B-complex vitamins. Fat-soluble vitamins
are stored readily in the body. These
are vitamins A, D, E, and K. An excess of these vitamins can result in a
toxic build-up, although this happens
rarely.

Daily need: The Food and Nutrition Board of the National Academy
of Sciences publishes a Recommended Daily Allowance (RDA) for
all vitamins and minerals. They now
have a separate category for people
over fifty. Nutritionists say the RDA
is a useful guide, but one with limitations. The RDAs have always been
recommendations for *average*, not *individual*, needs, and the over-fifty category is based on extrapolations from
the needs of *younger*, not *older*,
adults.

It's doubtful that our daily vitamin
needs decrease with age. It's highly
likely that they remain the same or
increase due to our bodies' dimin-
ished efficiency in absorbing nutrients
and the fact that in midlife we continue to be robbed of nutrients by alcohol, sugar, smoking, stress, air
pollution, and other hazardous chemicals in our water and food. Because
of the denatured, devitalized processed foods that make up a large part
of the average American diet, I believe it is important that we take *a
daily multivitamin supplement with
meals that provides at least 100 percent of the RDAs.* We may require
higher amounts of certain key vitamins in midlife. (See pages 208–17.)

?bers that help to slow the rate of
?ucose absorption and to keep the
?imination system healthy.

*Daily need: Most of your diet
?ould consist of complex carbohy-
?rates*—at least 60 percent of your
?tal daily calories. The average
?merican diet is typically *low* in
?omplex carbohydrates, while we
?ontinue to consume more and more
?mple carbohydrates.

Food sources: Complex carbohy-
?rates are abundant in all vegetables,
?ruits, legumes, seeds, and nuts; in
?hole grains like brown rice and
?lled oats, and in unsweetened cere-
?ls, pasta, and breads made with
?hole grains. Simple carbohydrates
?re found in table sugar, brown sugar,
?nd corn syrup. Blackstrap molasses,
?oney, and maple syrup are also sim-
?le sugars but contain some nutrients.
?e careful—*70 percent of the sugar in
?oday's American diet is hidden in
?rocessed foods* such as canned fruit,
?rankfurters, and most commercial ce-
?eals.

?INERALS

*Minerals are as life-sustaining and
?ital to your overall mental and physi-
?al well-being as vitamins.* We have
?inerals in all our body tissues and
?luids—the bones, teeth, muscles,
?lood, skin, and nerve cells. They act
?s catalysts for transmitting nerve
?essages, contracting and releasing
?uscles, producing hormones, and
?egulating the body's fluid balance.
?hey also work along with the vita-
?ins in food metabolism.

The major minerals present in relatively high amounts in the body are
calcium, magnesium, potassium,
phosphorus, sodium, chlorine, and
sulfur. The trace minerals present in
the most minute but equally essential
quantities are iron, zinc, selenium, io-
dine, manganese, copper, chromium,
fluoride, and several others.

Daily need: RDAs are available as
a guide for most minerals. As with vitamins, there's no sign that our mineral needs decrease with age.
Fortunately minerals are less fragile
than vitamins, and both the major
and trace minerals are rarely deficient
in the diet, with the exception of calcium, iron, and zinc. Women, for example, chronically get too little
calcium, which can result in osteoporosis in later years. However, minerals work together in an intricate
balance, so we should never take too
much of any one mineral. For instance, we need an equal amount of
phosphorus and calcium. Too much
phosphorus—which is abundant in
red meat, many processed foods, and
soft drinks—will deplete the body's
calcium. On the other hand, we need
about half as much magnesium as we
do calcium. Too much sodium, for
example, the most frequently used additive next to sugar, will deplete the
body's potassium in some people; this
in turn can alter the body's fluid balance, causing the retention of water
and increasing the risk or severity of
high blood pressure.

As with vitamins, the best insurance policy for getting your daily
minimum balanced mineral requirement is to take a *multimineral supplement with meals that provides at
least 100 percent of the RDAs.*
Mineral supplements are usually
already combined with a multivitamin supplement.

THE AGING EIGHT

1. MEAT

Meat is not without its virtues. It's a solid, rich source of complete protein, full of iron. Every once in a while I will crave your basic American hamburger and eat it with relish, literally and figuratively. But the benefits of eating meat and other animal proteins on a regular basis are unquestionably outweighed by the problems.

- Red meats are high in phosphates which, if taken in large quantities, drain calcium from the bones.
- Virtually all beef and poultry today come from animals raised in high-tech feedlots. Their meat contains synthetic hormones, toxic residues from pesticides, antibiotics, and other undesirable chemicals.
- Most meat and all whole milk products are very high in fat—especially in saturated fat and cholesterol, which are both associated with the fatty deposits on artery walls implicated in atherosclerosis and many of the major chronic diseases of the heart. (Dietary cholesterol is found exclusively in animal foods. In fact, every animal food contains some cholesterol; the highest quantities are in eggs, butter, and organ meats. I'll say more about cholesterol and fat shortly.)

Most of us eat twice as much protein as we need, most of it in meat. Ours has been a protein-centered society for a long time, convinced that only red meat can provide the protein we need, and the more the better. Now however, we know that too much protein is actually harmful, especially if it comes from meat or other fatty animal proteins. The right amount of protein *is* essential. In fact, the few long-term studies that have been done on nutrition and aging found that women with diets neither too low nor too high in protein lived the longest. But we don't have to eat large amounts of meat marbled with fat—and offering no fiber—to get it.

I recommend you *eat less meat, especially red, processed, cured, smoked, or charred meat—and also less liver.* Even though extraordinary for its A, C and B vitamins, liver is now out of my diet, and not just because of its high cholesterol content. The liver is the inernal detoxifier in animals just as it is for us, a kind of garbage dump for the chemicals to which cattle and chicken are increasingly exposed. Barbecuing or broiling fat-rich meats has been found to lead to the conversion of fat to potential pro-carcinogens. This is a problem with any burnt food that contains fat and protein together. Also, cured and smoked foods are full of nitrate and nitrite preservatives. The body converts these into nitrosamines, chemicals known to induce tumors in animals. Products like bacon, ham, and luncheon meats are not only high in these chemicals, but also high in fat and salt.

The alternatives you can turn to with confidence are *low-fat dairy products, fish, and combinations of plant proteins that complement each other.* I'm grateful to Frances Moore Lappé, who explains all of this so well in her ground-breaking and influential book, *Diet for a Small Planet.* In her latest revision, Lappé writes that getting enough protein without meat is even easier than she originally thought if we eat basically whole, non-junk foods—good news for those of us on low- or non-meat diets who don't want to get bogged down trying to keep track of amino-acid combinations.

As with vitamins and minerals, the protein we consume is not all *usable* protein. All nine essential amino acids are present in many foods, including some vegetables and fruits, but the amounts and proportions of all nine are what determine the *quality* of the protein in our diets.

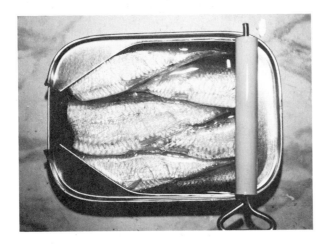

Sardines—rich in protein, calcium, iron, and vitamin A (but drain oil well).

Dairy products (such as eggs, milk, yogurt, and cottage cheese), fish, poultry, and red meat get A+ ratings on both the quantity and the usability of their protein. These are often called complete proteins for that reason. On the other hand, the protein found in plants—legumes (dried beans, peas, lentils), whole grains (rice, wheat, corn, oats, barley and cereals), seeds, nuts, some vegetables, and a few fruits—generally is lower in overall quantity. Most plant foods are weak in some amino acids while strong in others. But when two or more are combined, they too can merit A+ protein ratings.

The art of getting abundant and usable protein from non-animal sources is to combine one food's protein weaknesses with another's strengths. This can increase the usability of the proteins in both by 40 to 50 percent! Please be assured this is *not* as complicated as it sounds, and that if you eat a basically healthy, varied diet, you'll get all the protein you need. Patterns vary from food to food but, fortunately, there are good, predictable combinations; one of the best is *legumes combined with grains.* For example, beans with tortillas, or peanut butter on whole wheat bread provide an excellent protein balance. Of course, any time you add to vegetables, legumes, grains or fruit one of the dairy products, fish, or meat, you are maximizing the protein in those plant foods. Eating complementary proteins at the same meal works best, but you will also get the full value of the protein if you eat the beans at noon, for instance, and the tortillas a few hours later. Remember, *most* American diets provide way over the daily ideal protein allowance. If you're concerned about a protein deficiency you can watch for telltale signs like slowness in healing or unhealthy hair and nails.

Here are some of the ways I make sure Vanessa, Troy, Tom and I get the protein we need. By now, these are old favorites with us.

- *Yogurt and cottage cheese.* In their nonfat and low-fat forms, these are my main protein staples—sometimes a glass of skim milk and an occasional egg. I know a cup of plain yogurt will give me 20 percent of my daily protein allowance, and a cup of cottage cheese 60 percent. I add low-fat yogurt to just about everything—fruit, raw and cooked vegetables, salads. I also use it as a substitute for sour cream in sauces and baking. It's not only delicious—on a baked potato, for instance—but I can be sure the yogurt will maximize whatever protein is present in other foods. Yogurt, cottage cheese, and milk are also loaded with calcium and potassium. They may also have a cholesterol-lowering effect in some people.

- *New condiment-complements.* Yogurt is not the only surefire protein complement I use. Nonfat or low-fat milk on whole-grain cereals is one of the best combinations. I also add small pieces of fish or chicken (both without their skins) to brown rice, vegetables, or both. Low-fat cheeses like mozzarella are great on tortillas, vegetables, and salads.
- *Tofu and rice.* Called bean curd by the Chinese and tofu by the Japanese, this soybean product is the plant protein closest in quality to meat protein. Tofu and other members of the bean family, such as pinto (or kidney) beans, black beans, garbanzo beans (or chickpeas), provide inexpensive and excellent protein when combined with whole-grain rice—one of the highest-quality grains, and one of my favorites. Green or yellow vegetables, stir-fried or steamed, make this combination even more delicious and protein-rich. Tofu or beans can also be added to salads and soups. Somewhat lower in fat than mozzarella cheese, tofu is also an excellent source of iron and calcium and has been shown to lower blood cholesterol in some individuals.
- *Wheat germ—my favorite "additive."* Though it comes from grain, wheat germ is protein-strong where many plant foods aren't. It is also packed with vitamins and minerals. One to two tablespoons of wheat germ are an excellent protein maximizer for salads and vegetables like spinach, broccoli, collard greens, and mushrooms. (And mushrooms in combination with these dark green vegetables also provide good protein.) In addition, wheat germ complements potatoes, tofu, and grains such as rice, oatmeal, and cereals. I also add it to eggs, yogurt and the occasional hamburger we have, even though these don't need an added protein boost. And I use wheat germ in baking.
- *Seeds and nuts.* These are as rich as beans in protein, especially sunflower seeds and cashew nuts. They're also great protein complements to tofu, legumes, dark green leafy vegetables, and potatoes. And they're power-packed when combined with wheat germ and bran. Wonderful as they are, however, I use them sparingly because they're high in calories as well as fat.

191

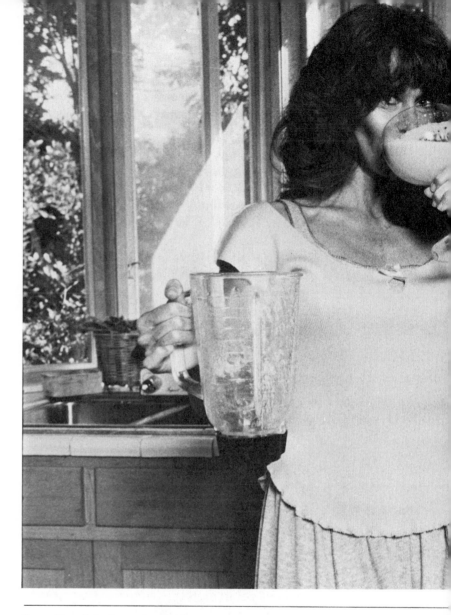

Jane Fonda's Protein Shake

Combine the following in a blender:

1 cup nonfat milk* or apple juice (when using milk, you might want to
  add ¼ cup apple juice as a sweetener)
about 3 or 4 fresh or frozen strawberries, or ⅓ cup blueberries or peaches
  (never with syrup!)
½ fresh banana
1 teaspoon wheat germ or bran
1 to 3 tablespoons protein powder, preferably made from milk and egg
  protein, with *no* sugar, artificial coloring or flavor added.

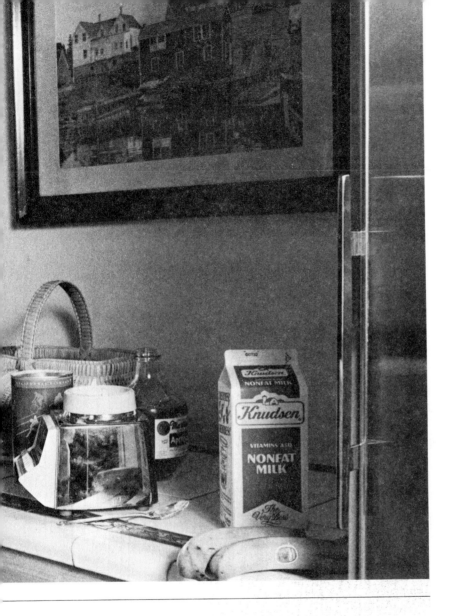

A few ice cubes if fruit isn't frozen
Optional: ¼ papaya (the more fruit you include, the more milk or juice you may want to add too)
Blend all of this together until smooth and thick.

---

* I advocate certified raw milk whenever you drink milk because pasteurization destroys many of the essential vitamins and enzymes in milk.

- *My protein drink.* If I'm going to be teaching several workouts, if I am under particular stress, or if I know I'm going to be on the run—more than usual—I'll be sure to have a breakfast protein drink before I leave the house in the morning—even if by the end of the day I may exceed my usual protein allowance. It assures me, at least, that I start the day having already gotten over half of the protein I normally need. It also gives me the sustained energy I need to keep going through the day.

2. FAT

Americans are reported to consume 130 pounds of fat a year. That's the equivalent of ten sticks of butter per person—*every week!* Meat heads the list of fatty foods, followed by whole milk, ice cream, whole milk cheeses, butter, margarine, and oils.

A high-fat diet is associated with the two leading causes of death in midlife women—breast cancer and heart disease. It is also implicated in high blood pressure, diabetes, and colon cancer, the second most prevalent kind of cancer in midlife women. The high calories in fat also contribute to our becoming overfat and overweight.

A high-fat intake limits the oxygen that gets to the cells, in essence suffocating them. It also impedes the metabolism of carbohydrates, our principal source of energy. Saturated fats, as you know, are associated with a high level of blood cholesterol. A certain amount of cholesterol is essential. For instance, it's a principal component of the sex hormones and every cell membrane. But the body is largely able to manufacture its own cholesterol for these purposes. An excess of cholesterol from animal protein in the diet is only harmful.

Unsaturated fats that come from vegetable oils, seeds, nuts and grains are preferable to the hard saturated fats. They contain the essential linoleic acid and help us to absorb the fat-soluble vitamins. Yet, even unsaturated fats are troublesome in excess. Polyunsaturated oils are known to be vulnerable to oxidative reactions, increasing the possibility of damage inside the body which many believe contributes to the process of aging, as I explained earlier.

I recommend that you *eat less fat of all kinds, but especially saturated fat.* These are the guidelines I follow.

- *Go for the lean.* In red meat, this isn't easy to do; you're better off eliminating it. If you can't, buy the leanest cut possible, trim all visible fat, and use meat more as a side dish than a main course. Eliminate lard altogether. In poultry, the white meat without the skin is the least fatty. In fish—among the leanest of animal protein sources—cod, lobster, shrimp, haddock, flounder, perch, red snapper, and sole are best; next are bass, halibut, crab, trout, pink salmon, and tuna (water-packed, if canned). Always remove the skin from fish as you do with chicken.

- *Use nonfat and low-fat dairy products*—milk, yogurt, and cheeses. The cheeses lowest in fat, in addition to low-fat cottage cheese, are feta and mozzarella. Incidentally, mozzarella is also relatively low in salt (though feta is relatively high). Ricotta and Neufchâtel are next best. I've taken butter, margarine (although it's cholesterol-free it's all fat and full of additives and preservatives!), shortening, sour cream, and cream cheese off my grocery list.

- *Vegetable oils, nuts, and seeds in moderation.* I make sure I get my daily requirement of linoleic acid by having one tablespoon of vegetable oil per day—usually as dressing in my salads. Safflower oil is richest, but corn, soybean, and sunflower oils are also excellent sources. A quarter cup of sunflower seeds is equally rich in this essential fatty acid, but with many more calories. In general I go easy on all vegetable oils, keeping them refrigerated, never letting them go rancid. Peanut, olive, and sesame oils, less liquid than the others, should be used even more sparingly, just to add flavor. All oils are 100 percent fat, nuts 85 percent, seeds 75 percent—each very high in calories (one tablespoon of oil = 120 calories).

- *Easy on the exotic avocado.* It's a fruit I love but it's 75 percent fat, even though unsaturated and rich in linoleic acid. High in vitamin C, but calorie-rich too.

- *Limit eggs.* Because of their cholesterol content, I try to limit my eggs to three each week, even though they are one of my favorite foods. In baking you can use just the egg white, which has no cholesterol. If you scramble more than one egg, you can leave out half of the yolks.

- *Eat less processed food.* Instant foods spell instant aging. A great deal of hidden fat is delivered in processed snacks and prepared foods like potato chips, crackers of all kinds, and luncheon

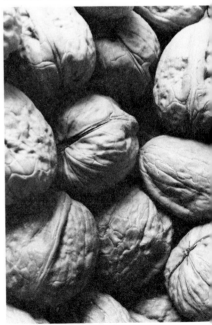

Walnuts—good protein, vitamin and mineral booster in salads.

meats. If you buy prepared foods like baked goods, with lots of added sugar, you can be almost certain they are loaded with fat as well. Commercially prepared granola is over 30 percent sugar—and contains equally as much fat. If when reading a label you see coconut or palm oil listed as ingredients—both saturated fats—pass on that item.

3. SUGAR

Sugar is like fat's twin. Both are tied to excess weight and to the overlapping list of midlife chronic diseases. If you look closely, you'll notice they inevitably appear together in most processed foods. *Sugar is the number one food additive.* At last count, the average American consumed 140 pounds of sugar a year. Think of it—that's 14 ten-pound bags! A TV network news story brought home to me recently just how hooked we are on sweet flavors. Congress received more mail protesting a proposed ban on the artificial sweetener saccharin than it did on the entire Vietnam War!

At any age, too much sugar wreaks havoc on us—creating blood sugar levels that are both too high *and* too low. Burning the simple carbohydrate of sugar for fuel is like burning newspaper for heat. Sugar ignites with a bright flame that quickly dies, necessitating that more "paper" continually be added. The rush of blood sugar, or glucose, causes the pancreas to secrete high levels of insulin, the hormone key that opens the cells to receive the glucose they need for energy. This surge of insulin causes the blood sugar level to drop quickly. In addition, the insulin then lingers in the blood, keeping the blood sugar down, so that we feel tired and crave more sugar—a vicious cycle. Less well known about insulin is that it also encourages our bodies to store fat! The more insulin we secrete, the faster fat is rushed to the cells and stored.

Scientists aren't completely sure why, but with age all of us seem to develop a mildly lowered tolerance for glucose. Insulin is still produced in response to the glucose broken down from both simple and complex carbohydrates, but the glucose or blood sugar isn't taken into the cells as well as in earlier years. This may be due to a decline in the number of insulin receptors on the cells—a condition which exercise can improve. It may also be that the insulin we produce is less potent. The exact cause is imperfectly understood. In children and young adults, blood sugar levels return to normal in a few hours after eating. In middle-aged and older adults, glucose may stay high in the blood for four to six hours. If we eat too much sugar (and also too much fat), this condition can cause trouble, even escalating into what is known as adult-onset diabetes. An extra load is put on the kidneys. The smallest blood vessels are damaged, circulation is impaired and as a result, the tissues that need life-sustaining oxygen and nutrients from the blood are ultimately adversely affected. We begin to store too much fat, and the more fat we have the less responsive we seem to become to insulin.

High levels of sugar in the diet are related not only to diabetes and weight problems, but also to an increased level of blood fats and therefore an increased risk of heart disease, urinary infection—to which we're also more susceptible in midlife—and tooth decay. In addition, at menopause many women also report that sugar is a trigger for hot flashes—and, of course, for depression. It also robs us of the B vitamins.

I recommend that you *eat much less sugar, especially the refined sugars.*

- *Take cane, confectioner's, brown and raw sugars off your shelves.* They are all sucrose, the simplest and most common sugar.
- If you have to have a sweetener, *substitute blackstrap molasses, honey, or maple syrup—but use **sparingly.*** Don't forget these are simple sugars as well. I notice, however, that I don't use them nearly as liberally as I previously used "the white stuff." The calories are more or less comparable teaspoon for teaspoon, but they're *twice as sweet* as table sugar so you tend to use less. Unlike table sugar, these also have some nutritional value. In fact, molasses, which is the residue from the sugar-cane refining process, is full of minerals. One tablespoon has more potassium, iron, calcium and magnesium than eight ounces of milk or a piece of chicken! It also has small amounts of all the most important B vitamins for midlife, which I'll talk about later in the chapter, and somewhat fewer calories than all the other sugars. Honey, regarded as the perfect food in some cultures, when uncooked and unfiltered has less sucrose than molasses and more fructose or fruit sugar, which is digested somewhat more slowly. It has small amounts of calcium, magnesium, potassium, iron,

Apples—fiber-rich satisfaction for a sweet tooth and excellent in salads too.

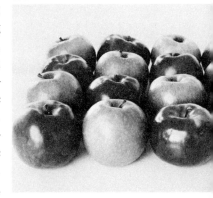

the B vitamins and vitamin C, and a trace of protein. It is also a mild laxative, a sedative, comes in many delicious flavors, and keeps for years without needing to be refrigerated. Maple syrup lies in between molasses and honey in terms of its nutrients and calories. But again, use very little of any of these.

- *Cravings solutions:* To satisfy a sweet tooth I turn to complex carbohydrates, which our bodies also break down into blood sugar, but more slowly than simple carbohydrates. They not only keep me from eating refined, high-calorie sugars, but I know they're energy- and nutrient-rich. Here are some of my favorites: nonfat yogurt with fruit or a little cinnamon; if I'm on the run, I always take an apple with me, like a tart green Granny Smith; slices of frozen honeydew melon in summer or frozen bananas any time of the year; and baked bananas or applesauce with cinnamon. If I bake bran or carrot muffins—both loaded with fiber—I use molasses or honey (and a minimum of vegetable oil). Fruit juice concentrates, such as apple, can be used to sweeten baked goods too.

- *Forget artificial sweeteners.* They *don't* help most of us lose weight. Americans are consuming more diet soft drinks than ever, but we're still gaining weight. Saccharin may be carcinogenic and the newest artificial sweetener, Aspartame, contains an amino acid whose effects in large quantities remain unknown. Usually these sweeteners come paired with other potentially harmful chemicals. In addition, artificial sweeteners allow you to cut calories, but they don't help you to overcome the need for a sweet taste.

- *Cut down the amount of processed food you eat.* Quantities of sugar come hidden in processed foods. You will find sucrose, dextrose, maltose, fructose, corn syrup, beet sugar, or invert sugar (50 percent dextrose/50 percent fructose) on almost every label. Read labels carefully: the closer the sugar additive is to the top of the list—and there are usually more than one in the same product—the more sugar present. Commercially prepared cereals are notoriously high in sugar. Sugar is also high in most canned fruits, some canned vegetables, yogurts with fruit, salad dressings, and many types of pickles, relishes, and other condiments.

4. SALT

Salt is our number two food additive. Too much sodium, the unwanted ingredient in salt, is the principal cause of high blood pressure, which has a tendency to increase anyway with age, and of water retention, which is implicated in depression and hot flashes at menopause. Fat cells can as easily fill with water as with fat, adding bloat and weight. Too much sodium also causes the body to excrete potassium. This makes extra work for the kidneys as well.

I recommend that you *eat less salt and salty foods.* We get plenty of sodium naturally in the unsalted foods we eat. We are far more in danger of getting too much sodium than too little.

- *No more salt shaker.* I never use salt in cooking and baking nor do I add it to the food on my plate. I just omit it. And I find that salt often covers up the true flavors in food.
- *Substitute "Veg-It," pepper, herbs, spices, and,* **in moderation,** *soy sauce.* "Veg-It" is a powdered herbal and vegetable blend that I use on just about every vegetable I eat—sprinkled in stir-fried vegetables or on a baked potato. I always have a peppermill for grinding fresh black pepper, and cayenne pepper is a staple. Soy sauce, made from soybeans, *does* contain sodium—but much less than table salt. It also has a stronger flavor, so you don't need to use as much. One-quarter teaspoon of soy sauce equals one teaspoon of salt in seasoning power. Shoya is a form of natural soy sauce that contains wheat. Tamari is another natural soy but without the wheat. There are also imitation soy sauces and some marked "mild" or "low-sodium."
- *Look for low- or no-sodium labels.* And always check the ingredients—anything with the word "sodium" has salt, for example, monosodium glutamate (MSG), sodium nitrites and nitrates (found in cold cuts, cured, and other meats as preservatives). Baking powder and baking soda contain sodium. Most cheeses are high in salt. Your best bet is cheese marked salt-free or low-salt. Some relatively low in salt are Swiss, Gruyère, Gouda (the one from Holland), mozzarella, and Neufchâtel (the last two are relatively low in fat as well). Even some bottled waters contain sodium, so look for those that are specifically labeled "salt-free." You might want to call your city water department to find out

the sodium content of your tap water. If it is high (over 150 parts per million), I recommend you drink bottled mineral, spring, or distilled water.

- *"Hold the salt. . . ."* Restaurants are becoming increasingly accustomed to hearing this request. Don't be afraid to insist that you don't want salt or MSG in your food.
- *Cut down on processed food.* Sound familiar? This means frozen, fast, and pickled foods; canned foods like soup; hot dogs, bacon, and sausage; salty snacks like pretzels and potato chips; and common condiments like ketchup.

5. PROCESSED FOODS

If you've read this far, you know why this is one of the Aging Eight. Just cutting processed foods from your daily diet would be a big step toward eliminating the fat, sugar, and salt trio. If you eliminate red meat as well and make the substitutions I have recommended so far, you'll have gone a long way toward covering your nutritional bases. At the same time you will be avoiding the major food toxins. We need to get our grains, vegetables, and fruits with *all*—or as much as we can—of what Nature has given them.

6. ALCOHOL

Excess alcohol works similarly to excess sugar as a stress-producer and as an antinutrient. It depletes us of vitamin C, many of the B vitamins, and, because of its diuretic effect, many of the essential minerals such as calcium, magnesium, potassium, and zinc. Alcohol has 7 calories per gram (more than both carbohydrates or protein) and has almost no nutritive value, with the exception of beer and wine, which contain traces of protein, carbohydrate and some minerals.

It's important to understand the whole complex of related effects that too much alcohol can have on our bodies. Alcohol is a well-known trigger for hot flashes, depression and insomnia; it's a potent oxidant once broken down inside the body—which, among other things, can lead to premature wrinkling, as I discussed earlier in my chapter on "The Skin"; it raises blood fats and blood sugars; it overloads the digestive system, the kidneys, and especially the liver, which can develop cirrhosis, a potentially fatal disease; it's a well-known risk factor in heart disease, cancer and diabetes; it causes accidents; and it's addictive. Unfortunately, midlife women who drink alcohol often also use prescription tranquilizers—compounding its negative effects. If you drink due to stress, I assure you that vigorous exercise can be a *powerful* and much more effective and long-lasting substitute.

There is some good news about alcohol. In *moderation* it has beneficial effects as a mild tension reliever, a mood elevator, and as a tonic for the heart. Alcohol relaxes the blood vessels and is believed to raise the level of "healthy" fats in the blood (called HDL for high-density lipoproteins), especially in people who exercise as well. One or two glasses of wine or beer a day, or a shot (1½ ounces) or two of hard liquor are considered moderate amounts. Remember, though, alcohol is a drug and even moderate amounts add 100 to 200 empty calories.

7. CAFFEINE

Found in coffee, tea, many cola soft drinks, chocolate, and some aspirin-type pain killers, caffeine is a drug and a diuretic that depletes us of vitamin C and many of the B vitamins, as well as calcium, potassium, and zinc. The tannin in tea, which has one quarter to one half less caffeine than coffee, depending on the variety, interferes with our absorption of iron as well.

Even though it constricts the blood vessels, caffeine is a known trigger for hot flashes, perhaps because it's also such a potent stimulant. It causes the adrenal glands to pump more adrenaline and the pancreas more insulin—raising and lowering blood sugar and encouraging fat storage. It also increases the appetite, arouses a craving for sweets, and stimulates the nervous system, which can cause insomnia, irritability, and finally, overall exhaustion.

Caffeine is one of a family of chemicals called methylxanthines which are associated in women with the development of fibrocystic breast condition, painful but benign lumpy breasts. This condition often subsides spontaneously in midlife, but it is also a possible risk factor for breast cancer. Eliminating all caffeine has been known to alleviate fibrocystic breasts dramatically (especially when accompanied by vitamin E), but it can take a year or more for symptoms to disappear in women after age forty-five (smoking can slow this down). Reducing dietary fat also helps.

During the writing of this book, I've managed to stop drinking coffee. It hasn't been easy. I love coffee. The smell of espresso in the morning used to be like a good friend. I had limited myself to a cup or two a day, in the morning only, but even then I began to notice that I was feeling tired again around 10:00 or 11:00 A.M. and wanting more. Somehow the more coffee I drank—and it's easy to do when you're working at a desk—the more I felt I needed to renew my energy. I had kicked the caffeine habit before so I knew what I was in for—headaches and a profound tiredness that would last about ten days. But this time I faced it as though I were going into battle. I knew it would be a tough battle but it was one I wanted to win. Now that I'm clear of it, I'm surprised how much better I feel. My energy is my own and I have more of it. My moods are more stable.

I've returned to one of the best natural energy boosters I know— three tablespoons of brewer's yeast flakes with a dash of cayenne pepper in a mug of boiling water. The cayenne cuts the flavor of the yeast. The many friends I've turned on to this energy drink find it tastes more like spicy chicken broth than the terrible yeast taste some of us remember from our childhood. I also drink herb teas in moderation, and enjoy their many flavors and healthful effects. Ginseng and chamomile are among my favorites. In addition, there are now decaffeinated coffees available that are both delicious and safe to drink. If you buy your decaf as beans or ground, be sure to ask for the water- or steam-extracted kind. If you buy your decaf commercially packaged, be sure the caffeine has been removed either by the same water-extraction process or, as the High Point brand does, by using ethyl acetate, the only caffeine-removing chemical that has proven safe thus far.

8.   SMOKING

The smoke inhaled from cigarettes doesn't go through the digestive system like alcohol and caffeine; rather, its residues enter the blood and tissues from the lungs. But smoking is no less a drug, and no less addicting. If there is a number one dangerous health habit, smoking may just be it. Unfortunately, more women are becoming heavy smokers and they are starting to smoke at an earlier age. I'll talk more about this later in Chapter Fifteen, "Planned Patienthood." But for now just a bit of what I've learned.

Smoking, even the smoke we inhale from others' cigarettes,

cigars, or pipes, depletes us of important nutrients: many of the B vitamins, vitamin A, and especially vitamin C. Like alcohol and caffeine, it may also have an effect on our calcium balance because it's a known risk factor for osteoporosis. It's also a potent oxidant. It accelerates the aging process, causing the cross-linking that can mean premature wrinkles, the stiffening of blood vessels and other connective tissues. Smoking constricts blood vessels and increases blood fats, affecting the whole circulatory system. One of its major toxins, carbon monoxide, reduces the ability of the red blood vessels to carry life-sustaining oxygen to the cells. Smoking is also a trigger for hot flashes and early menopause. People who smoke a pack or more a day are *twice* as likely to die from heart disease, emphysema, and lung cancer. Lung cancer, in fact, is about to surpass breast cancer as the number one killer of women in midlife! Fortunately, the health benefits begin almost immediately after quitting.

Before moving on, let's summarize the things you should cut down or cut out at midlife. Let this be your guide:

Less meat, especially red meat;
Less fat, especially saturated fat;
Less sugar;
Less salt;
Less processed food;
Less alcohol;
Less caffeine;
And NO smoking.

Now let's turn to the good news—the things you can *add* to your diet.

FOODS TO LIVE BY

When you minimize the things in your diet that take more than they give, that exhaust rather than rejuvenate, that damage rather than build—you've cleared your eating table for the really good foods you need, the *lifesavers* that are lower in calories and higher in quality nutrients.

1. COMPLEX CARBOHYDRATES

I've already told you about some of my own staples, many of which come from the large basic group of complex carbohydrates. These are the first and perhaps most important additions to your diet. Vegetables and fruits, dried beans and peas, seeds and nuts, whole-grain rice, pasta, cereals, and breads easily supplant the old red meats, butter, cheeses, salty processed foods, pies, and cakes. These complex carbohydrates are foods that have sustained whole cultures for centuries. They make up the largest part of my diet. The hardiest, leanest athletes eat the same way, as do the societies of the world known for their longevity.

Certain of the complex carbohydrate foods are good sources of the amino-acid building blocks, without the liabilities and calories that come with the fat in animal protein. Complex carbohydrates are gentle on the body too, digested more easily than animal proteins and more slowly than simple sugars. They are your energy base, loaded with vitamins and minerals, and your *only* source of fiber—the next essential ingredient in a diet for life.

2. FIBER

Fiber is the residue from plant cell walls which our bodies do not absorb. I think of food fiber as my natural insurance for a healthy digestive system and a kindly friend that helps me to maintain my weight. Fiber forms a gel in the gastrointestinal tract, which is known to slow the absorption of sugar, so your energy and your insulin levels are more steady. It also cuts down on the absorption of fats, so calories and stored toxins are moved speedily through the system. Because of all this, a high fiber diet has been proven to have a preventive effect on intestinal and breast cancer, diabetes, and heart disease.

There are two principal kinds of fiber, each with specialized functions. The pectins found mostly in fruits and vegetables are associated with reducing certain fatty substances like cholesterol in the blood stream. There is also evidence that the pectins help to keep blood pressure steady and, some believe, alleviate circulatory conditions like varicose veins. The cellulose found in whole grains, such as the wheat bran and wheat germ that come from the wheat berry, is the other kind of fiber. It tones the intestines for regular, quick elimination which protects against constipation, hemorrhoids, and

he more serious hazard of colon cancer, which is the third leading
cause of cancer death in midlife women.

A few raw carrots each day will give you plenty of *both* kinds of
fiber as will a diet that's generally high in complex carbohydrates. I
often add one or two tablespoons of raw bran to cereals, eggs, salads,
or soups and take a small supply with me when I travel to places
where fresh foods are scarce. I'm careful never to overdo this healthful additive, however. *Too much* bran can interfere with the absorption of key minerals like calcium, iron, and zinc, making them
unavailable to the body. And one last thing. This bulky fiber holds
up to five times its weight in water—that's why it works so well. If
you add bran to your diet, you'll need to take in more liquid as well,
which brings us to the next necessity of midlife—lots of H_2O.

3. WATER

Water is *the* primary nutrient—second only to oxygen as a pre-
requisite for life. The body can withstand the absence of food much
longer than it can the absence of water.

Water is present in each cell and constitutes two-thirds of your
body's weight. We must have water for virtually every body function. As the largest component of the blood, water is essential for
the easy transportation of nutrients and hormones to waiting cells
and for helping kidneys and bowels clean out their wastes. It also
regulates our body temperature through the cooling mechanism of
sweat, and keeps the skin and mucous membranes moist, as well as
the connective tissues such as the joint cartilage. Muscles alone are
75 percent water. If an athlete becomes dehydrated, her energy
takes a nose-dive and her performance stumbles.

Many of us, I think, go about our day sluggish because, unbe-
knownst to us, we're in some stage of dehydration, not realizing
we're but a glass of water away from feeling re-energized. But
usually we wait until we're parched with thirst before reaching for
water—by this time we may have lost a great deal of water from the
sweat of a workout, hot flashes, or just the heat of the day.

We also lose cellular water as we age—about 10 to 15 percent by
the time we're sixty-five. In addition, we are surrounded by water-
drainers. Caffeine, alcohol, and a lot of fat or sugar all draw water
out of the cells. And your reserves stay low if you consistently reach
for these or, to satisfy your need for liquids, reach for regular or diet

sodas—both high in sodium and caffeine. The secret is to remain hydrated all the time—healthfully.

If you are concerned about water retention, rest assured that drinking water is *not* a cause; on the contrary, it's one of the natural diuretic solutions I recommend to help flush water-retaining sodium out of the body. What I'm proposing is minimizing the unhealthful diuretics in your life and rediscovering water. It has restored my sense of well-being many, many times and helps to keep my weight down as well. If you tend to retain water, as I do, resist the temptation to cut down on your liquid intake. I try to drink six to eight glasses of water every day.

Some days I fill a half-gallon plastic water jug first thing in the morning with natural spring or distilled water (always use these, if you can, unless you know your tap water is free of questionable chemicals, pollutants and sodium)—this is the equivalent of eight eight-ounce glasses. It fits in the large tote bag I usually carry, so it stays with me at the office, on the set, or wherever I am, even at home. I make sure that by the time I turn out the light at night, that bottle is empty. Other times I'll fill a bottle half that size and make sure I get the rest in herb teas and bottled mineral, spring, or distilled waters, the kind with little or no sodium (club sodas are salty). The trick in all this is to make drinking water easy and convenient—between meals preferably, so your stomach enzymes are not diluted during digestion. Always have a jug of cold water in the refrigerator with lemons and limes for flavor nearby. Often it's water anyway, not food, that our body wants when we open the refrigerator door.

A great discovery about many of the foods I've been praising is how full they are of water (low calories and high water content seem to go together). Virtually every fruit is nearly 90 percent water—with watermelon, true to its name, even higher. Vegetables also contain lots of water, with the dark leafy green vegetables over the 90 percent mark. Dairy products are an excellent source, as are many fish. Oils, on the other hand, are by definition waterless, and sugars are nearly so.

4.   THE SUPERSTARS

I want now to venture into what has been fascinating nutritional territory for me and talk about the "micronutrients," the vitamins and minerals that enable the food we eat to go to work for us. These are essential in the formation of the body's hormones, enzymes, and nervous system chemicals. They also play a role in the body's ability to repair itself and, hence, may have a unique impact on the aging process.

We know that as we age, even though the need for calories decreases, our protein, carbohydrate, fat, fiber, and water requirements remain *constant*. Less is known about what happens to our need for vitamins and minerals as we age. Nutritionists are just beginning to look closely into this area. They agree that, at the very least, our micronutrient intake in midlife and beyond should stay the same as in earlier years. Their research may reveal that our requirements for vitamins and minerals actually *increase* as we grow older—especially because our bodies don't absorb nutrients as well as before. We have already learned in the case of calcium, for example, that women's calcium intake following menopause needs to increase. There is also some speculation that our need for vitamin B_6 becomes higher over time.

Until all the evidence is in on our requirements for each micronutrient at midlife and beyond, we should be sure, at minimum, to follow the existing Recommended Daily Allowances (RDAs)—while recognizing the limitations of these guidelines. The RDAs are based on how much the average person needs of each nutrient in order to avoid signs of deficiency, rather than on how much may be optimal for the individual. In addition, the RDAs listed for the over-50 age group are based mainly on studies of younger, not older, adults.

Whether we should take vitamin and mineral supplements in order to obtain these recommended daily dosages is one of the most controversial questions in nutrition today. Ideally, having a well-balanced diet is all most of us would ever need to ensure our getting a full range of micronutrients. And, in fact, our daily diet is always the place to start. No supplement can make up for inadequate food choices.

Rarely, however, do the daily eating habits of most Americans fit the ideal pattern—even with the best of intentions. If you see yourself in any of the following descriptions, you're likely to be running short on vitamins and minerals:

- You're single and tend not to cook for yourself and have little variety in your day-to-day diet.
- Single or not, you're on the go most of the time and tend to eat erratically and frequently settle for the convenience of fast foods.
- You're a casual vegetarian and tend to put little time into the planning and preparation of meals, getting most of your protein from eggs and cheese, getting little of your protein from other sources like beans, brown rice, or fish.
- You're always on a diet.
- You drink and/or smoke heavily.

Even when we manage to avoid these common scenarios, we can't always be sure how nutrient-rich the good foods are that we do select. It is widely known that vitamins and minerals are lost in the processing, storage, and preparation of food—and these losses can be considerable. In addition, it's impossible to make up for the nutrients that are lost when foods are grown in nutrient-depleted soils.

For all of these reasons, I've long advocated *taking a daily multivitamin and mineral supplement, one which gives you at least 100 percent of the RDAs*—regardless of your age. Doing so becomes even more important in midlife when we begin to consume fewer calories and, accordingly, fewer nutrients.

I take such a supplement every day. I have also begun to emphasize, in both my diet and in supplements, a select number of vitamins and minerals that I've come to think of as the *Superstars:* vitamins E, C, A, a number of the Bs, and, of course, the mineral calcium. These particular nutrients play a special role in midlife health and, potentially, in slowing an accelerated aging process.

There is evidence that some of these nutrients can increase our cells' ability to repair themselves and may help to protect against the damage that can result from abnormal internal oxidation, discussed in the chapter called "The Process of Aging." As you learned there, with age and with added stresses from outside the body, damage can outstrip the cell's own capacity for rejuvenation and repair. Vitamins A, C, E, B_1 (thiamine), B_6 (pyridoxine), and B_5 (pantothenic acid), as well as the minerals zinc and selenium, are dietary antioxidants that can shore up the body's internal repair machinery. Each works a little differently, so we need them all.

When I was researching this book, I was amazed at how often the Superstar vitamins and minerals were suggested for helping to solve problems with hot flashes, water retention, depression, brittle bones, and the wrinkling and drying of skin. Other circumstances may also increase our need for these nutrients beyond the amounts ordinarily recommended. Users of estrogen drugs, for example, need extra B vitamins. Heavy smokers need additional vitamin C. Stress, excess alcohol, fat, and salt, pollution in our water, food, and air—all of these nutrient-robbers may require us to take a little more of certain vitamins and minerals.

As one aspect of my own nutrition plan, I take dosages above the RDAs for many of the Superstar vitamins. As a midlife woman living in Los Angeles, one of the smoggiest cities in America, I want the extra protection I believe the antioxidant vitamins and minerals can give me. *Vitamin A* helps my skin in particular. *Vitamin E* is essential to utilizing vitamin A and is necessary for the health of all cells, hormones, circulation and even aerobic capacity. Vitamin E is also a healer of vaginal tissues and known to alleviate hot flashes as well in some women (this was discussed in the section "Is There Life After Menopause?"). *Vitamin C* helps both A and E in all of their functions. Vitamin C is essential for healthy collagen in the skin and in all connective tissues, both so susceptible to the process of cross-linking which causes the wrinkling and stiffening associated with aging. It's also essential in times of stress. The *B-complex* vitamins, equally important during times of stress, are essential for a healthy nervous system. The Bs and vitamin C are both important to healthy adrenals as well, glands critical after menopause for hormone production.

The following charts profile these vitamins and minerals. Whether you should take supplements as I do, beyond the basic multivitamin and mineral supplement already recommended, is a decision to be made after evaluating your particular nutritional and health status—preferably with a nutritionally informed physician. If there is little agreement currently about whether to take supplements in general, there is even less about what amounts to take. Until a consensus exists among nutritionists, a supplement plan has to be a matter of very careful individual assessment. Only the exact quantities are in question; that we need an abundance of these Superstars in our diets is undisputed.

SUPERSTAR VITAMINS AND MINERALS

	Vitamin A	*Vitamin E*
MIDLIFE IMPORTANCE	• Necessary for *healthy skin, hair, and eyes.* • Helps to maintain the *elasticity* and *smoothness* of the skin. • Protects against dryness and aids in the repair of the body's *internal soft tissues*—like those in the glands or lining of the digestive tract—and the body's *mucous membranes*, as in the vagina. • Contains key *antioxidant* properties.	• A major *antioxidant*, especiall protecting the body's fats and fa uble vitamins from the damag abnormal oxidation. • Provides essential most prote for every cell and cell membra the body, important for the nc *aspects of aging*, including m pause. • Necessary for the production health of all *sex and adrenal mones*, so important at menop and after. • Maintains strong, flexible cap walls, *improving circulation an ducing abnormal clotting* in blood that otherwise could lea heart attack or stroke. • Essential for *bringing oxygen nutrients to the body's cells*, in ing those of the heart and ske muscles, enhancing aerobic cap and endurance. • Helps to keep the *skin* smooth ducing itchiness that somet occurs with age; speeds healin the skin. • Vitamin E is known to alleviate *flashes* at menopause for s women. It may also be effectiv treating certain circulatory diso of the legs such as *varicose veins* cramping, and in playing a pre tive role against heart disease. ' min E has also been usefu treating *fibro-cystic breast condi* in some women, the somet painful and lumpy breasts that indicate a predisposition to b cancer.

Vitamin C

major *antioxidant*, especially in protecting the body's other vitamins and abundant connective tissues from the damage of oxidation.

essential for the formation and maintenance of healthy *collagen*, the protein that is the chief constituent of the body's connective tissue, which holds the *cells* together and makes up the walls of the *blood vessels* as well as the tissues of our *muscles, tendons, ligaments, cartilage, bones, and skin*. Together with the minerals zinc and selenium, vitamin C is also essential for the health of *elastin*, another key part of connective tissue.

necessary for the health of the *adrenals*, key glands at times of stress and for the production of estrogen after menopause. Most of the body's vitamin C is stored there.

stimulates the *immune system*, our body's principal mechanism of defense, which becomes increasingly vulnerable as we age and which is involved in fighting every threat to our health, from the common cold to cancer.

The B Vitamins

The eleven vitamins that make up the *B-complex* are all essential for *mental health*, an *active metabolism*, and *healthy skin*, particularly around the nose, mouth, and eyes.

Thiamine, riboflavin, niacin, pantothenic acid, pyridoxine, and folic acid are the most important B vitamins at midlife and necessary for:

* *Strong adrenal glands*, which require especially niacin and pantothenic acid
* *A healthy nervous system*, which requires especially thiamine, niacin, pantothenic acid, and pyridoxine
* The proper *conversion of carbohydrates* into the glucose we burn for energy, which requires especially thiamine, riboflavin, niacin, pantothenic acid, and pyridoxine

Thiamine (B_1) has *antioxidant* properties, especially when working in combination with vitamin C.

Riboflavin (B_2) is essential for *good vision* and *healthy skin, nails, and hair.*

Niacin (B_3), in addition to the roles mentioned above, is important for the formation and utilization of the *sex hormones* and helps to improve *circulation* and reduce blood cholesterol levels. It's also good for brittle nails.

Pantothenic acid (B_5) is an *antioxidant* and the most outstanding B vitamin in alleviating *stress*. In addition to its roles listed above, it may also aid in slowing the aging of the skin.

Pyridoxine (B_6) has *antioxidant* properties and is particularly important at menopause because of its effectiveness against *water retention* and *depression*. A natural diuretic, B_6 together with Vitamin C helps to form the brain chemical serotonin, associated with calm moods and necessary for sleep. It also helps to preserve high blood levels of the mineral magnesium, sometimes called "nature's tranquilizer." Lastly, there is interaction, still imperfectly understood, between B_6 and the hormone estrogen. Nutritionists now believe everyone's requirement for B_6 may increase over time.

Folic acid is important in the formation and utilization of *estrogen*. It is also essential for the division of body cells, the utilization of sugar, and the promotion of red blood cells in the

(continued on p. 213)

Calcium

* Essential for *healthy, strong bones and teeth* and for the *prevention of osteoporosis*.
* Necessary for *muscular contraction and relaxation*.
* Helps maintain *cell membranes and connective tissue*, especially of the skin.
* With magnesium, promotes the *proper working of the nervous system*, which can help relieve the nervousness, irritability, and insomnia sometimes associated with menopause—a natural tranquilizer.
* Helps to relax *blood vessels*, alleviating high blood pressure. It might also help to block cholesterol absorption.
* Calcium is the body's most abundant mineral, but is chronically underconsumed by women of all ages. Its RDA is now under review. Nutritionists believe our calcium requirement increases as we age.

	Vitamin A	*Vitamin E*
MIDLIFE IMPORTANCE		
POLLUTION PROTECTION	• Protects against the damage to internal tissues that can be caused by *smog* and also *smoking*—especially damage to the mucous membranes of the mouth, nose, throat and lungs.	• Protects against the damage to that can be caused by *smog, smo and radiation.* Taken with vitam it will help to protect the lung t in smokers. • Suppresses the tendency of sod nitrites and nitrates in food pres tives to form cancer-causing nit mines.
ENEMIES	• Smoking • Excessive alcohol	• Food processing destroys muc the vitamin E naturally occurrin grains and other foods. • Polyunsaturated fats call on F work overtime to help prevent process of abnormal oxidation polyunsaturated fats are know accelerate. The more fat of any that we eat the more E is necess • Smog • Iron will inhibit E's absorptio consumed simultaneously.
FRIENDS	• *Vitamin E* protects vitamin A from being destroyed. • *Zinc* helps to mobilize vitamin A out of storage in the body. • *Beta-carotene* is a water-soluble natural precursor or source of vitamin A.	• *Vitamin C* protects E from dest tion and helps to enhance its ac ity, especially in alleviating flashes and in keeping blood ves healthy. • The trace mineral *selenium,* itsel *antioxidant,* also enhances the act of vitamin E and often occurs na rally with E in our foods. • Vitamin E protects the fat-solu vitamins A, D, and K from dest tion.
RDA	• 4,000 IU, women (5,000 IU, men)	• 12 IU women (15 IU men)

Vitamin C	The B Vitamins	Calcium
	body. A deficiency of folic acid, which is not uncommon in older women, is related to anemia. Folic acid occurs chemically in combination with *PABA* (para-aminobenzoic acid), an *antioxidant* which may itself be a B vitamin.	
potent detoxifier, vitamin C pro- against many of the hazardous icals and effects of smog, cigarette e, pesticides, and radiation; sup- s the tendency of sodium nitrites nitrates in food preservatives to cancer-causing nitrosamines; and with the mineral zinc to prevent bsorption of lead into the body.		With magnesium, protects against the toxic metals lead and cadmium.
all the vitamins, C is the least sta- in heat, light, air, and water. erwashing fruits and vegetables deplete their vitamin C. oking—25 mg of vitamin C is de- yed for each cigarette smoked! aling another's smoke does the e. cessive alcohol og ess ffeine pirin trogen drugs	• Stress • Excessive sugar and refined carbohydrate intake • Excessive alcohol • Smoking • Estrogen drugs • Thiamine is the most vulnerable of the B vitamins to heat, air, and water, especially during cooking. Pantothenic acid and folic acid are similarly lost during storage and cooking. • Thiamine and pantothenic acid are also particularly depleted by the caffeine in coffee and tea.	• Smoking • Stress • High protein diet • High phosphorus intake—for example, from red meat and soft drinks • Caffeine and alcohol increase the risk of osteoporosis.
e *bioflavonoids*, often found natu- ly with vitamin C in fruit, protect amin C from destruction and en- nce its absorption and use. In par- ular, the bioflavonoids—which are o *antioxidants*—assist C in keep- g collagen healthy and capillaries ong. *tamin E* enhances the activity of amin C, while C in turn protects from destruction, as well as pro- cting A and the B vitamins. tamin C also greatly enhances the sorption of iron.	• All of the Bs work together and usually occur together naturally in foods. • *Vitamin C* protects the Bs from destruction.	• *Vitamin D* is essential for calcium's proper absorption and utilization. • *Vitamin C* also enhances absorption. • *Magnesium* balances the effects of calcium.
mg	• Thiamine: 1 mg • Riboflavin: 1.2 mg • Niacin: 13 mg • Pantothenic acid: No RDA; 4–7 mg is the estimated safe and adequate intake • B_6: 2 mg • Folic acid: .4 mg (or 400 mcg)	• 800 mg *SPECIAL NOTE*: Most nutritionists and physicians now agree that the present RDA is too low for women. The following is their revised recommendation for women's daily intake of calcium before and after menopause: • 1,000 mg *before* menopause • 1,500 mg *after* menopause

	Vitamin A	*Vitamin E*
SPECIAL PROBLEMS	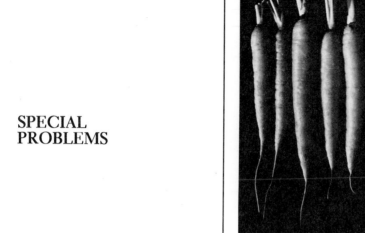	• *Menopause:* For the alleviatio. hot flashes, some physicians scribe taking vitamin E supplem in dosages up to 800 IU per day sometimes 1200 IU per day. P. cians advise increasing the do gradually, especially because e tiveness may be reached at a lo dosage for some women. (Vitam and B-complex vitamin supplem are often prescribed alongside enhance its effectiveness.) • *Fibrocystic breast condition:* Foi alleviation of fibrocystic bre some physicians recommend ta vitamin E supplements in dosage to 600 IU per day—always b sure to work up to this dosage gr ally.
SUPPLEMENTS: MAXIMUM ABSORPTION	• Vitamin A supplements should be taken with meals—once a day is fine. • *NOTE:* This is a fat-soluble vitamin that is stored in the body. Toxicity has been known to occur only from very large doses, yet a good policy is not to exceed 25,000 IU a day.	• Vitamin E supplements should taken with meals, preferably m containing a little fat, which hances the absorption of fat-sol vitamins. Once a day is fine. • The supplement should be a cor nation of alpha-tocopherol, the n studied and most potent of the se tocopherol forms of vitamin E, mixed tocopherols. A base of nat wheat germ oil or vegetable oi best. • Don't take vitamin E and iron plements or iron-containing med tions at the same time of day. will interfere with E's absorption • *NOTE:* Vitamin E is a fat-solu vitamin stored in the body. known level of toxicity has yet b found, but women with high bl pressure or rheumatic heart dise should consult their physicians may advise limiting daily intake 30 to 100 IU. • Taking selenium with your sup ment can enhance E's effectiven A good rule of thumb is 50 mcg selenium for every 200 IU of E— not to exceed 200 mcg a day, as lenium can be toxic at higher lev (continued on p. 2

Vitamin C	The B Vitamins	Calcium

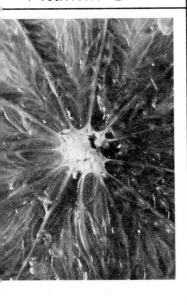

The B Vitamins

- *Menopause:* For alleviating hot flashes, some physicians may prescribe B-complex supplementation along with vitamin E. If so, be sure the niacin you take is in the form of *niacinamide*, which, unlike the niacin form itself, will not dilate the blood vessels. Such dilation can cause flushing, exaggerating the hot flash.
- *Water retention:* For alleviating water retention and the depression sometimes associated with it, some physicians prescribe vitamin B_6 supplements in dosages of 200 mg per day and up to 800 mg per day. Physicians advise increasing the dosage gradually, but *never* going beyond these amounts.
- *Estrogen therapy:* If you are on estrogen therapy, you need to be especially careful to get enough vitamin B_6 and folic acid. Discuss possible supplementation with your physician.

Calcium

- *Osteoporosis:* Physicians prescribe 1,500 mg per day calcium supplementation for women with osteoporosis.
- *Surgical menopause:* Physicians prescribe 1,500 mg per day calcium supplementation for women who have had their ovaries surgically removed.

Vitamin C

- *Vitamin C supplements* should be taken with meals.
- *Divide your daily intake into several doses.* This is a water-soluble vitamin. It is not stored in the body and is cleared from the blood every three to four hours.
- When you purchase your supplement, keep in mind the need for smaller dosages. In addition, for convenience look for a vitamin C supplement or a multivitamin that already contains the bioflavonoids, which may be listed as rutin, heseridin, or citrin.
- *NOTE:* If you have been taking a high level of vitamin C over a long period of time and then decide to decrease your dosage, be sure to do so gradually. Your body may otherwise perceive this change as a deficiency.
- *Ascorbyl palmitate* is a fat-soluble form of C which is also a strong antioxidant, able to penetrate areas of the cell which the water-soluble form of C can't.

The B Vitamins

- *Vitamin B supplements should be taken with meals.*
- *Divide your daily intake into several doses.* These are water-soluble vitamins not stored in the body.
- If you take any one of the Bs, you must be sure to take at least 100 percent of the RDA for the entire complex to maintain the correct balance of B vitamins.

Calcium

- *Calcium supplements should be taken in between meals,* either on an empty stomach or perhaps with a little yogurt, milk, or orange juice (the lactose and vitamin D in milk products and the vitamin C in citrus products enhance absorption).
- *Divide your daily intake into several doses,* saving the last for bedtime, because we tend to lose more calcium during sleep and also because calcium is a natural tranquilizer.
- When you purchase your supplement, read the label carefully to determine how much calcium is in each tablet and what kind of calcium is included. Calcium carbonate is the most concentrated form. Avoid dolomite and bone-meal products because of their high and potentially toxic levels of lead.
- Make sure you get the RDA of 400 IU of vitamin D each day, especially if you are not out of doors regularly.*
- Make sure your calcium dosage is always twice your intake of magne-

(continued on p. 217)

me supplements come already combined with vitamin D; be sure to watch, however, that you don't exceed 1,000 IU of D a day. In higher s D can have a *negative* effect on calcium, encouraging its excretion. In addition, vitamin D is fat-soluble and stored in the body, and can efore be potentially toxic at very high doses over a prolonged period of time.

	Vitamin A	*Vitamin E*
SUPPLEMENTS: MAXIMUM ABSORPTION		Supplements are available tha[t] ready combine E with seleniu[m] just make sure to note the selen[ium] dosage in relation to E's if you chase such a supplement.
FOOD SOURCES	• The *best* sources are *dark green leafy vegetables* like spinach, broccoli, collard greens, and parsley; *yellow vegetables* like carrots and sweet potatoes; *orange fruits* like cantaloupes, papayas, mangos, and apricots—especially dried apricots; and *fish oils* like cod liver oil. • Other excellent sources are nonfat and low-fat milk; ricotta, mozzarella, and Parmesan cheeses; eggs—but in moderation because of their high cholesterol content; and liver—in moderation if at all, because of the toxins that tend to be stored in animal liver. • Try red peppers, winter squash, and the spices paprika, cayenne pepper, and chili powder—all good sources.	• The greatest concentrations of v[ita]min E are in *unprocessed wh[ole] grains; unprocessed vegetable [oils]* especially safflower, corn and [soy]bean oils, and *dark green leafy v[ege]tables* like broccoli, spinach [and] parsley. • Among the best natural sources [are] *raw wheat germ* and *wheat germ*

Vitamin C	The B Vitamins	Calcium

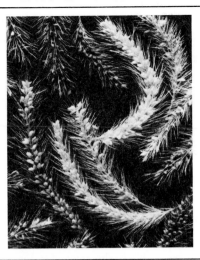

sium. Supplements are available which provide this proper balance as well as additional zinc, which may be absorbed less efficiently as more calcium is added to the diet.
- If you have a history of kidney stones, be sure to consult your physician, who may recommend keeping the dosage of your calcium supplementation under 250 mg a day. For most of us, however, supplementation even up to 2,500 mg a day, while unnecessary, is considered safe.
- Keep your phosphorus intake low; ideally it should never exceed your calcium intake. A deficiency is very rare.

Vitamin C

ll *citrus fruits and their juices* are ich in vitamin C, as are other fruits uch as cantaloupes, papayas, mangos, apricots, peaches, and strawber- ies.

qually abundant and sometimes nore plentiful in C are the *leafy, ark green vegetables* like broccoli, pinach, collard greens, and parsley. prouts, tomatoes, potatoes, and reen and red (especially red) pep- ers are also excellent sources.

he skin and white segments of all he above fruits, especially the citrus, re rich in *bioflavonoids* as well. (I on't advocate eating the skin be- ause frequently the skin is treated vith toxic chemicals.)

The B Vitamins

- The *complex carbohydrates*, which the Bs help to break down into glucose, come naturally supplied with many B vitamins. *Whole wheat and rice products, wheat germ, wheat bran, oatmeal, and dried beans* are all excellent sources of every B vitamin.
- Refined carbohydrates and sugars, on the other hand, are barren of Bs and actually increase our need for them.
- *Brewer's yeast* is the richest natural source of every B vitamin with the exception of B_{12}.
- *Liver, eggs, nuts, and seeds*, particularly sunflower seeds, are also rich sources—but eat them in moderation, especially liver, as noted elsewhere.
- *Niacin* is found in many foods in addition to the above: poultry and fish, especially chicken and tuna; leafy, dark green vegetables like raw broccoli, collard greens, parsley, spinach; corn, mushrooms, potatoes, and sprouts, as well as cantaloupe and oranges.

  The foods rich in Bs are also rich in the amino acid *tryptophan* which the body is able to convert to niacin (60 mg of tryptophan = 1 mg of niacin).
- *Pantothenic acid* is also found in many additional foods, especially broccoli, mushrooms, and yogurt.
- B_6 is also found in chicken, tuna, and bananas.
- *Folic acid* is also found in chicken and tuna, and in spinach, collards, and parsley.

Calcium

- All dairy products are rich in calcium. Among the best are nonfat and low-fat milk, nonfat dry milk, buttermilk, nonfat and low-fat yogurt, and low-fat cottage cheese. Whole milk and whole milk cheeses are excellent as well, but should be consumed in moderation because of their fat and cholesterol content.
- Leafy, dark green vegetables are also abundant sources of calcium: collard, mustard, and turnip greens, kale, and broccoli.
- Fish: canned sardines and salmon are good sources when you also eat the bones.
- Tofu, corn tortillas, and molasses (in moderation) are also excellent sources.
- Vitamin D is usually added to milk and is found in limited amounts in yogurt and the same green vegetables and fish that are rich in calcium.
- Calcium is found nicely balanced with magnesium in all the leafy, dark green vegetables (it's actually part of chlorophyll), tofu, molasses, and tortillas.
- See also the "Best Calcium Foodstuffs" chart on p. 108.

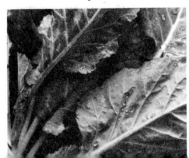

IRON

The most abundant of the trace minerals found in the body, iron is present in every cell and often associated with robust health because of its role in *keeping the blood oxygen-rich.* The average diet is low in iron, so deficiencies are common, especially in women. If you're iron-deficient, your tissues can't get enough oxygen and you become anemic—fatigued, more vulnerable to stress and illness.

Nutritionists believe that iron deficiency takes a back seat to calcium deficiency in women past the age of forty, especially after menopause when women stop menstruating. I still make sure, however, that I get my minimum *18 mg* a day—some in my multimineral supplement, most from the foods I eat. Foods rich in protein are frequently also rich in iron: poultry, eggs, whole grains, cereals (especially oats). But my favorites are wheat germ and bran, tofu, raisins, spinach, and parsley—all very high in iron. The leafy, dark green vegetables and sprouts rich in iron also contain vitamin C, which *triples* the absorption of iron when consumed at the same time. (If you drink lots of coffee, tea, or red wine on the other hand, these can interfere with iron absorption.) Sunflower seeds, garbanzo beans, and blackstrap molasses are also rich sources—in moderation. Cooking your food in iron pots will add to your iron intake.

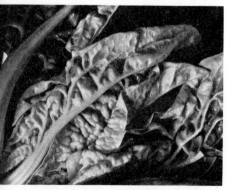

ZINC

The second most abundant trace mineral, zinc also has strong *antioxidant* properties (the only other antioxidant mineral is selenium). Zinc is thought to be just as necessary and just as scarce in the average American diet as iron. White spots under your fingernails may suggest you are deficient in zinc.

This mineral promotes healing in the body's *skin*, including the *face and vaginal tissues.* In fact, 20 percent of our zinc is stored in the skin. Zinc helps to transport vitamin A, the skin vitamin, to skin cells. It also intensifies the action and absorption of other vitamins, especially the Bs. Zinc is a component of the enzymes involved in the breakdown of food and in metabolism, as well as the enzymes that protect the body from internal oxidation. It is also a part of the hormone insulin, and is involved in the building of protein in the body.

While I master learning which are the zinc-rich foods, I rely on a multimineral supplement to assure that I get the *15 mg* of zinc I need at minimum each day. (A good rule of thumb is not to exceed 40 mg a day, however—you *can* overdo minerals.) Protein foods are usually good sources of zinc, as they are for iron: chicken, fish, eggs, yogurt, milk (especially nonfat dry milk); mozzarella cheese is especially good. Whole grains, beans, sunflower seeds, and mushrooms are also good sources.

POTASSIUM

One of the major minerals neede our bodies along with calcium magnesium, potassium is importan the proper working of the *nerves muscles.* Tired, cramped muscles sometimes be a sign that your p sium stores are getting too low. P sium also normally regulates the *balance* in the cells, helping to keep *blood pressure* stable as well. If have an excess of sodium, you'll a matically lose potassium, which m a disruption of this fluid bala Water will be retained and b pressure will go up. You also lose tassium when you sweat, whether f exercise or hot flashes; when you g a crash diet of the high-protein/ carbohydrate kind which causes a of water; and if you use diuretics, as alcohol, caffeine, or prescrip medications.

Fortunately, potassium is abun in virtually all vegetables, especially leafy, dark green kind; in fruits, d beans, seeds, whole grains, and d products. My potassium staple is banana—which also gives me a lo magnesium and vitamin B_6. Sunfl seeds, garbanzo beans, and dried cots are among the richest sources, again, use them sparingly. A baked tato with the skin and a little yo added is a potassium bonanza. thing with blackstrap molasses, in s of its sugar content, will have a g portion of potassium.

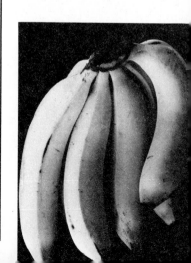

5. THE SUPERFOODS

Even though I consider a supplement plan an essential part of my diet, *food always comes first*, as it should for you. If money is tight, supplements go to the end of your shopping list. Your daily greens, beans, dairies, and grains are your natural vitamin pills; fresh fruits and vegetables are your natural antioxidants.

What I've noticed is that at midlife it's the *humble* foods of life that become the *champions*:

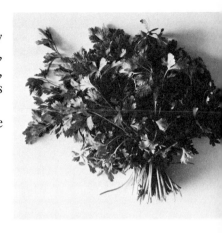

> Broccoli, Bran, and Bananas . . .
> Papaya, Parsley, Potatoes, and Peppers . . .
> Carrots, Cantaloupe, and Collards . . .
> Tofu, Tomatos, and Tortillas . . .
> Lemons and Legumes . . .
> Spinach and Sprouts . . .
> Yogurt and Yeast . . .
> Wheat Germ and Watermelon . . .

All of these are low in calories, but *packed* with nutrients—especially with what I call the midlife superstars. They are also generally low in fat and sugar, but high in fiber.

Let's do a little nutrient analysis of a *salad*—another daily staple in my life. First, the lettuce. Iceberg has a little of most midlife vitamins and minerals, as well as some fiber and *a lot* of water. The greener romaine variety has double the nutrient value and many more times the vitamin A. But spinach! This lifelong friend has 25 times the vitamin A, 9 times the vitamin C, 6 times the iron, 5 times the calcium, and 3 times the potassium of iceberg lettuce. In addition, spinach offers vitamin E, some of the Bs, and a little protein—all for a pittance of calories.

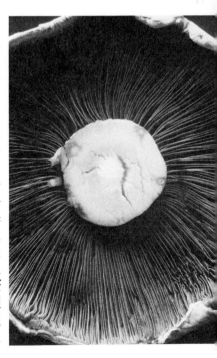

If we add tofu to our spinach, we add more protein too, while increasing the usability of the protein in the spinach. Tofu also supplies more calcium and iron. Some wheat germ can maximize spinach protein even more while contributing more Bs, vitamin E, and some selenium. The additions are endless. Mushrooms mean more potassium. Alfalfa or mung bean sprouts bring more iron, Bs, C, and protein. A few seeds or garbanzo beans, perhaps in place of tofu, add protein, potassium, iron, and even some calcium, zinc, and B vitamins. A few orange slices, delicious with spinach salad, will give more C, which can triple the absorption of the iron in spinach.

Using lemon instead of vinegar in our dressing will do the same. Finally, a little bit of safflower oil to bring out all these flavors will give us a good dose of vitamin E, as well as the essential fatty acid, linoleic acid.

This is not to denigrate iceberg, romaine, or any other kind of lettuce. We don't want them to go the way of the oft-maligned potato (which, by the way, has never left my own diet). We need *all* these vegetables, which brings me to the importance of variety.*

6. VARIETY

Taking in a variety of all kinds of foods is absolutely essential. Without it, your palate and body become indifferent and bored—and you also risk missing the full range of vitamins and minerals you need. So be sure to experiment with the possibilities and to mix and match foods the way I did with a simple spinach salad.

Now, let's take a moment to review the nutritional pluses that merit center stage at midlife:

More complex carbohydrates
More fiber
More water
More of the Superstar vitamins and minerals
More of the Superfoods
More variety
And, ALWAYS, balance and moderation.

The last guideline on this list is perhaps the most important of all—and at the heart of what I want to talk about next.

A WORD TO CHRONIC DIETERS

Everything I've written about eating—eating for the long haul—is my way of giving my body the best to work with, especially now that I'm a woman in midlife. It's also how I maintain my weight.

---

* We all need to be aware that two of the superfoods, spinach and bran, can interfere with calcium absorption in the body. Don't eliminate these, though. Just be sure you consume your major daily supply of calcium-rich foods or your calcium supplement at another time during the day.

Emphasizing some foods and de-emphasizing others helps me to stay where I want to be—without chronically being on a diet.

A chronic dieter usually tends to go on binges as well. The two go hand in hand, as I know from painful years of eating disorders. The problem for many of us is setting ourselves an unrealistic, unattainable goal for what we want to weigh and how we want to look. This prompts us to start on an unhealthy crash diet that is impossible to maintain—impossible because the human organism isn't meant to endure long-term deprivation.

In my twenties I often subsisted on 500 calories a day and wondered why eating one apple would cause me to retain water and put on weight. There was also a constant unsatisfied hunger that made me tense, anxious and, understandably, preoccupied with food. Now I understand how *counterproductive* my extreme dieting actually was—physically as well as psychologically.

Earlier in the "Middle-Age Spread" chapter I explained how crash-dieting causes us to lose as much lean muscle as we do fat, which results in a lowered metabolism. In addition, I talked about how your body will fight back if you are repeatedly or chronically undernourished. It will hold on to all the fat it can, slowing down your metabolism even further if necessary. That's why in those years when dieting was a way of life for me, the thinner I'd get the more easily I would put on weight.

I had to learn the hard way that we can't go on thinking we can drop ten pounds or so any time we want, fast, and with no consequences. Not only is it harder to lose weight if that has been our pattern, but it can cause damage that, with age, is harder and harder for our bodies to repair.

Striving to be thin might very well be an undesirable and unrealistic goal for you. In attempting but failing to attain it, you will hate yourself and feel very guilty and depressed—as though not achieving that visualized ideal of thinness proves you are worthless and lacking in discipline. As we all know, these are the very emotions that can send us off on a binge cycle which lowers our self-esteem even more.

I beg you to stop thinking "thin" and start thinking "balance and moderation"—a concept that assumes ever more importance in midlife.

Let's take that approach in looking at both maintaining our weight and losing weight at this time in our lives. Changes to our muscles and metabolism that occur with age, also described in the chapter "Middle-Age Spread," necessitate to some degree, sooner or later, that all of us cut calories. The *average* woman in her forties *may* have to cut 100 calories from her daily diet, another 100 in her fifties, and more as she moves into her sixties, seventies, and eighties. This might mean doing without a bran muffin, or a tablespoon of oil in your salad dressing, or a little daily bread. It's not a crash diet. It's a slight readjustment, a reorientation. If you translate the 100 calories into exercise, you don't need to cut down at all—another mile jogged or briskly walked will keep your weight steady! You'll *burn* the surplus.

Only one word of caution on exercise before we go on. A compulsive dieter tends to also be a compulsive exerciser, list-maker, and workaholic. What we should strive for is to reduce all our compulsions. Don't replace extreme dieting with extremes of working out. Remember, balance and moderation.

If you want or need to lose pounds, here's my advice:

1. *Use the gradual method,* not cutting more than 500 calories a day from your ideal diet. This is the best because it's the least stressful to your body, most sparing of your muscle, least likely to trigger a binge and therefore easiest to maintain.

2. *Cut especially from the fat and sugar categories,* next from certain of the higher-caloried complex carbohydrates, such as fruits, beans, seeds, nuts, and breads. The largest part of your diet should still be complex carbohydrates, but with the emphasis on vegetables. Don't increase or decrease your daily protein allowance—but emphasize nonfat dairy products. You want to avoid the high protein–low carbohydrate diets that cause a quick weight loss, because the pounds dropped won't be just fat—they'll be largely water and muscle. And they're the pounds that you put back on immediately—but minus the muscle. Besides, you *need* the vitamins and minerals and energy that come with the complex carbohydrates.

3. *Exercise regularly.* I can't emphasize this enough as a companion to cutting calories. Cutting another 500 calories by burning them is ideal for losing weight safely and more quickly. (See p. 82 of the "Middle-Age Spread" for my Exercising to Lose Weight guidelines—and the next chapter, "Hitting Our Stride," devoted entirely to exercise.)

The benefits of exercise, however, go far beyond thinness. A main goal of exercise is to like yourself more. Exercise can help you feel better about yourself and your looks. Whatever girth you have will become more muscular and better proportioned. You'll have better skin tone and there will be a smooth, solid feeling to your flesh. And you will have more energy than you imagined possible! Don't forget too that exercise improves our ability to cope with stress. So if you exercise, you will be less apt to binge when you feel pressured.

4. *Try to eat your final meal of the day before 6:00 P.M., or as early as possible.* In one well-publicized study, a group of people were fed one meal a day consisting of 2,000 calories, either as breakfast, lunch, or dinner. Those who ate all these calories for breakfast lost weight, those at lunch maintained, and those at dinner *gained*—the difference was up to two and a half pounds!

5. *Don't skip breakfast.* If you want to skip a meal skip dinner. Breakfast sets the tone and gives you energy for the day. Several studies have even revealed that eating breakfast regularly may be a factor in a longer life.

6. I've often expressed my belief in the importance of *eating when hungry,* forgetting that for chronic dieters and those who suffer from eating disorders hunger has no meaning. You may no longer know when you're hungry, especially if your eating patterns have been distorted by too much tension and anxiety. What's important in this instance is to establish *regular eating habits:* three meals a day at routine intervals composed of a healthy variety of foods, including solid, fibrous foods you must chew.

—Eat slowly and chew well so digestive enzymes begin to work *before* the foods reach the stomach.

—Don't eat absentmindedly while talking on the phone or watching TV (and try not to eat your lunch at your desk if you work in an office).

—Take the time to savor and enjoy what you are eating.

—If you feel a binge coming on, take a walk, an hour-long one, if possible.

MY KITCHEN

I like to cook and do so as often as I can. Over the years I've tried to learn to shop smarter and to store and cook food in such a way that my family, frequent guests, and I get the most out of whatever feast I've prepared—whether it's a salad, a sandwich on whole-wheat pita bread, or a whole dinner spread complete with fruit and yogurt for dessert. What follows are some of the culinary customs that have evolved at our house.

The Basic Equipment

- **A good, heavy wok,** one of the most versatile and basic cooking utensils in my kitchen. This is an ancient Chinese pot that can be used to steam, stir-fry or deep-fry. The iron variety is best because it distributes heat evenly. Most woks will come with instructions for proper care—essential to learn and easy to do.
- **Steamers** are the next essential. I use the bamboo kind that are stackable so that foods which cook faster can be added later and removed individually. The single-layered stainless steel kind is also excellent.
- **Thick stainless steel or enamelware pots and pans** to which food doesn't stick are the best and can last decades. Teflon, as long as it's undamaged, is also good to use. (Avoid aluminum utensils which can release aluminum oxide into food.)
- **A blender,** usually used daily in our house.
- **Good, preferably carbon steel knives** for cutting vegetables and meats.
- **A lettuce spin-dryer** may seem a luxury, but it can help you to use much less oil in your salad dressings. When tossed about thirty times, one tablespoon of safflower oil can coat a huge bowl of salad greens if they are nice and dry.
- **Vegetable brushes,** for scrubbing vegetables without the need for paring off nutrient-rich skins.
- **A garlic press,** for fresh garlic.
- **A peppermill,** for fresh pepper.
- **Lots of canisters or glass jars** with airtight lids for storing. Save large plastic bottles for freezing vegetable cooking-water to use later in soup stocks.

Shopping

- Have a **list** in order to avoid impulse buying.
- **Shop along the walls of the supermarket** where the fresh fruits and vegetables, dairy products, fish, and poultry are. Here you

can improvise—see what's in season and what's freshest. Look for the bright greens, reds, and yellows. Always pick up some lemons and limes and fresh herbs. Frozen is second best to fresh, and canned produce the last choice.

- **Stick to your list in the middle aisles** that usually stock the soft drinks, sweets, and processed foods. Learn the location of dried herbs and spices, dried beans and peas, rice, whole grain cereals and breads, wheat germ and wheat bran.
- **Shop with an eye to getting the most nutritive value for your food dollar and your calorie currency.** A baking potato, for example, offers far more nutrition than a bag of potato chips. It also costs less, and has far fewer calories and almost no fat.
- **Don't buy foods containing "empty" calories**—that is, foods high in calories but bereft of nutrients.
- **Read the labels** and remember that the ingredient appearing first on a label is present in the greatest quantity and all the others in diminishing amounts. Be careful to avoid preservatives, artificial colorings, sugars, fats, and sodium.
- If you're worried about your weight, don't shop when you're hungry.
- **Locally grown produce** is always the best if you have that option (don't buy fruits and vegetables that have been sitting in the sun, however; this depletes their nutrients).
- Try not to buy too much fresh fruit and vegetables at one time. They begin to lose half of their vitamin C after just two or three days in the refrigerator, and even more quickly if stored at room temperature. Even potatoes lose their vitamin C if stored for a long time.

Storing

- In the art of storing foods properly, **it's not what we're keeping out as much as what we're keeping in that's important**—life-sustaining vitamins and minerals. The goal is to buy and keep foods as *fresh* as possible. (Vitamins are more vulnerable to air, light, and heat than minerals, especially vitamin C and the Bs.)
- **Refrigerate fresh fruits and vegetables promptly.** Don't wash or cut them before putting them into a crisper or airtight plastic containers. Never soak or store them in water. Asparagus, green

beans and lima beans can be frozen fresh without losing flavor or nutrition. Mushrooms do best in a brown paper bag that sits inside a plastic bag or container.

- Dried raw grains, beans and seeds can last eight to ten months in airtight glass containers. They'll last indefinitely if refrigerated. Any fresh, whole foods keep better in cool, dry, dim places.
- Once opened, vegetable oils, wheat germ (raw or toasted), and soy sauce (when it comes without preservatives) can spoil and should be refrigerated. For this reason, it's best to buy these in small quantities even if they cost a few cents more.
- Whole-wheat flour will also last longer if kept refrigerated, or even frozen. It contains the vitamin E and oil that's been processed out of white flour and, therefore, has a shorter shelf life.

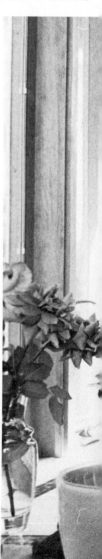

- Don't store fruit juices or leftovers uncovered in the refrigerator or in open lead-soldered cans.

Cooking

- **Stir-frying** is the best cooking method for preserving nutrients. Exposing highly nutritious vegetables to high temperatures for a short period of time will not cause as much nutrient loss as the long-term exposure of baking, boiling, and regular frying. And if you use a wok, only small amounts of vegetable oil are required. Corn and peanut oils are the best for cooking at higher temperatures.
  Method: The idea is to have a hot wok and hot oil. First heat

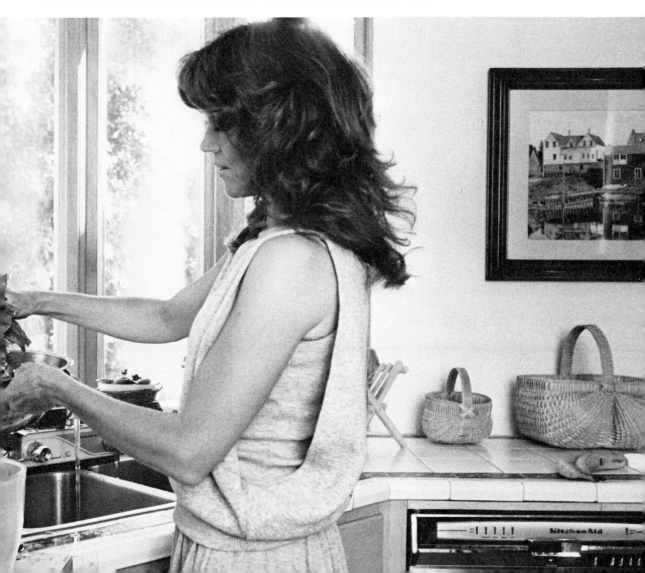

your wok, then add 1–3 tablespoons of oil (usually 1 tablespoon for your complement and 3 tablespoons for your main dish). You'll know it's very hot if a scallion or green vegetable leaf burns immediately. Stir-fry the ingredients separately and toss together later. The stir time is usually no longer than 2–3 minutes.

You can also water-sauté in your wok, though I find it hard to cook without the oils that so nicely enhance the flavor and give body to the food I'm cooking. A few drops of sesame or olive oil can add even more flavor.

- **Steaming** food over boiling water is the next best method. Vegetables steamed *al dente* retain their crispiness and brilliant color. Heat always takes a toll, so remember, even in steaming, fastest is best. And always keep lids on tight. Save the water for soup stocks.
- **Microwave** cooking is safe and preserves nutrients. Although microwave ovens cook at a high temperature, they do so in a very short period of time.
- Boiling is probably the **worst** cooking method, but if you do need to boil vegetables, save the water and freeze it for later use in soups. If you boil potatoes, leave the skins on to help to hold nutrients in.
- **Don't soak or overwash vegetables and fruits.** Scrub, rather than peel carrots and potatoes, for example. The skin contains nutrients and also protects against vitamin and mineral loss in cooking.
- **Try not to cook more than you need.** Leftovers are a poor substitute for freshly cooked foods.
- When cooking fish and chicken, **always remove the skin first.** Trim any visible fat on any meat. Stir-fry, broil or bake, in that order, rather than pan or deep frying.
- **Avoid regular frying** generally—too much fat and too much time. Bake rather than fry potatoes, for instance. Broil rather than fry meat. Bake or steam rather than fry tortillas.
- Toast bread lightly, if at all, in order to preserve the nutrients.
- Without salt, it takes a real knack to cook delicious soups, which are great for keeping your weight down and full of nutrition. Use the freshest vegetables possible, concentrated vegetable broth powders (look for no- or low-sodium products), whatever cook-

ing water you've frozen and saved for homemade stock, and some of the seasoning suggestions below.

- I seldom bake, but when I do I look for recipes that call for little fat or sugar. I make a practice of cutting the sugar in half and preferably substituting honey for table sugar. I omit all salt. I never use shortening, margarine, or butter. If necessary, I'll substitute a vegetable oil. I always use whole-wheat flour, sometimes a mixture of whole wheat and unbleached white flour. Adding nonfat dry milk, soy flour, or wheat germ is a great protein booster.
- *Here are some of my regular substitutes:*
  —Nonfat, low-fat, or buttermilk for whole milk
  —Nonfat or low-fat yogurt for sour cream and mayonnaise
  —Egg whites for whole eggs or egg yolks (you can feed the yolks to your pets)
  —Wheat germ for bread crumbs

The Art of Seasoning

This is a skill I'm still learning, but here are my alternatives to salt, sugar and unhealthy condiments.

- **"Veg-It"**—a powdered vegetable and herbal salt substitute.
- **Pepper**—fresh-ground black (here's where your peppermill comes in), lemon pepper, crushed red pepper flakes (these are hot), and cayenne pepper. Cayenne should always be added last in cooking because heat lessens its potency. I often pepper chicken before cooking (sometimes also adding rosemary and garlic).
- **Natural soy sauce**—in moderation, usually without preservatives. I look for those marked low-sodium, though they're harder to come by.
- **Garlic**—and the whole garlic family of onions, shallots, chives, and leeks. Fresh is best (this is where your garlic press counts), but powders and dried forms are okay too. Garlic is not only one of the most potent seasonings, but it is said to be medicinal— good for the digestion and for reducing blood fats. (Don't use garlic or onion salts; these have sodium in them.)
- **Cinnamon**—my great sugar substitute that is wonderful on yo-

Henry Fonda's Salt Substitute

3 oz. powdered vegetable broth
¼ teaspoon garlic powder
⅛ teaspoon oregano
¼ teaspoon dill weed
¼ teaspoon paprika
¼ teaspoon honey fructose
¼ teaspoon marjoram
½ teaspoon powdered kelp
⅛ teaspoon ground celery seed
¼ teaspoon Five-Pepper blend
½ teaspoon dry mustard
Grated lemon peel to taste

Mix all ingredients and store in closed container in dry place. This blend of seasonings is low in sodium but not completely sodium-free, so be sure to sprinkle on lightly for flavor.

gurt. It's also good on applesauce, baked bananas, in baking generally and even in some exotic chicken dishes. Cinnamon contains vitamin A, vitamin C, calcium, iron and even some fiber. (Nutmeg and mace are also good sweet spices.)

- **Chili powder, paprika, and cayenne**—all three are extraordinarily rich sources of *vitamin A* (just one teaspoon of paprika has 1,273 IU; chili 908 IU; cayenne 749 IU). They also contain significant amounts of vitamin C and potassium. All are very good with tomatoes and tomato dishes, especially Mexican cuisine. Essential for salsa. Additional cumin and ground coriander, components of chili powder, will add even more flavor.
- **Oregano, basil and bay leaf**—also good with tomatoes and tomato dishes, especially Italian cuisine. (Oregano, cloves, the minty herbs rosemary and sage, and the flavoring vanilla are all *antioxidants*. In fact, many spices and herbs were our original natural food preservatives.)
- **Ginger**—a common spice in Chinese and Japanese cooking, excellent with stir-fried vegetables and chicken dishes.
- **Curry powder**—an Indian spice, best used independently on vegetables and chicken.

- **Parsley**—very high in nutrients, especially when fresh, and a good natural diuretic.
- **Poppy seeds**—a good substitute for high-calorie sesame seeds.
- **New condiments**—Yogurt, salsa, wheat germ, bran, lemons, limes. Try yogurt or salsa on a baked potato or with baked tortilla chips. Spike sparkling water or salt-free tomato juice with a slice of lemon or lime.
- **Flavored vinegars**—As you're cutting down on oils in your salad dressings, add more flavored vinegars, like rice vinegar and various herb vinegars. Lemon is a great addition or substitute for vinegar in salad dressings too.
- **Fresh herbs** are always best because they contain minerals *and* vitamins. Dried herbs have generally lost their vitamins, but these are often all that's conveniently available. One tablespoon of fresh herbs is roughly equivalent to one teaspoon of dried.

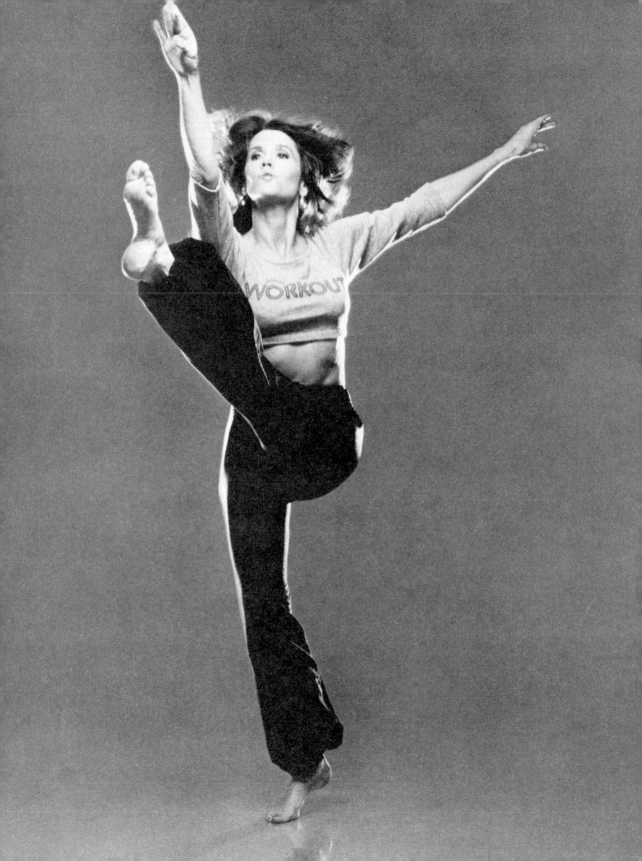

CHAPTER *14*

HITTING OUR STRIDE

There is no drug in current or prospective use that holds as much promise for sustained health as a lifetime program of physical exercise.

Walter M. Bortz, M.D.
"Disuse and Aging"

THIS MORNING I climbed the last grade at the end of my run feeling the kind of satisfying exhaustion that comes with a hard workout. Anticipating the exhilaration of reaching the top, I thought about the irony of a woman nearing her fifth decade forging *up* hills on a regular basis when she should, by tradition, be "*over* the hill." And I'm far from being the only woman for whom such vigorous exercise is the road now taken in midlife.

I've spoken with many women who are beginning to exercise seriously in their thirties, forties, fifties, and sixties—the years when it's so important to be fit and to feel positive about ourselves. These women aren't lamenting the loss of what they were able to do in years gone by. Rather, they're discovering physical abilities they never knew they possessed. Becoming physically active in your middle years, you may see your muscles for the first time, and be surprised your body is responding to your workout as you'd always been told it would, surprised to find you have better color and more energy than you did as a young adult. If you're returning to exercise, even after a decade, your previously trained muscles will come back fast. They seem to have a kind of memory so that all you've done before still counts. We're not starting out at zero when we resolve to resume an exercise program, the way we often are when we resume an abandoned diet. And it's *never* too late.

BREAKING THE AGE BARRIER

• The American Women's Himalayan Expedition placed the first American flag on Annapurna, the tenth highest peak in the world. *More than half* of the team members were in their middle years! None showed the fitness changes usually associated with their age. All measured 40 percent *above* what is considered normal fitness for other midlife women. Out of the entire team whose youngest member was twenty, those with the lowest body fat and the strongest aerobic power were the women in their forties.

• Another group of active women, all in their forties, were studied for fitness changes associated with age. Over a six-year period, they maintained a level of cardiovascular endurance *comparable*, and in some cases even *higher*, than that of average twenty-year-olds.

• Several women who were members of the 1980 All-American Masters Swim Team were found to have the same percentage of body fat as women in their early twenties. They also had an aerobic power *twice* that of their own age group and comparable to that of young athletes. These swimmers were *women in their seventies!*

This is Irene Miller, 42, one of the American Team who first climbed Annapurna.

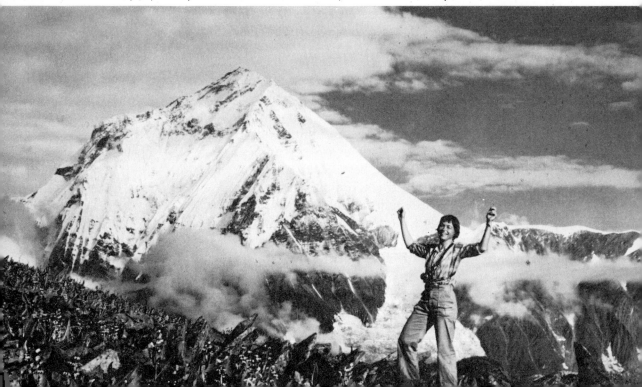

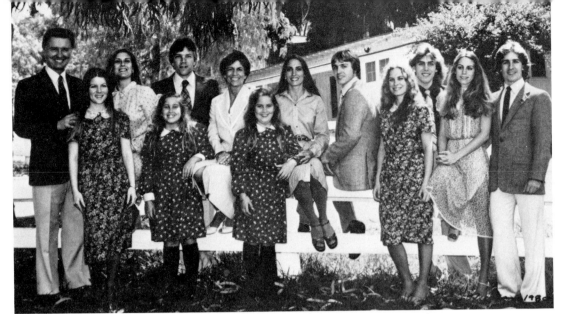

That's Pat Walters, sixth from the left, fifty pounds lighter. Nine of these shining faces are her children, including the twins in the front!

Until recently the common assumption has been that the need for exercise decreases through life. The risks of vigorous exercise have been greatly exaggerated and our physical ability in the middle and later years tremendously underrated. But now we know that *age is no deterrent to exercise,* including aerobic endurance training, when it is done sensibly and regularly. For every decade after thirty it takes us longer to adapt to exercise and longer to progress, yes, but the benefits of exercise for people in midlife and beyond are the same as for younger people. No matter what your level of fitness, you can *improve* with age. If you've been sedentary a great deal of your life, you can be even more fit in your middle years than you were in your *twenties!* Physiologists who specialize in exercise and aging are just beginning to document this inside the lab. I know dozens of women who are in better shape at midlife than they ever were at any other time. Pat Walters, fifty-two, is a classic example. She says,

At forty, I was on my way to becoming the classic Italian matron. I'd had nine children. I loved being a mother and still do. But I was fifty pounds overweight, unhealthy and inactive. I was in the habit of the daily coffee klatch with other women in the same boat. Over a cup of coffee and a couple of cigarettes, we'd spend hours talking about our kids and husbands. Misery loved company then.

By midlife, Pat had already had surgery for kidney stones. She also suffered from high blood pressure and high levels of blood fats, depression and terrible headaches. She took tranquilizers on a regular basis. She had problems with water retention and her weight was up to 170 pounds. After her children left home, she tried going back to school. She also tried working, thinking that might help her overall state of non-well-being. Then in her mid-forties she decided to investigate the nearby Pritikin program that offered what back then was still considered a new-fangled approach to fitness: aerobics and low-fat eating. After that visit, Pat told us, she went "cold turkey"—no more red meat, no pills, no cigarettes, no caffeine. She also began thirty minutes a day of aerobic jumping on a mini-trampoline. "I climbed the walls at first," she remembered laughingly. "Giving up coffee was the hardest. But I felt better in a month. My headaches were completely gone. The fleshy bags under my eyes slowly went away. Within a year I'd lost fifty pounds. Now I'm never sick. I'm up every day at 5 A.M. I'm strong. I'm happy. I love to walk. And I've learned it's okay to sweat. I grew up in a time when women were 'ladies' who didn't sweat—they perspired occasionally on a warm day, yes, but would never sweat." With a partner, Pat now works as the principal fitness and health consultant to a thriving private health spa in California.

Pat's "secrets" for feeling and looking great are finally becoming well understood in this country. But her nutrition and exercise program has been around for centuries.

Throughout the world people who are active and follow low-fat diets live in good health well into old age. Three such societies have been carefully studied by the distinguished Harvard gerontologist Alexander Leaf. He found that people from the village of Vilcabamba in the Andes Mountains of Ecuador, the province of Hunza in the Karakoram Mountains of Pakistan, and the district of Abkhazian in the Caucasus Mountains of the USSR commonly live exceptionally long, active, and robustly healthy lives long into their eighties and nineties. After visiting these cultures Dr. Leaf reported, "I returned from my three surveys convinced that vigorous active life involving physical activity (including sexual activity) was possible for at least one hundred years, and in some instances longer."

In spite of the fact that these mountain valley communities are separated by thousands of miles, their ways of life are remarkably similar. The inhabitants in all of them participate in strenuous outdoor activity, follow wholesome moderate diets, and maintain as well a lifelong community involvement. Their daily lives are organized around the hard work of farming, often on steep mountainsides. Their food intake is between 1200 and 1900 calories—compared to our average 3300. Except for the Russian group, animal protein and fats make up *less* than 5 percent of their diet—compared to our 40 percent. Each group has its own alcoholic beverage—but there is no alcoholism. And because there is no retirement as we know it, women and men in these societies remain active in their families and communities until they die. Their social status actually increases with age.

As a whole, we in America are as sedentary as these remote peoples are vigorously active. Our more urban culture has viewed exercise as an *option* even though it's as essential to our health and well-being as good food. Many Americans go through their daily lives feeling run down without recognizing what they're suffering from is *exercise deficiency.*

The absence of consistent physical activity will cause changes similar to those caused by aging itself—and at a dramatically faster rate! The body of a young athlete, for example, forced to rest for even a few weeks will begin to mimic the aging process. His or her blood pressure rises and the metabolism slows down. The heart and lungs become less efficient, the joints less flexible, and both the nervous and immune systems more sluggish. The muscles and even the bones atrophy, as a broken limb does when immobilized in a cast. Compared to the decline caused by inactivity, the lessening of physical fitness due to age alone is actually quite minimal.

Athletes who work out through midlife give us a glimpse of what pure aging would be if we didn't speed the process by becoming less active. After the age of thirty, for instance, a marathon runner will lose just two minutes a year on her best finishing time—if she continues to train. And this relatively small decrease is due to those gradual changes to our muscles, heart, lungs and blood vessel network that I spoke of in the chapter on "The Process of Aging." But we don't have to match the maximum performance of an athlete to keep these changes to a minimum. We *do* need to be consistently active. Exercise plays a far more important role in determining our health and vitality in midlife than our actual age. The right exercise

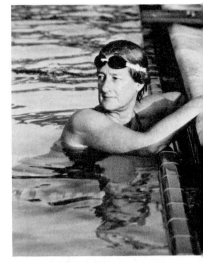

Anne Adams, 55, helped found the Masters swimming program in Southern California.

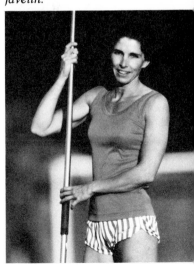

Dr. Frances Conley, 42, brain surgeon, holding her javelin.

program can even reverse some of the body's degeneration due to disuse. From the tiniest cells to the largest muscles, from the capillaries to the heart and lungs, exercise tones your whole body, inside and out.

But we also have to be realistic. Even the most rigorously followed exercise program cannot completely eradicate the signs of having had babies, or nursing, and of plain old gravity. We can tone it up and tune it up but we'd best make friends with those little signs of life's journey and not expect the impossible. Yet regular exercise remains Nature's best hormone treatment, tranquilizer, aphrodisiac, facial, diet pill, sleeping pill, laxative, joint lubricant, muscle massager, bone builder, back protector, and antidote to the chronic fatigue for which so many women can find no solution.

AN EXERCISE PRESCRIPTION

To achieve all the benefits that exercise can bring to midlife, does it matter what kind of exercise we do? Yes, it absolutely does matter.

- We need exercise that works *the whole body.*
- We need exercise that sustains or improves our *strength, flexibility,* and *aerobic power*—the three unchanging components of total fitness that I talked about in my first book and that form the bedrock of both the Workout and Prime Time, the new program for midlife women introduced in this book.

Balance

The body, even the middle-aged body, thrives on being pushed—though not compulsively. Once again, the concept of balance steers us in the right direction. If you develop a muscle's strength, you must increase its flexibility as well. If you work the lower body, you must not neglect the upper. If you work the outer thigh, do the inner. If you work out hard, you must also work out easy. You need balance in every aspect, otherwise you're setting the stage for injury.

Without intending to, we sometimes strengthen some muscles while others remain weak. For example, many people get shin splints when they have strong calf muscles in the back of the leg but

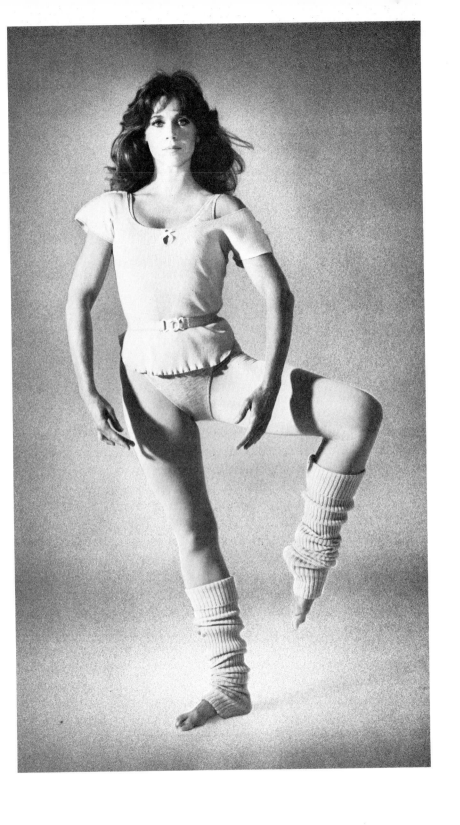

THE EXERCISE EFFECT—SLOW AGIN

Lasting Aerobic Fitness

- **A stronger heart and blood vessel network**
  - —The heart muscle becomes more powerful, so it can pump more blood with less effort—when your body is both at work and at rest.
  - —Miles of capillaries are added to the blood vessel system, enabling more oxygen and nutrients to be carried to cells throughout the body.
  - —Arteries open up, so that blood pressure decreases.
  - —The ability of the blood to dissolve harmful clots is increased.
  - —Levels of harmful fats in the blood are decreased while the more healthful high-density lipoproteins (HDL) are increased. These substances speed fats and cholesterol through the blood.

- **Stronger lungs**
  - —The size and elasticity of the lungs is increased lowing more oxygen to be taken in and held.
  - —The diaphragm and other muscles used in breat are strengthened, which means an improved cap for deeper, slower breathing.
- **Greater maximum breathing capacity—the true si vitality**
  - —As the heart, blood vessels, and lungs get tuned your aerobic power is increased—one of the prin measures of your fitness at any age.
  - —The body's interconnected system for getting w oxygen, and food to the cells improves, so the w body benefits.

NO MIDDLE-AGE SPREAD

- Muscles increase in size, strength, and tone—even in midlife.
- Building calorie-burning muscle means reducing fat tissue and developing a metabolism that functions better, both during exercise and at rest.
- Combined with a moderate diet, exercising is the fastest and smartest way to burn calories and to lose both weight and inches.
- The appetite is suppressed for several hours following exercise.
- The urge to consume too much coffee, tea, tobacco, alcohol, sugar, and other harmful stress- and pound-producers is reduced.
- The body finds its true contours and a positive body image is strengthened along with the muscles.

VIBRANT SKIN

- The skin receives the benefits of a natural facial.
- The connective tissues are strengthened, making the skin thicker and more elastic.
- Circulation to the skin is improved, which cleanses, gives a more even tone, and even helps to remove bags under the eyes caused by edema.

STRONGER JOINTS, BACK, AND BONES

- The supporting muscles for joints, the back, and the bone strengthened, so you become injury-prone during exercise as well as during everyday ac ties.
- The connective tissue of the c lage, ligaments, and tendons comes thicker and more resil
- Cartilage is also nourished by pumping action of the jo primed by exercise.
- Posture, body alignment, and ance are improved.
- Bones become more dense.

Easier Menopause

tuned-up hormonal system
Both the production and the use of estrogen and other sex hormones are believed to be maximized. The hormones produced are in greater equilibrium. The adrenal and ovary glands are healthier. Tissues are more receptive to hormone messages. A well-functioning endocrine system may ease the entire physical and the psychological experience of menopause.

the alleviation of hot flashes
The reduction of stress and improved regulation of body temperature through sweating may lessen the occurrence, intensity, and frequency of hot flashes.

sexual fitness
-The increased circulation of hormones, oxygen, and nutrients helps to keep sexual tissues moist and elastic.
-The general musculature is stronger, the joints more limber, and aerobic stamina greater—which can mean a better sexual experience. A PC muscle toned by Kegel exercises, and toned stomach, hip, and thigh muscles are especially important.
-Senses are heightened and you can be reawakened to your body if you've been closed off to it. You'll feel more conscious of yourself as a sexual person.
—Exercise increases levels of testosterone, the hormone associated with sexual desire.

- **Greater mental health**
—Pent-up energy is released, which leaves you feeling calmer.
—As the body develops an increased efficiency and ability to tolerate stress, we also conserve energy, feel less fatigue and more vitality.
—An increased blood supply carries more oxygen and energy-rich nutrients to every cell, including those in the brain, where many of our natural mood elevators reside. Exercise is known to increase the production of several of these brain chemicals, such as the endorphins.
—Unneeded water and sodium are excreted, reducing the fluid retention that can cause depression.
—Healthier adrenals are not only important for their production of estrogen, but also for their critical role during times of stress.
—The ability to fall asleep quickly improves, as does the capacity for more restful sleep.

...tter ...

digestive system
-The whole digestive tract, which breaks down food and moves it through the body, is tuned up.
-The absorption and utilization of nutrients improves, including the metabolism of glucose.
-The elimination of wastes is more efficient, making gentler work on the kidneys and combating constipation.

immune system
-The immune system is strengthened in fighting all diseases—from the common cold to cancer.

- **Nervous system**
—Memory, the ability to react quickly, and other intellectual functions improve.
—The nervous system remains in a state of preparedness that thrives on physical activity. This means being trained away from sedentary tendencies. Activity itself and the good feelings derived from exercise generate the desire for more activity. *In this way exercise tends to perpetuate itself.*

weak muscles in their shins in front. The weaker muscles try to compensate by overpulling as they move the leg, so they become strained and painful. Also, if you concentrate on a single sport you may work one group of muscles to the point of overuse and breakdown. If you swim often but get no other exercise, you may strain the muscles in your shoulders, or if jogging is your only exercise, your knees may suffer.

Incorporating more than one sport or an all-over body workout like Prime Time into your exercise plan will protect against such imbalances, and also keep you from being bored. Your body likes variety too! If you are just beginning to exercise you may feel the desire to master one area before moving on to another, but eventually you will want to add other dimensions to your workout. No matter what you do, your exercise program must include the fitness ingredients that follow.

Strengthening

You can develop a great deal of strength and muscle tone by performing repeated muscle contractions against your body's own resistance, such as the leg lifts or abdominal exercises found in my Prime Time program. These deep muscular contractions should be followed by stretching and relaxing. Your muscles will grow stronger and firmer, as will the connective tissue of joint tendons, ligaments and cartilage. This in turn stimulates stronger bones.

You can vary your strength-building program by using weight machines, but never more than two or three times a week; your muscle fibers need at least forty-eight hours to recover from that kind of workout.

Stretching

Stretching is really the other side of strengthening. It often happens, however, that one is emphasized at the expense of the other. Muscle-bound body builders frequently can't touch their toes. Bodies limber as rag dolls are sometimes as limp. The goal is to attain strong *and* supple muscles, firm *and* flexible joints.

Slow, sustained stretches like those we do in Prime Time

lengthen and warm the muscle fibers, without going beyond the range of their elasticity or that of the joints. If the stretch is forced, the exact opposite will happen. The muscles will contract and tighten up. Muscles work best at their greatest length but can be injured if you don't warm up first. To avoid musculoskeletal injuries, try to be as relaxed as possible when you stretch, breathing all the while, concentrating on lengthening the muscle you're working and releasing its muscle tension.

It's often thought that because stretching is slow, it's too easy and doesn't do much for you. But this is far from the case. The slower you work, the more control you have; therefore, the more intense and challenging the stretch. Dancers have learned this. Yoga masters too know the power of stretching. As you stretch one group of muscles, you're contracting their opposites. When you stretch the back of your legs, for instance, you're strengthening the front at the same time; when you lengthen the muscles of the lower back, relieving spinal column compression, you're strengthening your abdominals.

Aerobics: *The Heart of the Matter*

Though it is just one part of the fitness triad, aerobic exercise is its foundation. Aerobics require us to take in a rich supply of the oxygen that enables the muscles and other cells of the body to produce energy. How much oxygen our lungs inhale, how much oxygen-carrying blood our heart pumps, and how much oxygen your muscles use when you're exercising vigorously is the best measure of our overall fitness.

After age thirty, we all gradually lose some of our aerobic power because of the normal aging changes to muscles, heart, lungs and blood vessels. But as you've learned, we can profoundly minimize these changes through exercise—aerobic exercise. Maintaining or improving your aerobic fitness will affect you profoundly, physically and mentally, because the cardiorespiratory system is central to the vitality of the entire body. Being strong and flexible will enable you to do your aerobics safely, playfully, and enthusiastically.

Aerobic exercise uses the body's largest muscle groups—the legs and the buttocks. These are our "second lungs and second hearts," the endurance muscles that in rhythmic continuous movements

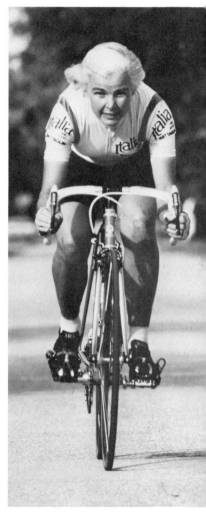

Joan Paul, 50, cycles every morning at 4:30.

make us breathe deeply and send blood coursing through the body. If you get the upper body working too, all the better. The heart, lungs and blood-vessel network all get stronger. If you are in good condition your heart will become so efficient that it can pump in 45 or 50 beats the same amount of blood in a minute that the average person's heart can pump in 70 or 75 beats.

To be most effective, *aerobic exercise must be brisk*—raising the heart and breathing rates. Remember first, however, we want to drink in oxygen, so the exercise can't be so fast we're gasping for air and have to quit after a short burst of effort. If you begin to pant and are unable to carry on a conversation comfortably, you'll know you're exercising *an*aerobically, that is, *without oxygen*. The muscles are demanding oxygen faster than your cardiorespiratory system can deliver it. Without sufficient oxygen, the muscles will quickly fatigue and your exercise session will be cut short as a result. To avoid this, we have to find the proper balance of briskness. The exercise can't be so intense we have to stop, nor can it be so easy we don't call upon the cardiorespiratory system to improve.

This balance is also essential for those of us who rely on exercise for losing or maintaining our weight. Exercise that's very high in intensity or anaerobic, like sprinting or weight-training, uses stored carbohydrates or glycogen as its only fuel. Exercise that's moderate in intensity or aerobic, like brisk walking or studio aerobics, uses fat as its major fuel. As I explained earlier in Chapter Five, "Middle-Age Spread," fat is burned only in the presence of abundant oxygen. If we want to become fat-burners—and the body gets better at this with practice—and if we want to burn as many calories as possible, the goal in exercise should be to *go longer*, not faster, at an aerobic pace.

The ideal aerobic intensity gets our hearts pumping significantly above their resting rates but still somewhat below their maximum. You want to aim for reaching *75 percent* of the maximum number of times your heart can beat in a minute. This is called your *training heart rate*. This should be your *goal*. To arrive there safely, begin your exercise program at a *60 percent* training rate. (Exercise below this level will give your heart and lungs little conditioning.) Maintain this minimum range for a month or two. After six months build to your ideal 75 percent training heart rate. After six months or more, depending upon how fit you've become, you can progress up to 85 *percent*—if you wish. Going that high, however, is *not* necessary for staying fit.

You'll find a standard formula for calculating your own training heart-rate in the chart on page 246. Notice that it gradually decreases as your age increases. This happens because we lose about one beat a minute in our maximum heart rate for roughly every year after thirty.

How do we know if we're exercising at the ideal training rate for us? By the pulse, at rest and immediately after exercise. This is our internal coach that tells us whether we need to work harder or to ease up. The pulse is our best, most convenient clue to how much blood and therefore how much oxygen is being pumped by the heart and used by the muscles. In the beginning I suggest you take your pulse frequently, learning what your resting rate is and regulating your exercise rate. As you get stronger, your resting rate will lower and you will push to the upper end of your training range. Eventually, you'll just know when you're exercising at the ideal intensity, though periodic pulse checks are always a good idea.

To be most effective, *aerobic exercise must be steady and sustained for at least 15 to 30 minutes* depending on the intensity of the aerobics you are doing. *Very brisk* aerobic exercises like running, cross-country skiing, hiking uphill, stationary bicycling and studio aerobics can easily work you to the upper range of your training rate, so 15 minutes for these is a good minimum. *Mildly brisk* aerobic exercises like walking, cycling, swimming, calisthenics and rebounding on a mini-trampoline don't work your heart quite as strenuously, so a longer period of 30 minutes is the best minimum. Optimally, these sessions can be *increased* to 30 minutes for the very brisk and an hour for the mildly brisk aerobics. These suggestions are only guidelines, however. Checking your pulse rate immediately upon finishing is the best way you can measure the intensity of the aerobics you're doing. Whether very brisk or mildly brisk, at these longer durations you will burn *at least* 300 calories a session, a level highly recommended by exercise physiologists. Don't forget to plan for additional time to warm up and cool down.

The Pulse: Your Coach Within

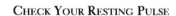

FIND YOUR TRAINING RATE

Your target training range is 60–85 percent of your maximum heart rate. The ideal training goal is 75 percent.

To find your maximum heart rate, subtract your age from 220 beats a minute, which is everyone's maximum heart rate in early adulthood.

Now multiply this number by 60 percent, 75 percent and then 85 percent to find the lower, middle and upper ranges of intensity for your aerobic exercise.

CHECK YOUR RESTING PULSE

Take your pulse for a full 60 seconds. The best time is in the morning before you get out of bed. If you check it weekly, do so the morning following your day of rest from vigorous exercise.

CHECK YOUR TRAINING RATE

Immediately after exercising, take your pulse for 6 seconds. Multiply this by 10 to calculate how many times your heart has been beating per minute during exercise. Use either the pulse in your wrist or the carotid artery in your neck.

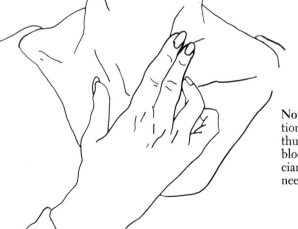

Note: A few high-blood-pressure medications lower the maximum heart rate and thus the training rate. If you're taking high-blood-pressure medication, call your physician to find out if your exercise program needs to be adjusted.

Aerobic exercise should be regular and consistent—at least three times a week to *maintain* your aerobic fitness and up to six times to *improve* it.

Depending upon how fit you were when you started, after six months to a year of brisk, sustained, regular aerobic type exercise, you will have laid a solid foundation of fitness. You do *not* need to exceed 30 to 60 minutes of these aerobics to continue to improve your cardiorespiratory health. If you want to go *beyond* these levels, you should know that your risk of injury will increase; you'll need to be especially sensible. The only reasons why you might want to exceed the standard regimen, I think, are if you are training for an athletic event such as a marathon, if you particularly need the extra mental "lift" aerobic exercise can give, or if you need to drop excess fat pounds faster. As I explained in the chapter on "Middle-Age Spread," aerobics are unparalleled for burning stored fat, for building lean muscle, and possibly for lowering the set-point that some believe regulates the amount of fat our body likes to store. We may eventually find that higher levels of aerobic exercise are better for bones as well, but we wouldn't want that to be at the expense of the joints. Incidentally, some good news—the heavier or bigger you are, the more calories you'll burn during exercise.

Time Off

You should add a final component to your fitness package—*rest*. What I've learned over the years is that the body grows strong with exercise through a process of breakdown and recovery. If building is done in reasonable graduated stages, we recover each time at a higher level of fitness. This is how we *improve*. But the body needs time to recover. This means we must create a balance between rest and exercise in order to reap the maximum benefits. This is especially important in midlife when it takes somewhat longer for the body to rejuvenate itself.

At minimum, you need one day every week *without* vigorous exercise. A leisurely walk, by all means; running, no. Enjoy your time off without guilt because you know you're doing something good, essential in fact, for your body and yourself. While you're resting, your body is doing its internal repair work.

FOOT POWER

When I wrote my first Workout book I had just discovered running. Four years later, I have now added walking and hiking to my exercise repertoire. I discovered their benefits while walking three or four miles of precincts a day during my husband's campaign for the California State Assembly. The intensity of campaigning didn't allow me time for my usual Workout, but an unexpected and welcome byproduct of walking precincts was that I dropped several pounds, maintained my level of aerobic fitness, and trimmed my legs and hips. Walking and hiking are the most natural forms of aerobic exercise. And along with running, I find walking to be the most exhilarating and convenient of the aerobic sports. Both take you out-of-doors and let you explore your community—its flats and hills, its rainy and sunny days, the early morning fog, the evening sunset. You encounter other walkers, joggers and friendly well-wishers.

Brisk walking is an ideal outdoor exercise for midlife. Its benefits match those for running—you just have to do it longer. Every mile walked, for instance, burns essentially the same number of calories for every mile run—about 100. Walking faster, or running faster, increases only slightly the calories spent. Going farther and for a longer period of time rather than speeding up, is what counts if you want to maximize the benefits in any aerobic sport. Aerobic aficionados refer to this as LSD, or long-slow-distance—all done at your training rate, of course.

Walking is good for everyone, from beginners to athletes suffering from injuries who need "active rest." It's an excellent alternative exercise to do between hard workout days, or to take a longer break from the stresses of other sports. Walking places little pressure on the joints and lower back, so there's rarely a chance of injury. In fact, walking is the perfect introduction and preparation for running and other more vigorous aerobic sports. It greatly strengthens muscles, tendons, ligaments, and bones, giving them the chance to get used to supporting the entire body in aerobics. It calls upon muscles which are used for both pulling and pushing motions, unlike running, which employs primarily the pushing muscles.

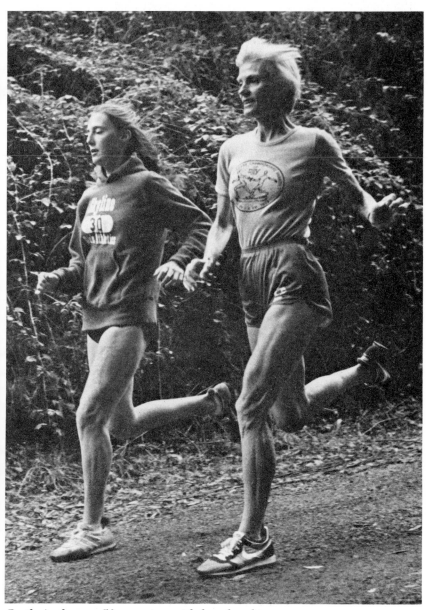

Ruth Anderson, 50, running with her daughter.

Walking is my alternative to running on days when I want a slower pace, a supplement to my exercise program, or simply the time to savor the beauty of the outdoors. Walking any old way won't do, however, if you're walking for fitness as well as for nature. Here are a few of the basics I follow.

Walkout

- **Walk briskly.** To get the aerobic benefits of walking, your pace is important. A desirable and realistic goal is to be able eventually to walk four or five miles in an hour. This is equivalent to a 12- or 15-minute mile.
- **Walk with weight slightly forward.** Push off from the back toes instead of grabbing with the front heel. The feet should point as straight ahead as possible and legs should be aligned with your hips.
- **Walk in long, stretching strides.** This picks up the pace and helps the rhythm of your walk, working your legs and buttocks to their maximum. The stronger you become from walking, the better your stride will become. Moving out from your hips will increase your stride as well.
- **Walk tall.** Think of keeping your chest lifted, back flat, and head up—if your path is smooth enough so you needn't watch your steps. Imagine the top of your head lifting and feel the sensation of stretching your neck and lower back, held erect but not rigid.
- **Walk your arms.** Swing them vigorously, wide and free like a pendulum. Don't carry anything; you want to be as unencumbered as possible.
- **Walk relaxed.** Your legs should roll easily out of your hip joints; the knees and ankles relaxed. Your arms should swing easily from the shoulder joints, your elbows and hands relaxed, your face soft.

With legs and arms pumping in tandem, you may be as surprised as I was at how quickly you work up a sweat. Walking hills will add to the intensity of your Walkout even more. Inclines are known for building endurance and strength, especially for the quadriceps, the front thigh muscles that help to keep the knee joint stable. Going downhill, while easier aerobically, puts more stress on the joints, so remember to stay loose and don't speed up. If it's an especially steep descent, you may even want to slow down a little.

Once you've mastered the basics and your body is adjusted, adding weights to the wrists or waist will also increase the challenge of walking. Even a few pounds will greatly increase the demand on the aerobic system. (You can add as much as 20 percent of your body weight, but remember to do so *very gradually*. I don't recommend using weights on the ankles when you walk because they can put too much stress on the knees.) I tend to favor light weights that wrap snugly around the wrists or that fit into specially designed weight gloves. Both will work the upper body more. I use these from time to time in running as well, because the foot-power sports strengthen the lower body much more than the upper.

A slow walk before and after an aerobic walk or run is a good way to warm up and cool down. But because walking, like running, tends to strengthen the back of the legs more than the front, unless there's a *lot* of hill work, I often do five or ten minutes of gentle stretches before walking (and *always* before running). I emphasize stretching the calves and the back of the thighs or hamstrings. And I repeat this afterward too. (For examples of calf and hamstring stretches, see pp. 337–45 of the Prime Time exercises.)

If you've been sedentary for a long time and want to run, not walk, I strongly suggest a period of walking first, followed by a period that alternates walking with running, slowly increasing the duration of the running until the walking is phased out. When you run, always make sure you can still carry on a conversation—this will ensure you're running at a comfortable pace. If I can talk without being out of breath, I know I'm working with a good balance between taking in and letting out oxygen, which is the basis for building aerobic endurance. Land on the heels rather than on the balls of your feet to minimize the strain on the feet and lower legs; push off with your toes. Again, take care in going downhill. And, remember, the first few miles are the *hardest*, not the easiest as one would imagine. It takes a while to break out of our resting inertia and to get the blood flowing. These are the miles that make us the most fit. The rest comes easier. If you don't feel right after 10 to 20 minutes of running, you're straining too much.

A POUND OF PREVENTION

Injuries are most likely to occur in the first six to eight weeks after you begin an exercise program. The most common are injuries to the muscles and to the tendons, ligaments, and cartilage of the joints. These often result from exercising too hard and too long after being inactive, or from not being familiar with some of the nuts and bolts of exercise. Prevention is the most powerful medicine.

The *surfaces* on which you walk or run can make the difference between being sidetracked with injury or moving smoothly forward injury-free. The best surfaces are even and soft; having both is ideal. Always avoid concrete if at all possible. This goes for the concrete floors often covered by rugs in exercise studios as well. Carpets are not enough for protection; you want a wood floor at best or mats at the very least.

Asphalt is a little less stressful than concrete for walking and running. Sometimes it's even preferable to a dirt path that's rocky or uneven. The sloping sides of roads are also best avoided. Walking or running on such uneven surfaces tugs the joints at unusual angles. This is frequently the cause of the infamous "runner's knee." The patella, or kneecap, supposed to ride smoothly in a groove at the end of the thighbone, is pulled toward the side, resulting in friction and irritation to cartilage under the kneecap. Repetitive running on hard surfaces sends stresses back up through the legs, as high as the hips. This is frequently one of the main causes of stress fractures and shin splints, a soreness or mild chronic strain in front of your shins. You can avoid shin splints by stretching out the calves and heels, by shortening your stride, by making sure always to land heel first, and by wearing good running shoes.

The *shoes* you wear for walking, running, and even studio aerobics can to some extent compensate for hard and uneven surfaces. But even on ideal terrain, protective shoes are a priority. They're expensive, but this is not the place to economize. An inexperienced walker or runner will often skimp on shoe gear in the beginning, waiting to see if she takes to the exercise or thinking she's not doing much mileage. But this is just the time you need the most protection, when your feet and lower body are adapting to the new stresses of the exercise. An injury early on might be the very reason you give up. So, please, wear your worn-out duds if you want, but no worn-out shoes.

Finding an excellent running shoe, which is what you want for walking too, is a simple matter these days. Go for the top brands that have made the design of athletic shoes a science. You want to pay attention to these features in the shoe you buy: *cushioning, stability,* and *good toe-box room.* A well-cushioned shoe will protect

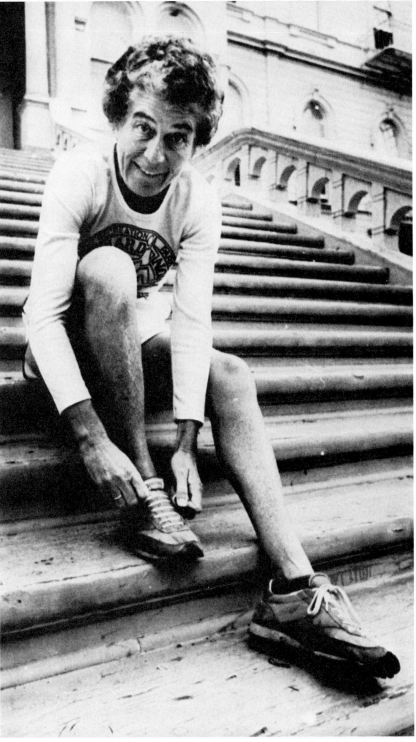

Sister Marion Irvine, 54, began running at age 48. She holds the world record for the over-50 age group in the half-marathon and marathon.

the muscles, bones, and joints of the legs from hard surfaces and from the pounding of running. But softer is not always better; moderately soft shoes are more stable. A very firm, reinforced heel can minimize the side-to-side rocking motion that is so hard on the knees and hip joints. You want enough room so your toes don't rub against the front of your shoe in walking and running, whether flat or downhill. Make sure you get training shoes—not those made for racing, which tend to have less cushioning and reinforcing materials in order to keep them lightweight. The waffle sole is for dirt paths and tracks; the ripple sole for asphalt. I tend to run and walk on both surfaces and use the rippled variety.

Your shoes will get dirty; they'll get wet. You'll be out in all kinds of weather, and most likely all kinds of paths. So don't hold back on your running in order to keep your new shoes looking bright. Most of the best brands have a removable insole for easy drying and airing out. Plan to replace your shoes as the cushioning becomes compact and loses its bounce, and as the outer soles wear down, especially if they wear unevenly as they do for so many of us.

If you're contemplating hiking on trails or rough terrain, I recommend the new lightweight hiking boots that have more traction, durability and ankle support than a running shoe. They're also usually waterproof, or nearly so. Make sure the socks you wear are thick and preferably of a wool or cotton-synthetic blend (the all-cotton ones hold onto moisture and can cause blistering); a special thin "wick" liner sock will help keep your feet dry. For running and walking, a light cotton sock is fine.

The *clothes* you wear are important not only for comfort and the boost you get from looking good. They're also important for keeping your body temperature stable, essential for a good exercise session. In order for sweat to succeed in cooling the body, it has to be able to evaporate. As it evaporates it cools the blood closest to the surface of the skin; this cooler blood then returns to the body's inner-core tissues. So don't wipe away sweat. On hot, humid days wear a minimum of light, loose-fitting clothing. Wear fabrics that "breathe." And avoid rubberized or plastic suits, and, on hot days, heavy sweatshirts and sweat pants. They won't help you to lose weight faster by making you sweat more; the weight you lose in water will be replaced as soon as you drink fluids again. They can also cause dangerously high body temperatures. On cold days, if you're exercising outdoors, wear one layer less of clothing than you normally would. Several layers are better than one. Use old mittens or gloves to protect your hands and wear a hat, since 40 percent of your body's heat is lost through your neck and head.

A good sports bra is a worthwhile investment for an active woman who wears more than an A cup, especially if she runs. You want to look for a bra that fits snugly, and is strong enough to hold you firmly for any type of physical activity, but of a fabric light enough to also breathe. Cotton blends are best for their absorbency and fewer seams. Make sure the straps don't slip off your shoulders and that no fasteners or rough elastic that could chafe are touching the skin.

While the rest of your clothing should be as nonconstricting as possible, elastic support stockings are a must if you have varicose veins. (Incidentally, all exercise that gets the legs moving, especially walking and the bicycle exercise, is excellent in alleviating the discomfort and complications of varicose veins.)

To complete these guidelines for preventing injury, let me briefly repeat several absolute rules for safe exercise that I first introduced in "Body Mechanics":

1. **Always warm up before exercise and cool down afterwards.**
   Warm flexible muscles, unlike tight, short, or cold muscles, are resistant to injury.

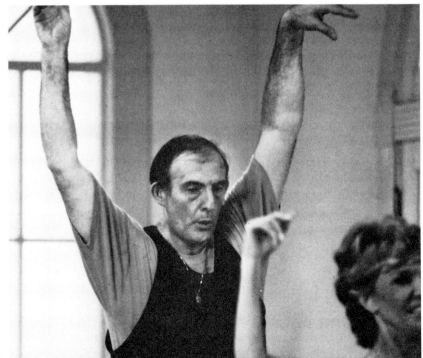

Prime Time class is for men too.

255

2. **Always make sure you're hydrated.** Drink lots of fluids a while before and also after exercise. Water is best. Dehydration can dramatically reduce performance.

3. **Always observe signs of overdoing.** These can be fatigue, loss of motivation, or a higher resting heart rate. Any pain that gets worse during exercise is a signal to stop. Not heeding this warning causes 80 to 90 percent of all injuries. Pain that continues for several hours after exercise, different from the normal stiffness and soreness that can come with exercise, is a sign to cut back.

4. **Always pay attention to form when you exercise.** Keeping the joints and the back in proper alignment through good posture will reduce abnormal pulls.

5. **Always exercise on an empty stomach (and empty bladder).** If you've just eaten, avoid strenuous exercise for at least one hour. Otherwise, the blood needed for digestion will rush out of the stomach to the muscles, which may leave you feeling nauseated. If you have been exercising vigorously just before eating, try to wait at least twenty minutes after stopping before going to the table. If you want the appetite depressant effects of exercise, exercise no more than two hours before eating.

A "Medical" Opinion

Most of us needn't see a doctor before beginning the kind of gradual, sensible exercise program I'm advocating. However, if you say Yes to any of the following conditions, a medical checkup is very important before you start.

1. You or your family has a history of heart or coronary artery disease.
2. Your blood pressure is high.
3. You experience extreme breathlessness after mild exertion.
4. You have bone or joint problems.
5. You are over age sixty and not accustomed to vigorous exercise.
6. You have some medical condition not mentioned here that you think needs special attention in an exercise program.

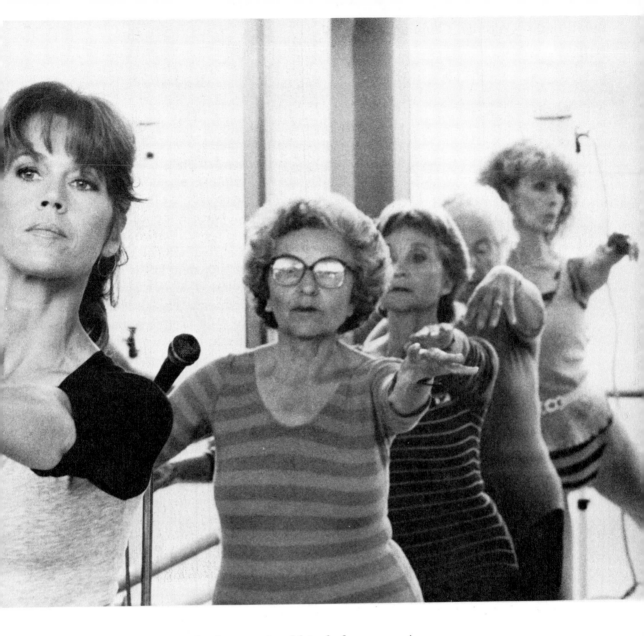

A complete pre-exercise medical exam should include an exercise stress test. This will measure your heart's ability to deliver oxygen-containing blood to the muscles as they work harder and harder while you work out on an indoor exercise treadmill or some other equivalently challenging exercise. Make sure your physician is equipped to do this kind of test.

GETTING STARTED

The first principle of beginning exercise in midlife is starting slowly—no matter what program you've chosen to embark upon. You should think of the entire first month as a warm-up month. You've got years in which to improve, so enjoy this first phase when your body and mind adjust themselves to the rigors of regular work-outs. You can go all-out later if you wish, once every part of you is strengthened, limber, and up to speed. Remember, you're building for the long haul. You want a lasting relationship with exercise.

Progress is quickest and most apparent at the start. You may experience a beginner's high, a sense of elation and accomplishment that nothing can take away from you. This can last months, often years. It's a wonderful time, in spite of little setbacks or how hard day-to-day individual workouts can be. Down the exercise road, as you get closer to being in top form, you'll find that improvements at a more advanced level come more slowly. "Personal bests" are always harder to come by when you're already near your full potential. That's why shaving seconds off of world records requires such athletic prowess. It's helpful to know in advance that eventually you'll come to an exercise plateau. But don't think this means you'll be sliding backward. It's just that you reach a level of physical fitness that's easier to maintain than it was to achieve. The honeymoon period, the thrill of fast improvement and quick results, can't last forever. But your reshaped body *can* endure—if you continue to exercise regularly. It's at this point that we recognize exercise as a lifelong process. There will be more peaks of progress ahead and more plateaus as well.

In the initial stage of your exercise program, the best rule of thumb to assure steady but gradual progress is never to increase beyond 10 percent of your previous day's workout—whether it's in repetitions, weights, miles, hills, or speed. The body is built to respond to overload by becoming stronger, but in well-measured and reasonable doses. If the goals you've set for one week or longer tire more than energize you, repeat them before building up. This is very common. Progress is an upward curve, yes, but never steadily so. You'll have your good days and your bad days. Just don't stop. Try not to let two days go by without having exercised. But if you miss a session, don't fret needlessly. It's the big picture that counts. If you miss a week or more, resume at just a slightly lower level. Don't throw in the towel. Remember, "a journey of a thousand miles begins with one step."

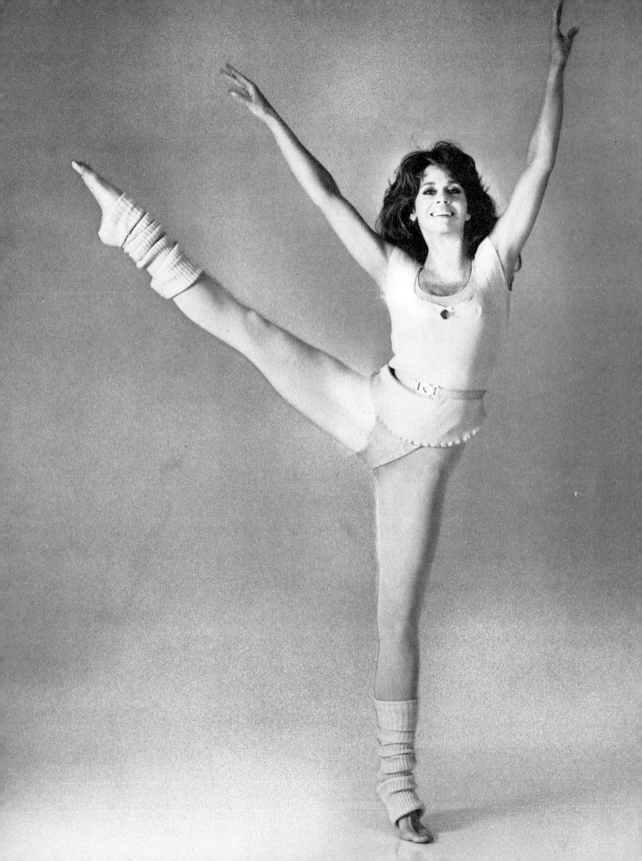

PART FIVE
Prime Time Workout

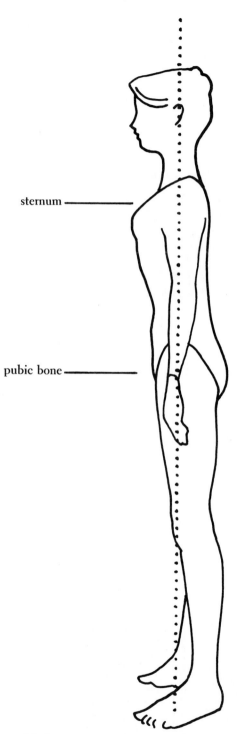

sternum ——————

pubic bone ———————

Curl your pubic bone up toward your navel. Stomach should be pulled in, chest is lifted, neck is long, head is lifted, shoulders are pressed down and back, weight is slightly forward.

THE PRIME TIME WORKOUT is designed for midlife women, and for all those who want a comprehensive exercise program but find the Beginners' and Advanced Workout in my first book too difficult. It's also for anyone who does the regular Workout but simply wants a change of pace, as well as for people who have never exercised, who are overweight, or who may be suffering from back problems, arthritis, or injuries from overuse.

This does not mean that Prime Time will not challenge you. It will. And it will increase your strength, muscle tone, flexibility, circulation, and cardiorespiratory fitness.

Prime Time works the entire body, head to toe. It strengthens and lengthens every major muscle group. It tones the arms, waist, stomach, hips, thighs, legs, and even the neck and chin. Every joint will be strengthened as well. The shoulders, wrists, hands, fingers, ankles, and feet will be put through their full range of motion. Special emphasis is given to protecting and strengthening the neck and lower back. Prime Time even includes exercises for the internal pelvic muscles.

Please join my stepmother, Shirlee Fonda, in this new Prime Time Workout. I'm proud to have her as the model of what midlife women can accomplish.

HOW OFTEN?

I'm often asked how frequently we should work out. Three times a week is minimal in order to see results. Six days a week is optimal, but don't be compulsive about it or feel guilty if you miss a day or two. Listen to your body. When you are tired, rest. If you are able to set yourself a consistent exercise schedule, before long you'll feel tired much less often.

Regularity is the key. It's also the hardest part. You must find a set time that belongs to *you*. Like so many women, you've probably spent a good part of your life worrying about everyone else. Give yourself a break. Isn't it time you invested a little time in yourself?

Some people, myself included, prefer to exercise in the morning. If I work out early, it's out of the way and I begin my day with elation and vigor. For some, evening exercise is beneficial—there's no question it can help rid you of the stress and tension that build up during the day and perhaps keep you from overeating at night as well. For others, the lunch break is the more convenient time. When I'm not filming, I take a late morning class at my Workout Studio. If a filming schedule requires me to be at work at 6:30 or 7:00 A.M., I'll do a 5:00 A.M. workout at home. This means I'll go to bed the night before when my son does, at 9:00 P.M., since I try never to sleep less than seven or eight hours a night.

Choose the time that's best for you and stick to it. This is most difficult in the beginning as you adjust to the addition of this 45-minute commitment to your schedule. If you're determined, however, it will become an automatic and welcomed part of your day.

HOW TO GET READY

1. Turn the phone off before you start.
2. Empty your bladder.
3. Select an area for your workout where there is no draft and where you can swing your arms and legs without hitting anything.
4. Find a sturdy chair whose back comes up to about your hip bone. You will use this for support during the "barre" exercises.
5. Have a glass of water or diluted juice standing by to keep you hydrated.
6. Keep an exercise mat, towel, or blanket ready to cushion your back and hips during the floor work and to keep dust and carpet fibers out of your nose and hair.
7. Try to have your stereo or tape player close by in order to minimize the time it will take you to replay or change your music.
8. Wear the kind of comfortable and absorbent exercise clothes

I talked about in the previous chapter. Don't try to exercise in blue jeans or slacks.

MUSIC

Make music a part of your exercise routine. The time will go faster. You'll also have more fun and be more apt to move rhythmically.

I have made a videotape, record, and cassette of the Prime Time Workout. (Information on where you can find these is given in the Resource Guide.) In each of these, I give instructions and count the repetitions to music. To work from this book, you will need to choose your own music with a variety of rhythms, an easy-to-follow driving beat, and cuts with a long enough running time so you won't have to keep interrupting yourself to start the music over. It's fun to experiment and find songs that inspire you to keep going and to work harder.

HOW TO DO IT

The Prime Time Workout is divided into sections. Do them in the sequence given. The exercises within each section should flow gracefully from one to another. In the beginning, it will seem awkward and mechanical as you try to learn what to do and when to breathe—while at the same time referring to your book. Do not rush it. Go over the instructions carefully—it is important to do the exercise correctly. Otherwise you risk getting hurt and you won't be getting as much as you should from your efforts.

Try to memorize the exercise series as soon as possible so you can go with the music and move smoothly from one exercise to the next. Stick to the beat. If you feel up to it, add more repetitions.

Try to avoid any interruption to your workout. It's a lot easier to be distracted when you're working out at home, so pretend you're in a class—that you *can't* stop. Momentum is crucial. For one thing, that's what keeps your pulse rate up and burns the calories. For another, if you stop to answer the phone or the doorbell, for example, your muscles will cool down and be more susceptible to injury when you start up again.

BREATHING

I describe proper breathing in many of the exercises. It is important to inhale and exhale as instructed. You may find you have a tendency to hold your breath, especially when an exercise is more difficult. Don't. You need to get oxygen into your bloodstream and out to your muscles. Without sufficient oxygen your muscles can't function properly. And you need to exhale in order to eliminate waste products and toxic gases. In general, you should breathe out when you are making the most effort and breathe in when you ease up. One final thing: Try to remember during the exercises to make a conscious effort not to tighten your jaw and to keep your face relaxed.

And now . . . let's get started!

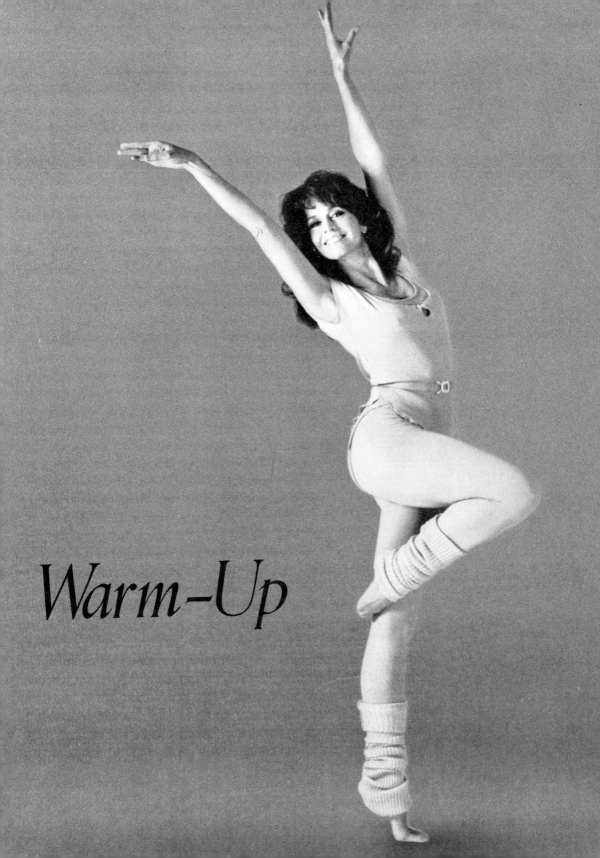

Warm-Up

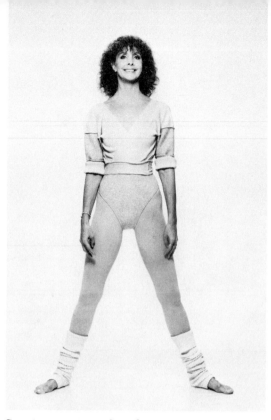

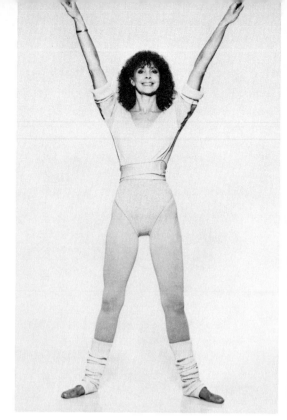

1

Starting position: Standing erect, place feet a little more than hip distance apart, slightly turned out. Stretch your torso up, chest lifted, taking weight off the lower back, which should be flattened. Stomach should be pulled in, pubic bone lifted, shoulders down, arms at sides. Maintain this posture throughout. Inhale through your mouth, then exhale.

Inhale again while lifting arms above your head palms down . . .

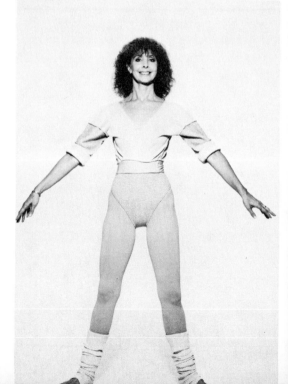

then exhale while bringing arms back down again.

2

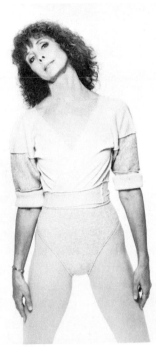

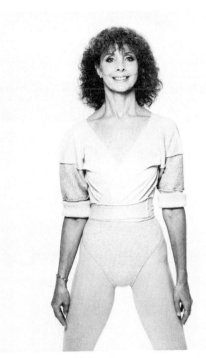

Inhale, then exhale as you press your right ear toward the right shoulder and stretch for 4 counts. Feel the stretch in the left side of your neck. Be sure your shoulders are pressed down.

Bring your head back to center position in 2 counts as you inhale.

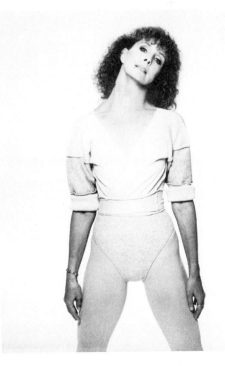

Exhale as you reach your left ear toward the left shoulder and stretch for 4 counts.

Return to center position in 2 counts as you inhale. Do this sequence 2 times.

3

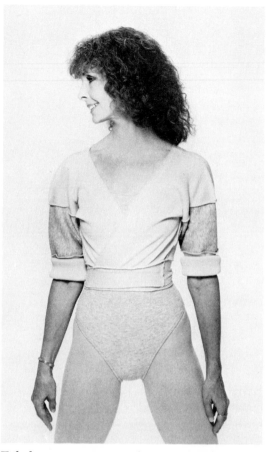 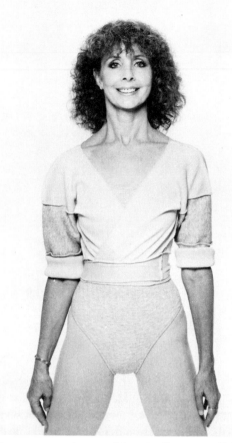

Exhale as you turn your head to the right for 4 counts. Try to lengthen your spine as you turn your head. Be sure your shoulders are pressed down.

Return to center position in 2 counts. Inhale.

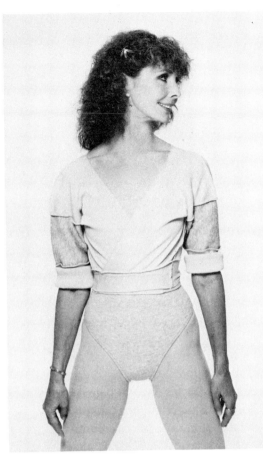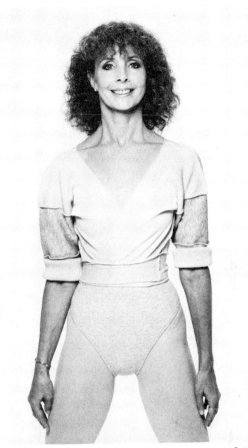

Exhale as you turn your head to the left for 4 counts.

Return to center position in 2 counts and inhale. Do this sequence 2 times.

4

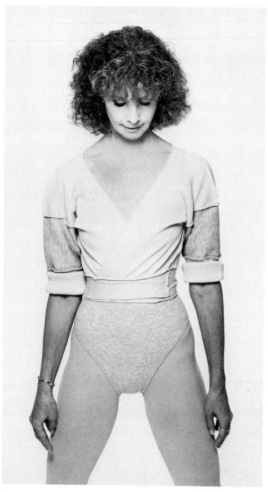

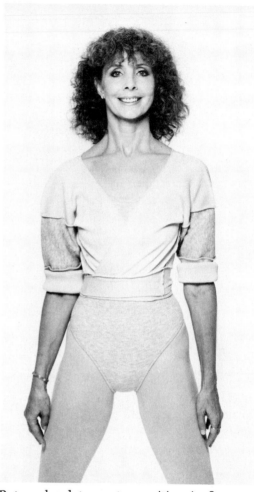

Bring your head forward for 8 counts. Keep your shoulders back and down. Continue to pull up from the hips, taking the weight off your lower back.

Return head to center position in 2 counts. Breathe normally.

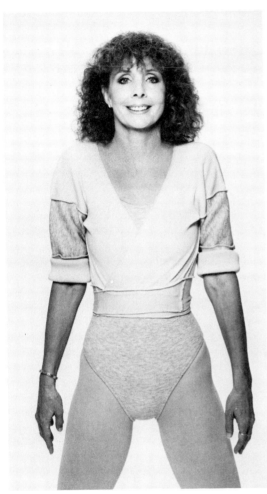

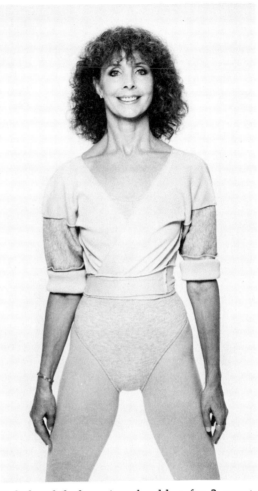

Inhale while lifting shoulders up for 2 counts.

Exhale while lowering shoulders for 2 counts. Resist the movement as you lower shoulders. Do the entire sequence 2 times.

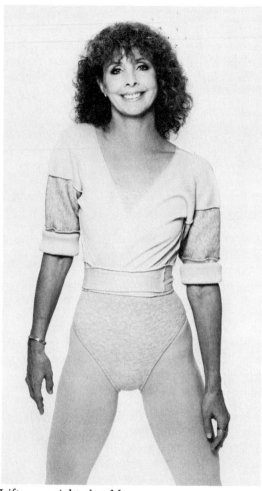 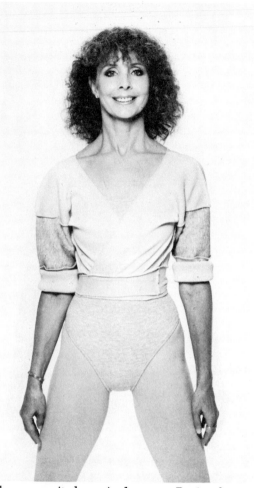

5

Lift your right shoulder up . . .

then press it down in 1 count. Resist the motion as you lower shoulder.

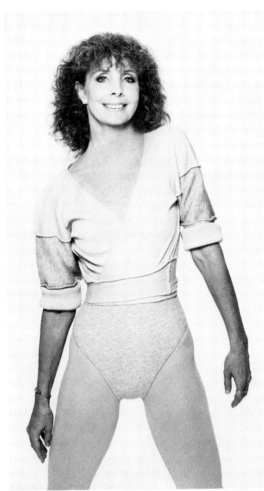

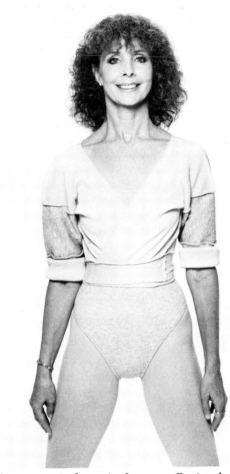

Lift your left shoulder up . . .

then press it down in 1 count. Resist the motion as you lower shoulder. Do this sequence 4 times.

6

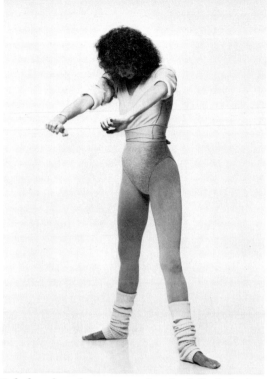

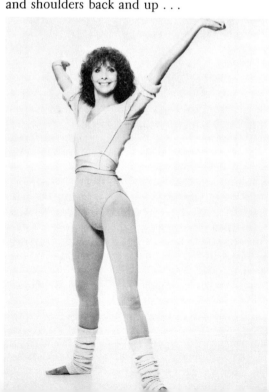

Inhale, then lower your head while bringing your arms and shoulders forward . . .

Exhale and continue to circle your arms and shoulders back and down, without arching your back.

then lift your head as you circle your arms overhead.

Now reverse: Inhale while bringing your arms and shoulders back and up . . .

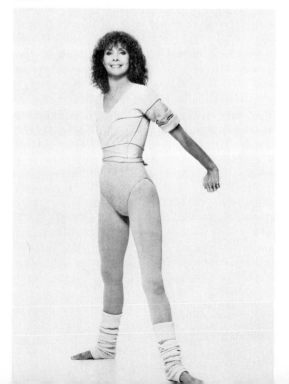

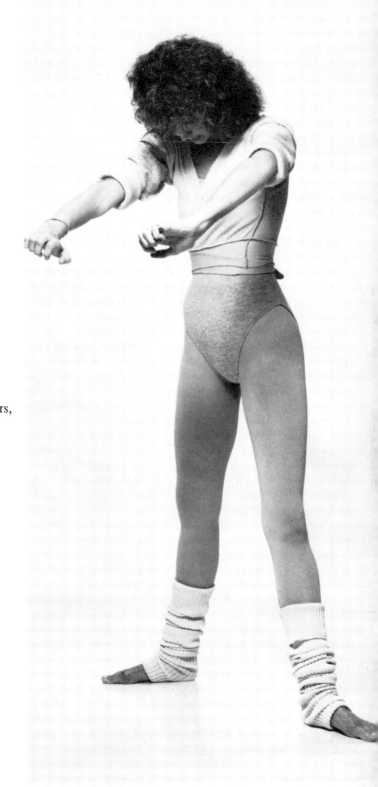

then exhale while circling your arms, shoulders,
and head forward and down.
Do entire sequence 3 times.

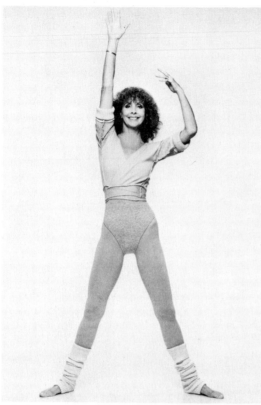

Inhale and bring both arms above your head. Exhale as you reach your right arm as far toward the ceiling as you can. Feel the stretch up your right side. Inhale.

Exhale as you reach your left arm as far upward as you can. Feel the stretch up your left side. Repeat, reaching right and left, for a total of 8 sets. Inhale as you change arms. Reaching right and left makes one set.

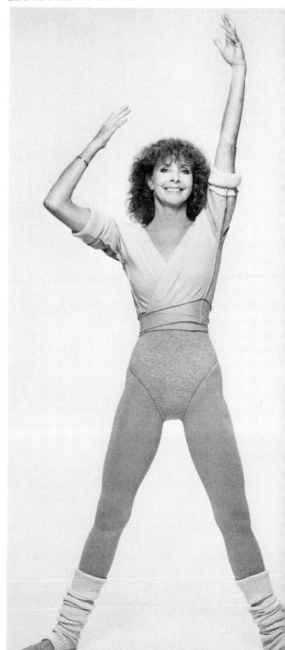

Take your rib cage to the left and stretch for 8 counts. Feel the stretch along the left side of the rib cage. Repeat right and left for 4 counts each. Alternate in single counts, moving to each side 8 times.

NOTE: If you feel at all breathless with your arms overhead, please lower your arms for a few counts, relax, and continue from there.

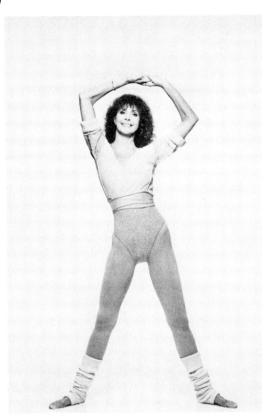

Clasp your hands over your head and, trying not to move your hips, reach with the rib cage to the right for 8 counts. Be sure your shoulders are pressed down. Feel the stretch along the right side of the rib cage.

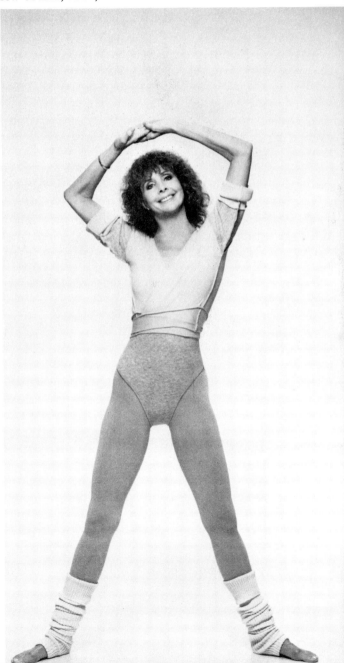

9

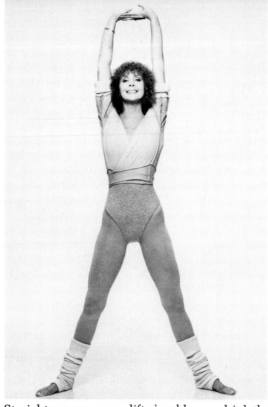

Straighten your arms, lift shoulders and inhale while reaching to the ceiling with arms and shoulders.

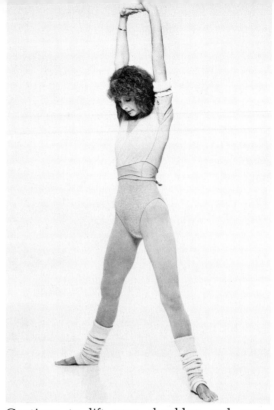

Continue to lift your shoulders and arms, pressing them back as you press your chin to your chest. Stretch up in the back, lengthening your spine, and press your hips forward.

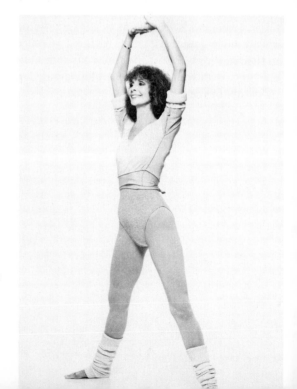

Exhale as you bring your head up and press your shoulders down. Keep spine lengthened.

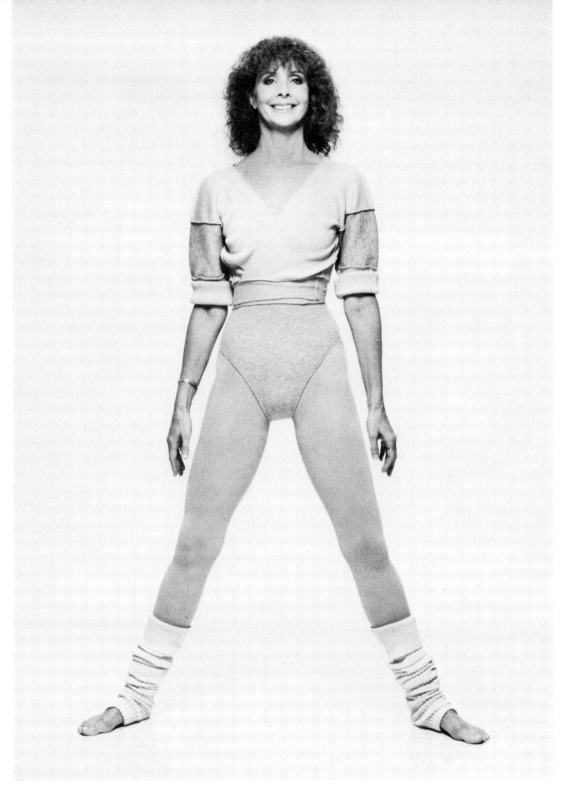

Bring your arms down to your sides.

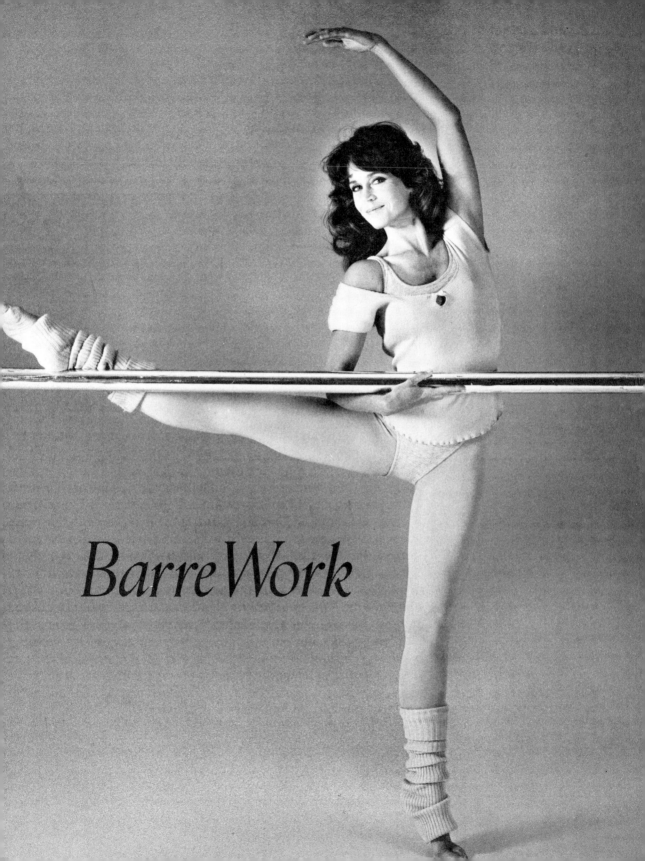

BarreWork

1

Your support can be a chair, table, or railing. It should be sturdy and reach approximately to your hip bone.

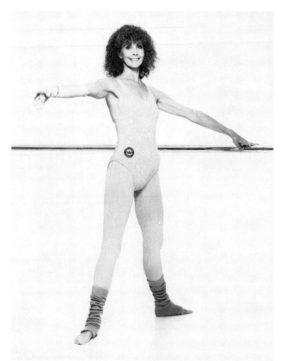

Starting position: Hold on to a support with your left hand. Place turned-out feet a little farther than hip distance apart. Take right arm out to the side. Keep weight evenly placed on both feet, pulling up tall from the hips, pubic bone lifted.

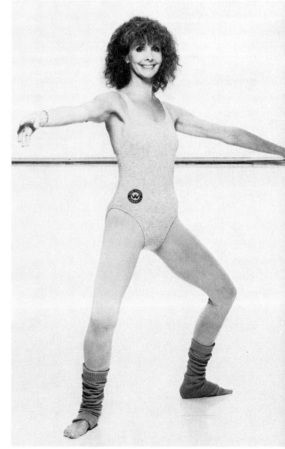

Bend knees in 2 counts, pressing knees apart in alignment with the toes. Keep the hips tucked under, back straight, stomach pulled in. Keep lifting away from hips as you bend your knees. *Don't let your ankles roll inward. Try to keep the weight centered with knees over your feet.* Then straighten knees in 2 counts, resisting the upward movement. Do 4 sets. Repeat movement, bending and straightening in a single count for 12 sets.

2

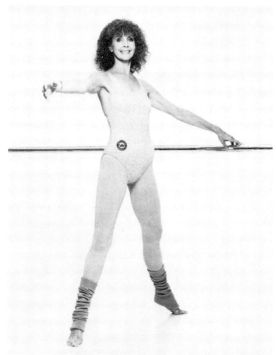

Keeping weight distributed evenly, press up onto your toes. Keep hips and back in a straight line, your weight slightly forward.

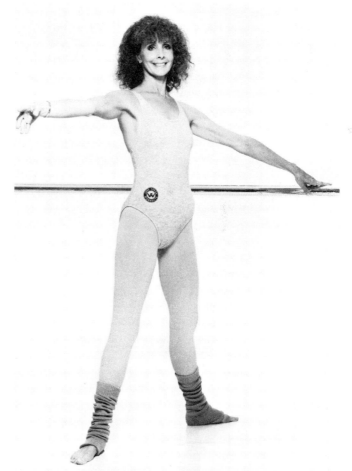

Resist as you lower your heels down to the floor, pressing heels forward as you come down. Do 8 sets. *Breathing:* Exhale as you lower your heels.

3

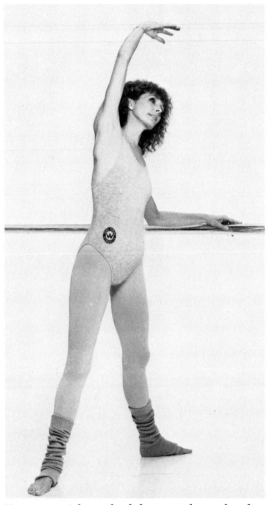 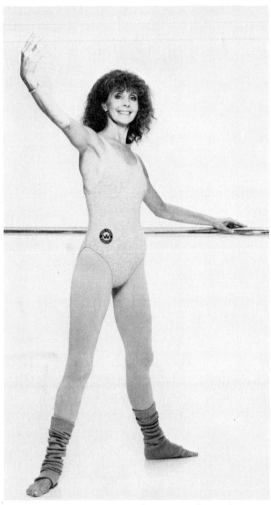

Keeping weight on both legs, reach overhead to the left with your right arm for 6 counts. Hips are square to the front, the pubic bone lifted. Don't arch your back.

Open right arm up and out to the side in 2 counts.

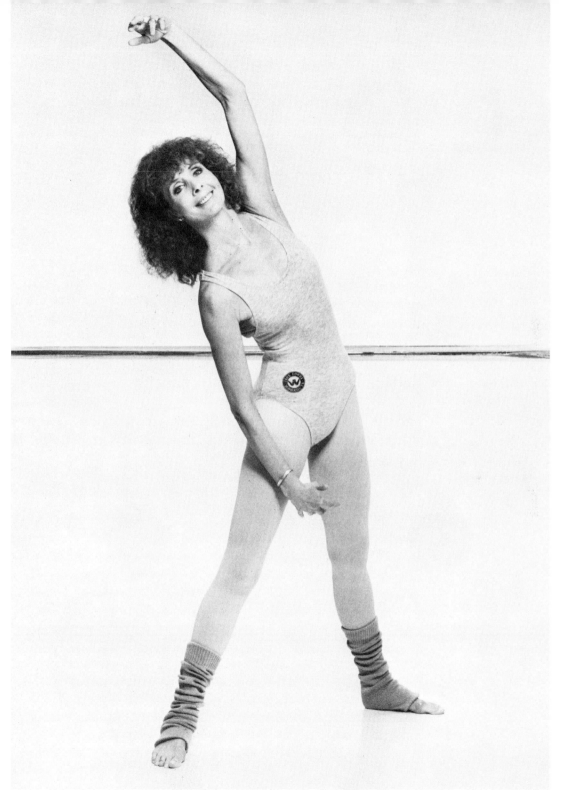

Take left hand off support and lift left arm overhead, reaching to the right for 6 counts. Pubic bone is lifted, back is straight, arm is directly over your ear. Then open arm and come back to center in 2 counts. Stretch tall in the torso, with abdominals pulled in. Breathe normally.

4

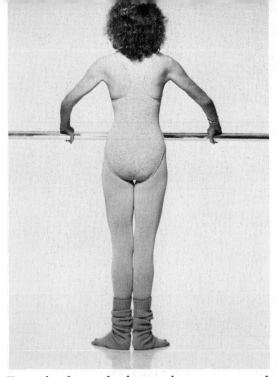

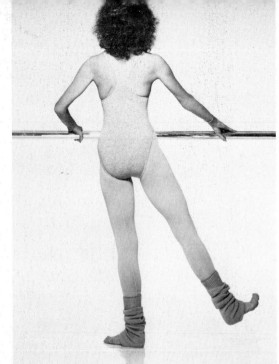

Face the barre, heels together, toes turned slightly out. Pull up tall, pubic bone lifted, keeping hips and back in a straight line.

Take right leg out to the side, slightly forward, and circle foot outward (circling clockwise) 4 times . . .

. . . then circle foot inward (circling counter-clockwise) 4 times.

Bring heels together.

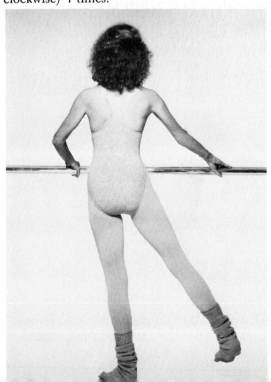

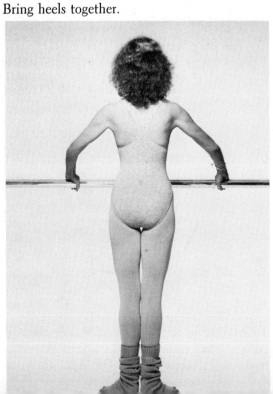

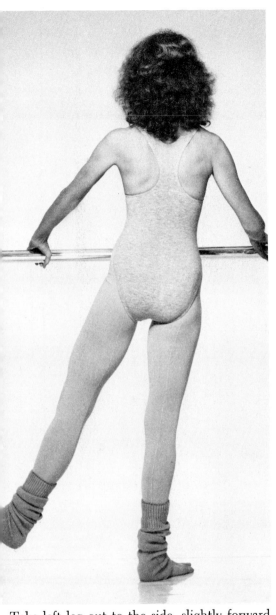

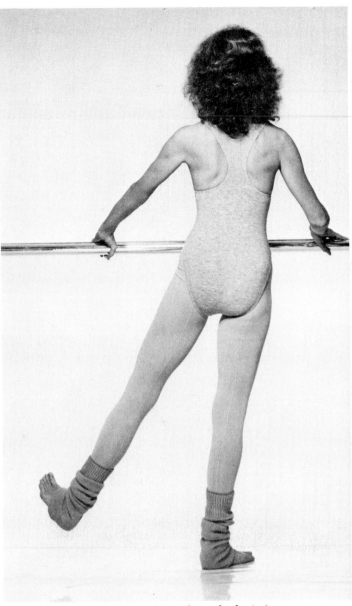

Take left leg out to the side, slightly forward, and circle foot outward (circling counterclockwise) 4 times . . .

. . . then circle foot inward (circling clockwise) 4 times. Breathe normally.

5

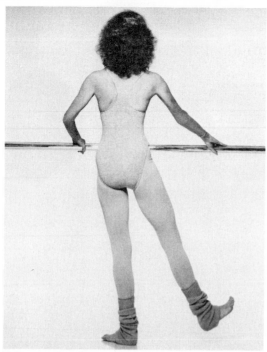

Bring right foot out to the side, slightly forward. Flex foot . . .

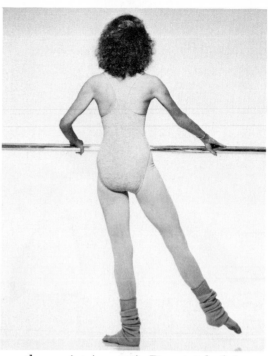

. . . then point (one set). Do a total of 4 sets.

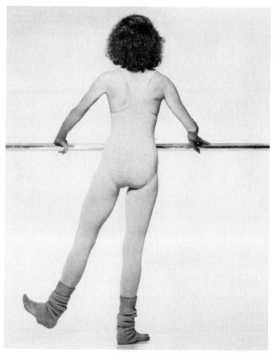

Repeat 4 sets with left leg.

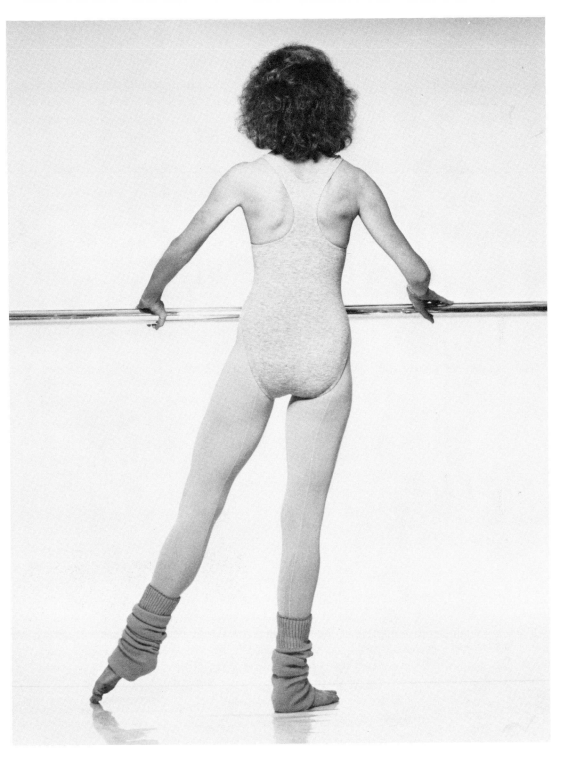

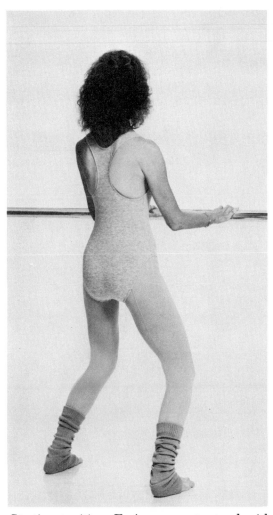 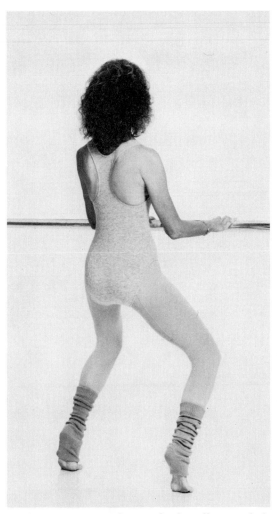

Starting position: Facing support, stand with your feet parallel, slightly more than hip distance apart. Keeping back and hips in a straight line, pubic bone lifted, bend your knees over your toes. Be sure your heels stay on the floor.

Making sure your knees don't roll in, inhale and press your heels over toes as high as you can. Be sure to keep your weight evenly balanced over both feet.

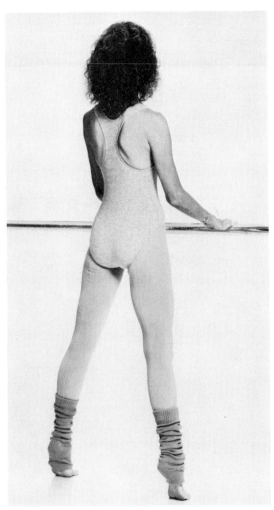

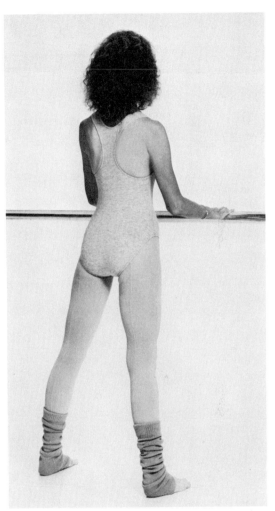

Keeping your hips and back in a straight line, straighten your legs, staying up on toes.

Lower heels to floor and exhale. These four movements make up one set. Do 4 sets. Then reverse the movement: come up on toes, then bend knees, then lower heels, then straighten legs. Do 4 sets.

7

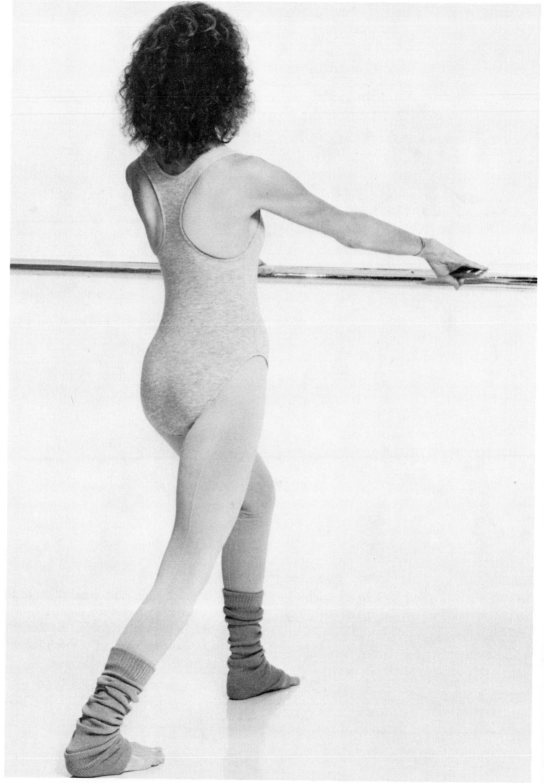

Bring your left leg forward, your right leg back. Bend both knees and press right heel into floor for 8 counts, stretching right calf.

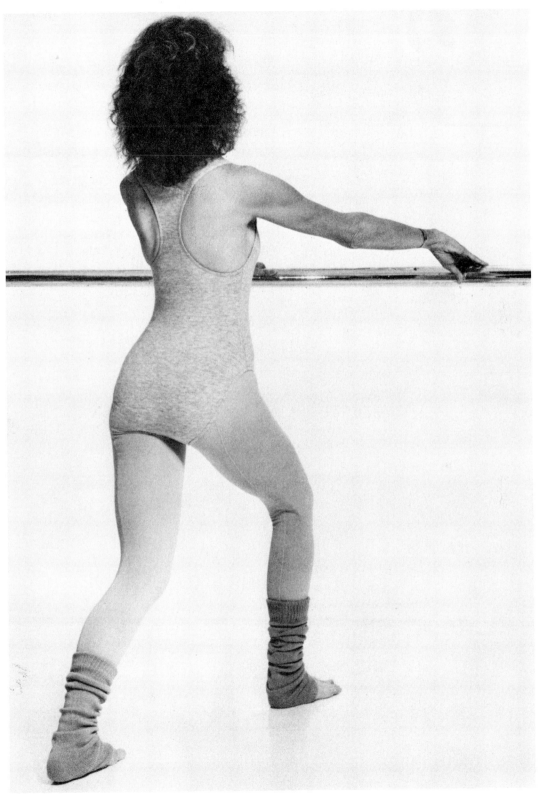

Change feet and stretch out left calf for 8 counts.

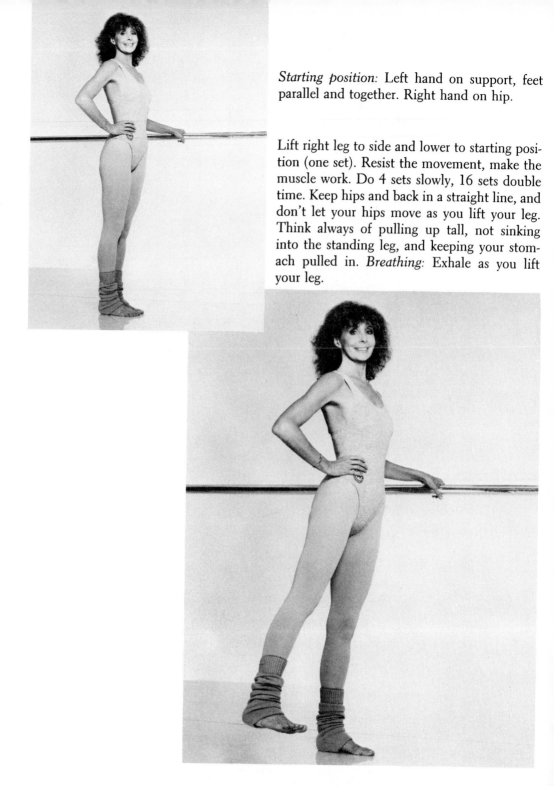

8

Starting position: Left hand on support, feet parallel and together. Right hand on hip.

Lift right leg to side and lower to starting position (one set). Resist the movement, make the muscle work. Do 4 sets slowly, 16 sets double time. Keep hips and back in a straight line, and don't let your hips move as you lift your leg. Think always of pulling up tall, not sinking into the standing leg, and keeping your stomach pulled in. *Breathing:* Exhale as you lift your leg.

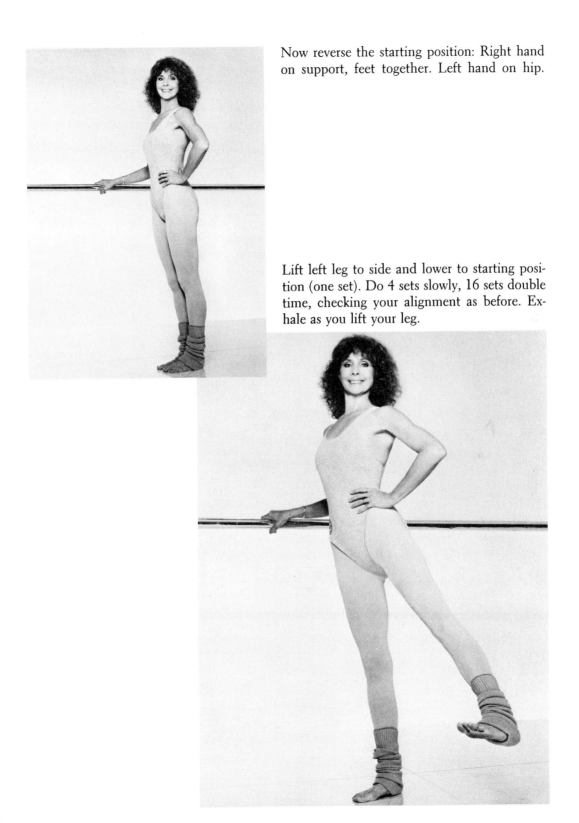

Now reverse the starting position: Right hand on support, feet together. Left hand on hip.

Lift left leg to side and lower to starting position (one set). Do 4 sets slowly, 16 sets double time, checking your alignment as before. Exhale as you lift your leg.

9

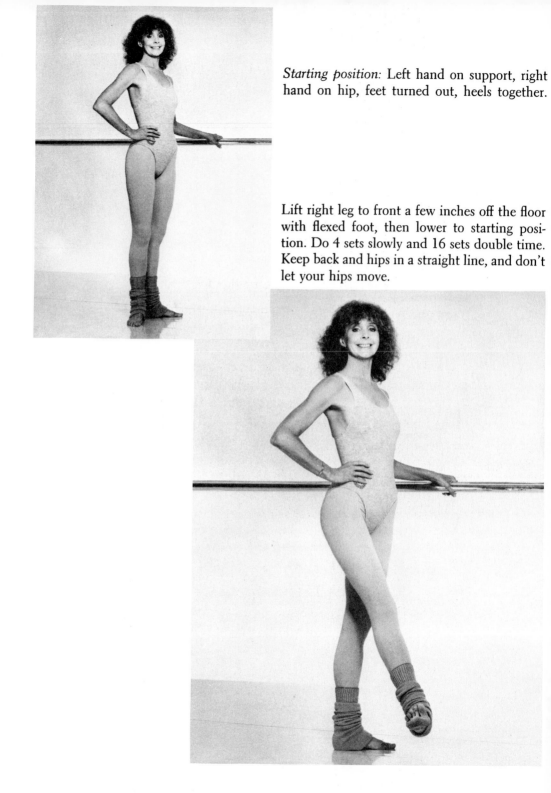

Starting position: Left hand on support, right hand on hip, feet turned out, heels together.

Lift right leg to front a few inches off the floor with flexed foot, then lower to starting position. Do 4 sets slowly and 16 sets double time. Keep back and hips in a straight line, and don't let your hips move.

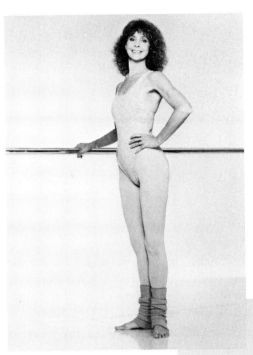

Reverse the starting position: Right hand on support, left hand on hip, feet turned out, heels together.

Lift left leg to front with flexed foot, then lower to starting position. Do 4 sets slowly and 16 sets double time. Keep back and hips in a straight line, and don't let your hips move.

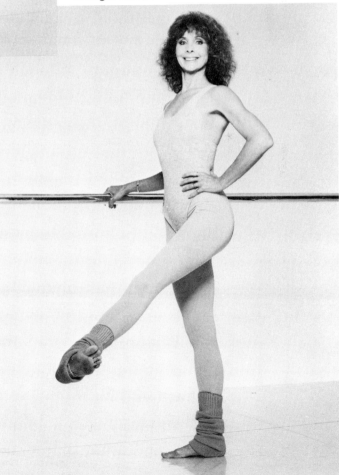

10

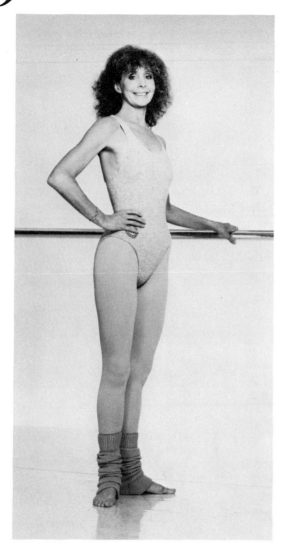

Starting position: Left hand on support, right hand on hip, feet turned out, heels together.

Lift right leg to the back and lower it to starting position (one set). Do 4 sets slowly, 16 sets double time. Be sure to keep your pubic bone lifted. You must not arch your back.

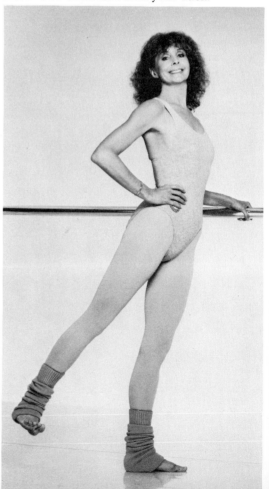

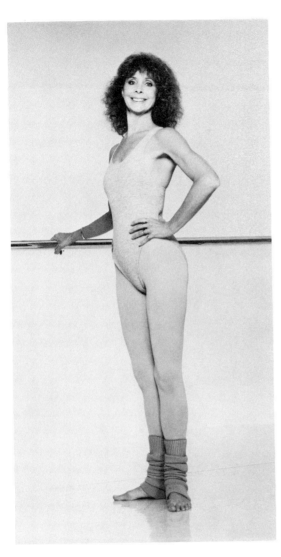

Reverse the starting position: Right hand on support, left hand on hip, feet turned out, heels together.

Lift left leg to the back and lower it to starting position. Do 4 sets slowly, 16 sets double time. Be sure not to arch your back.

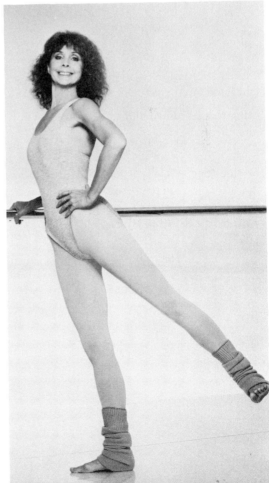

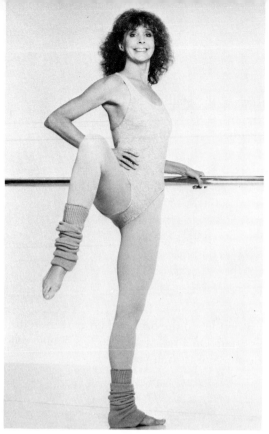

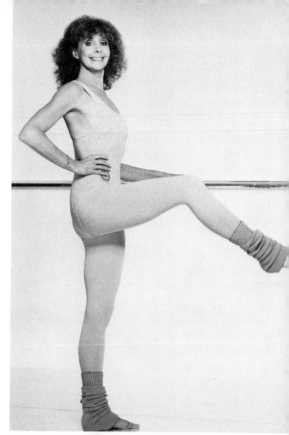

Starting position: With left hand on support, right hand on hip, lift bent right leg to the side.

Swing this leg down and up as you cross it toward the support . . .

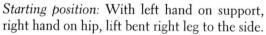

. . . and then swing it down and out again to the side (one set). Do 4 sets. Stand up tall on supporting leg, keeping your back and hips in a straight line. *Breathing:* Inhale as leg crosses front, exhale as leg opens to side.

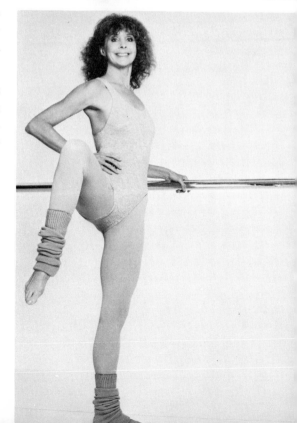

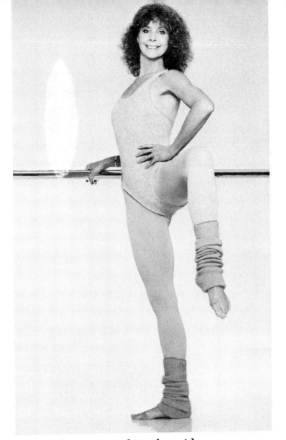

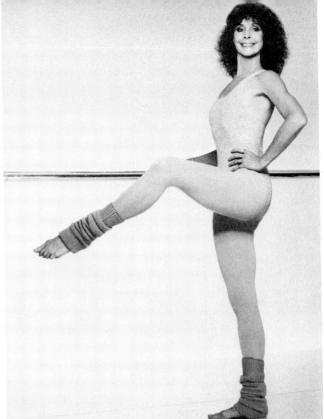

Turn and repeat to the other side.

With right hand on support, swing the left leg. Do 4 sets.

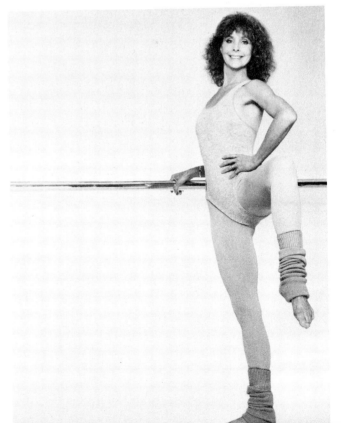

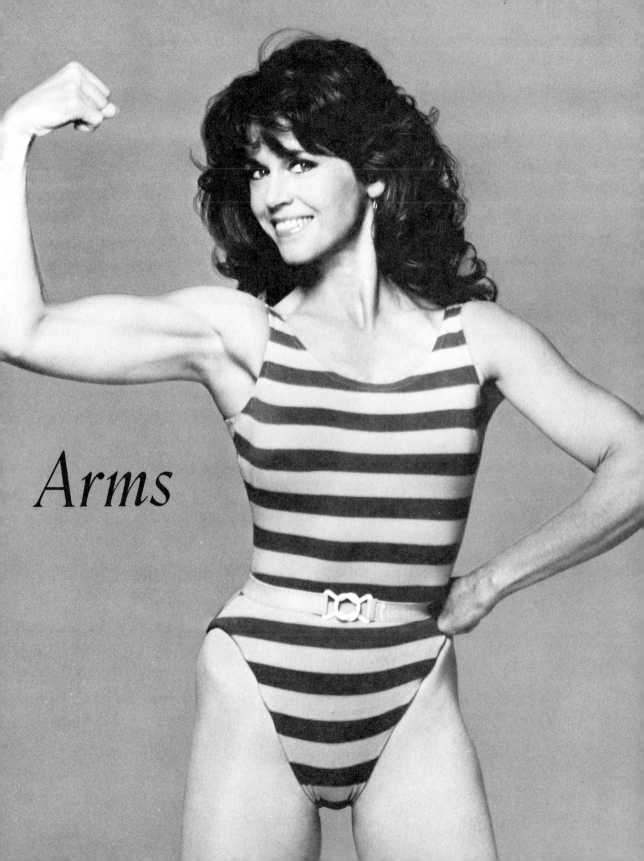

Arms

1

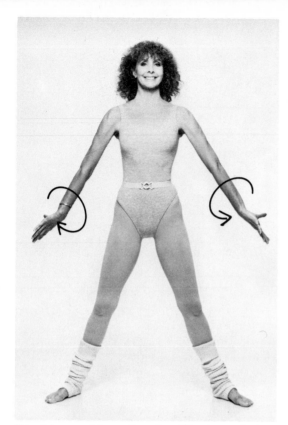 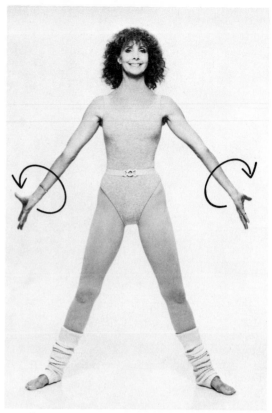

Starting position: Stand with feet slightly turned out, a little more than hip distance apart. Squeeze your buttocks and press hips forward as you stretch up tall. Keep your shoulders down. Open your hands and rotate the entire length of your arms inward, turning them from the shoulders and wrists . . .

. . . then rotate the entire length of your arms outward, turning them from the shoulders and wrists. Be sure your hands are open and fingers extended. Rotating in and out makes one set. Exhale as you rotate arms in. Do this exercise slowly for 8 sets, then repeat 8 sets at double time.

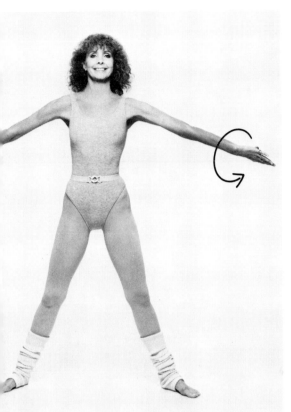

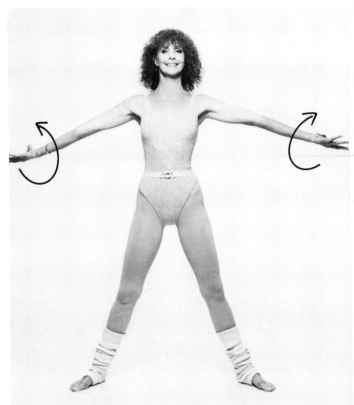

Continue rotating while raising arms out to the side, taking 8 sets to lift to just below shoulder level.

Keeping arms just below shoulder level, continue to rotate arms for 8 sets.

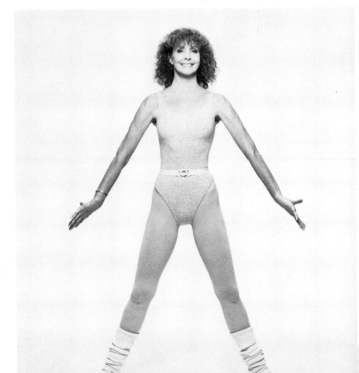

Continue to rotate while lowering arms, taking 8 sets to lower.

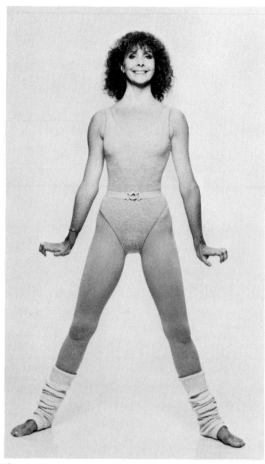

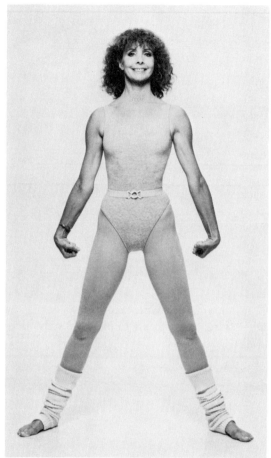

2

Flex your hands and press the heel of each hand in toward your body as you inhale . . .

. . . then make a fist and press your knuckles down and in toward your body while you exhale. These two movements make one set. Be sure to keep your shoulders down and your arms straight and taut. Do 8 sets slowly. Repeat 16 sets double time. If you feel any heaviness or discomfort in your legs you can gently bend one knee, then the other.

3

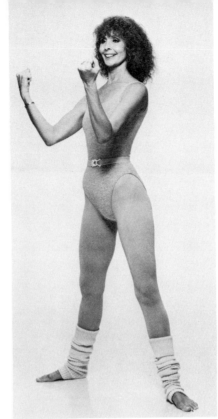

Starting position: Bring your arms forward, parallel to each other with elbows bent, fists clenched, palms facing you.

Inhale and swing elbows back. Be sure to keep your elbows in close to your body and your fists below your waist.

Extend your arms forward as you open your hands palms down . . .

. . . and exhale as you press straight arms as far back as you can, palms facing back. Be sure to keep your arms straight and taut and your hands open with fingers fully extended. Return to starting position to repeat. These two movements, the bent-elbow swing and the straight-arm press, count as one set. Repeat this exercise for a total of 8 sets.

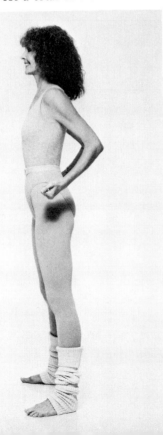

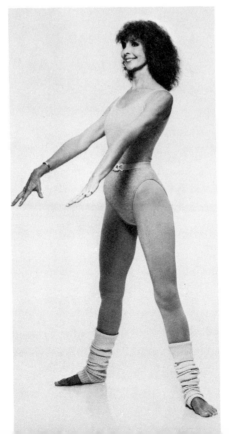

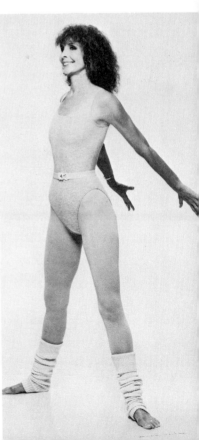

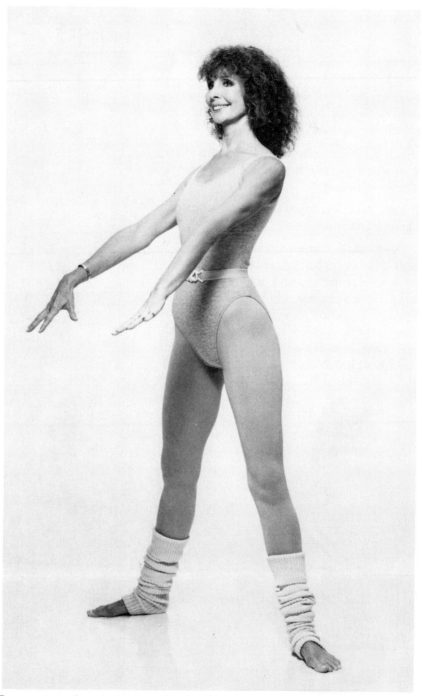

Repeat just the straight-arm press. Keeping your arms straight, hands open, and palms facing down, bring your arms forward . . .

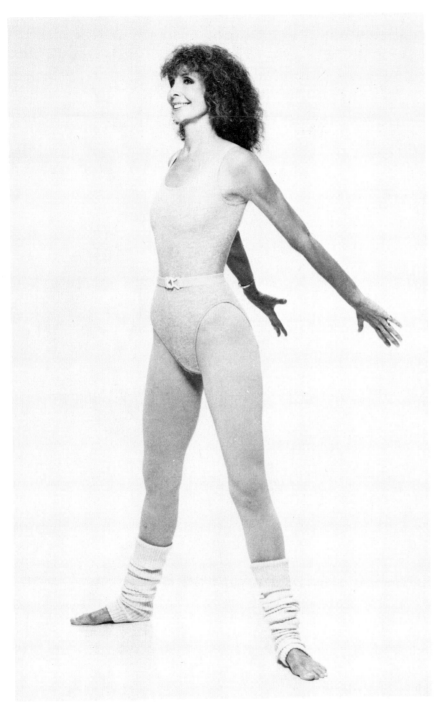

... then press them as far back as you can. Do 24 sets.

5

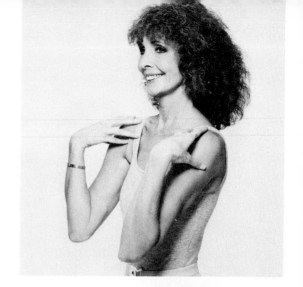

Place your hands on your shoulders with your elbows down . . .

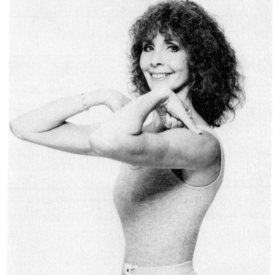

lift your elbows to the front up to shoulder level . . .

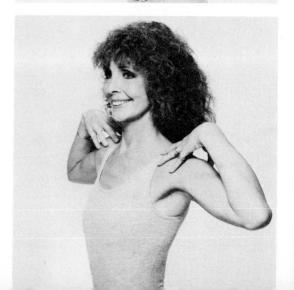

then open your elbows to the side by lifting and placing elbows in the open position.

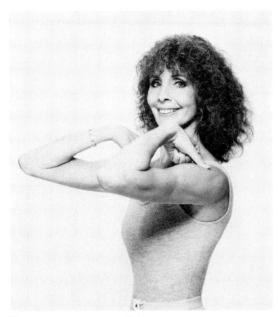

Return to center position . . .

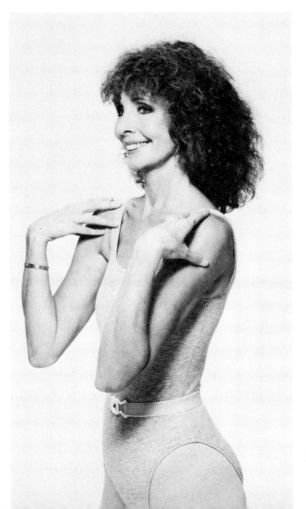

and press elbows down.
Repeat entire sequence 4 times.
REMINDER: Squeeze buttocks tight, pull stomach in, flatten back and pull up in the waist.
Breathing: Exhale as you open elbows to side. Inhale when you bring elbows back to center.

6

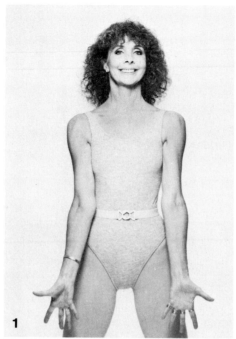

1

Bring your arms down to your sides and open your fingers, palms forward.

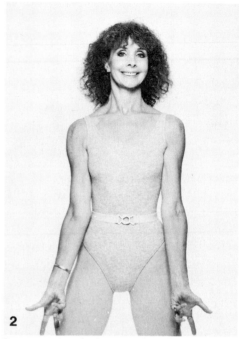

2

Beginning with the little finger,

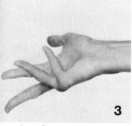

3

fan fingers in one at a time, and close hands completely into a fist.

Flex fists in toward you and bend your elbows . . .

then bring fists to shoulders as you raise your elbows to shoulder level.

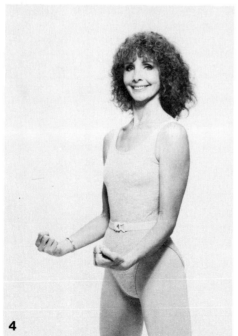

4

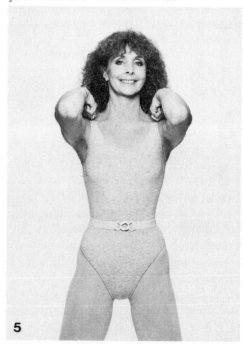

5

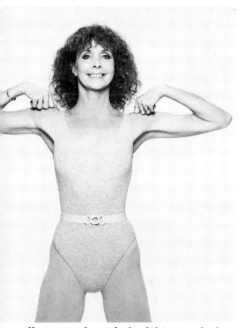

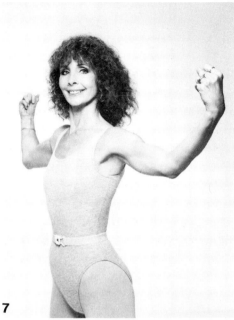

7

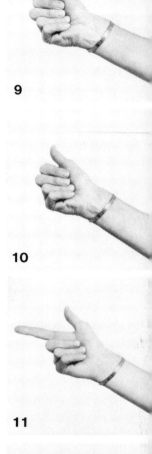

9

10

11

our elbows to the side by lifting and plac-
ws in open position . . .

unfold your arms to the side, keeping
elbows up . . .

d extend your arms completely, fanning fingers open one at a time beginning
th your thumb . . .

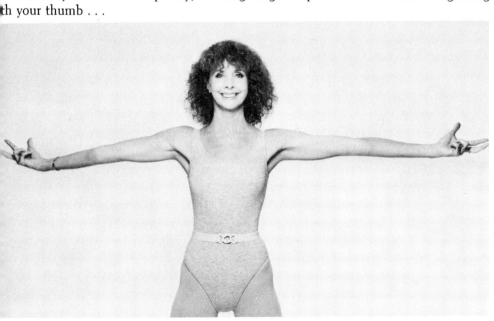

12

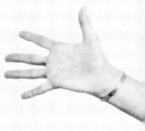

13

(continued on next page)

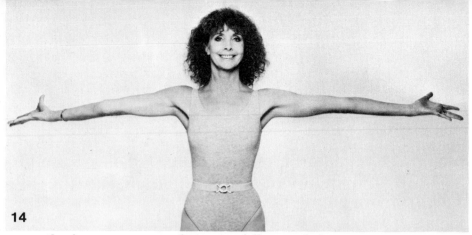

14

. . . until palms are open to ceiling, arms fully extended.

15

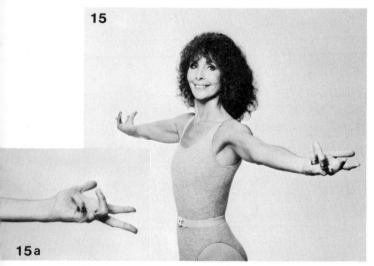

15a

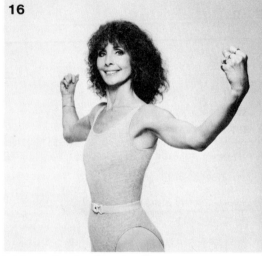

16

Now reverse the movement. Fan your fingers inward one at a time, beginning with your little finger.

Make a fist, bend your elbows . . .

and bring fists to shoulders, elbows lifted to the side.

Bring elbows to the front . . .

17

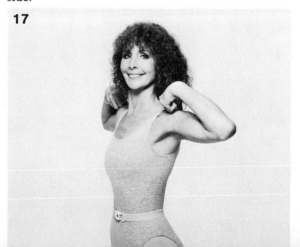

18

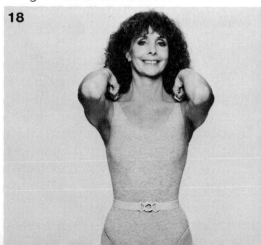

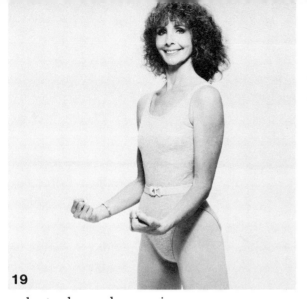

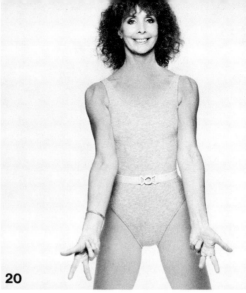

19

20

and extend arms down again . . .

as you fan your fingers out one at a time beginning with your thumb . . .

. . . until your arms and hands are fully extended and you feel a good stretch.
Do this entire sequence one time slowly. Then do 6 sets, using 2 counts to bring fists to shoulders, 2 counts to bring elbows to the side, 2 counts to extend arms and fingers to side; and 6 counts to reverse the movement.

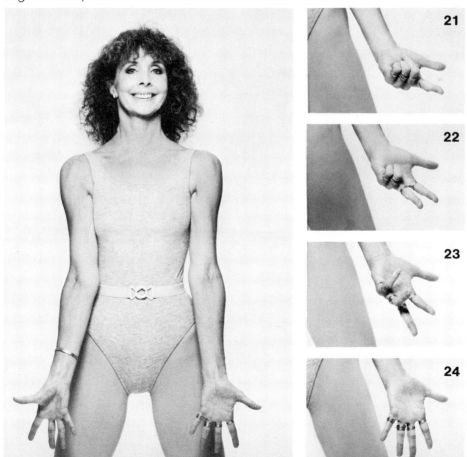

21

22

23

24

317

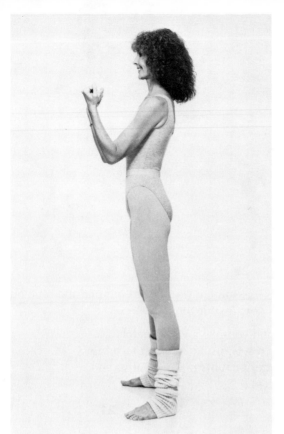

Relax your arms by swinging them forward and back . . .

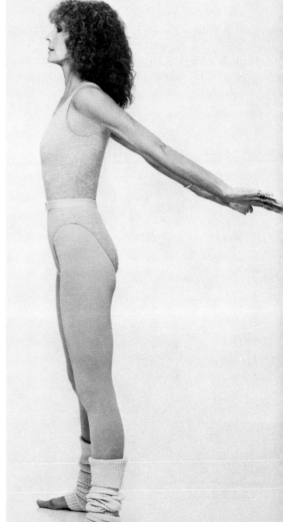

as you inhale and exhale deeply. Do this 8 times.

Starting with your arms down at your sides, circle your hands outward, rotating from the wrists, as you bring your arms to shoulder level in 4 counts, one hand circle per count.

REMINDER: You can bend and straighten knees as you do all these arm exercises, especially if you feel any discomfort in your legs. Bending and straightening will increase circulation and warm up the leg muscles.

Now circle your hands inward, rotating from the wrists . . .

as you lift arms over your head in 4 counts, one hand circle per count. Breathe normally.

. . . and we'll go right into the waist section.

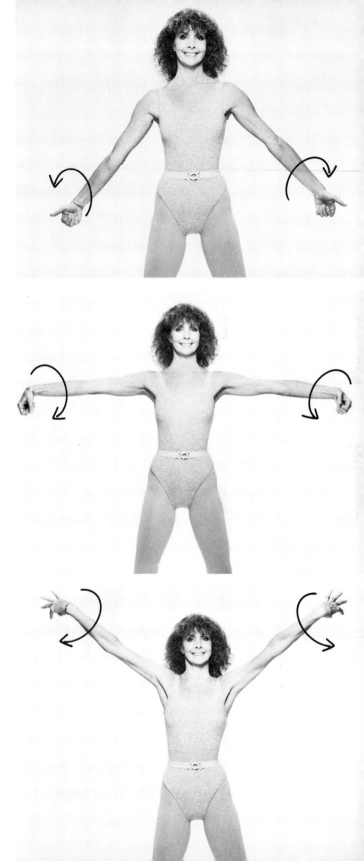

Waist

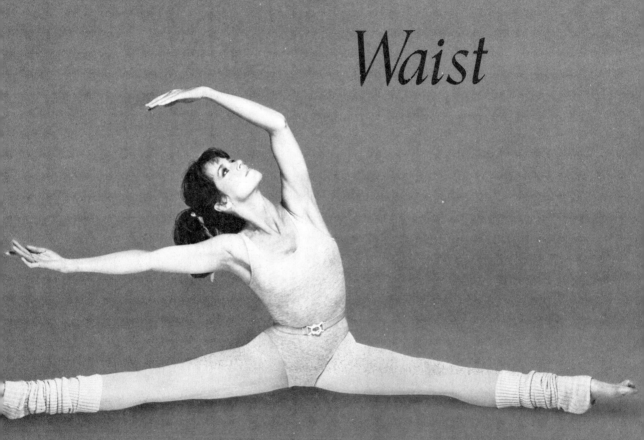

1

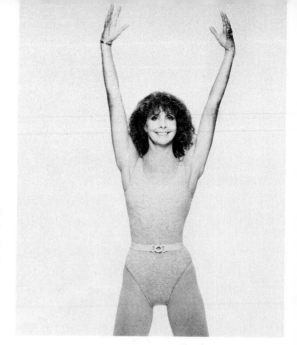

Starting position: Stand with feet slightly turned out and placed wider than hip distance apart, stomach pulled in, buttocks tight and arms overhead.

Lower your right arm and reach over to the right, extending your left arm directly over your ear. Gently pulse as you reach for 14 counts. Be sure to keep your hips facing front and your weight slightly forward and evenly distributed on both feet. Stretch up and out. Don't let the right side collapse. Breathe normally.

Come back to center as you open both arms to the side in 2 counts . . .

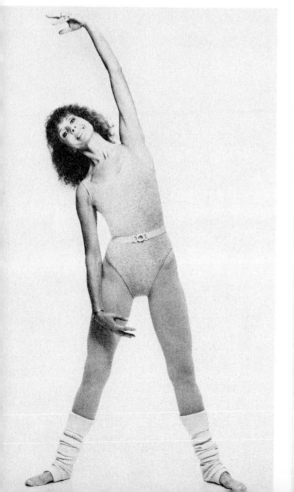

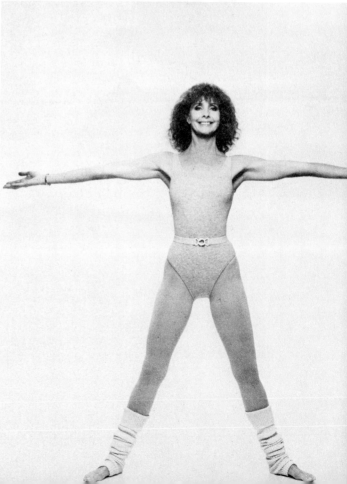

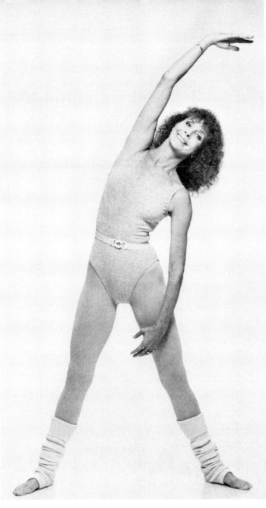

. . . and repeat to the left side, reaching your right arm over to the left, pulsing gently for 14 counts. Don't lean back.

Come back to center and open both arms to the side in 2 counts.

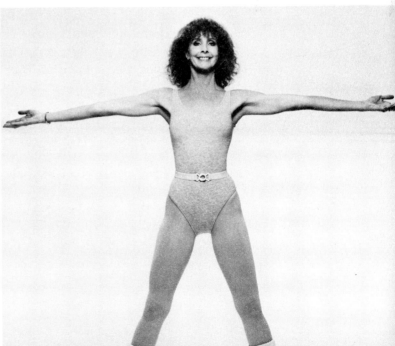

2

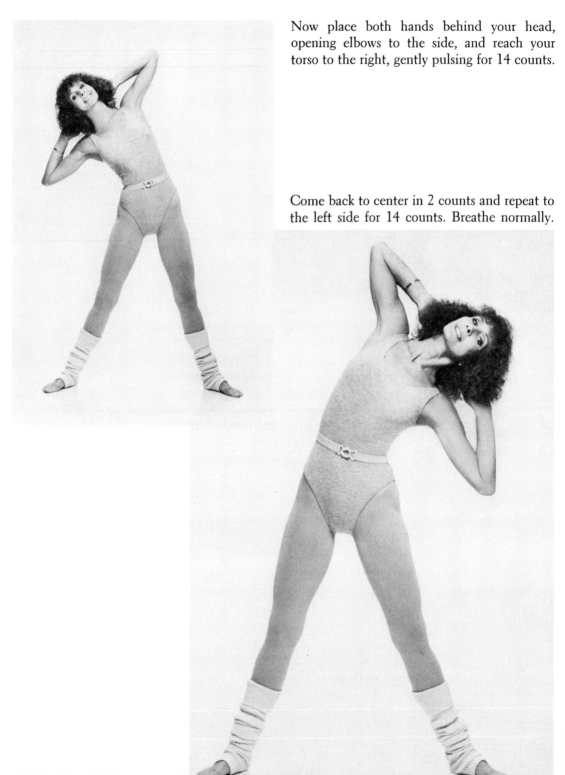

Now place both hands behind your head, opening elbows to the side, and reach your torso to the right, gently pulsing for 14 counts.

Come back to center in 2 counts and repeat to the left side for 14 counts. Breathe normally.

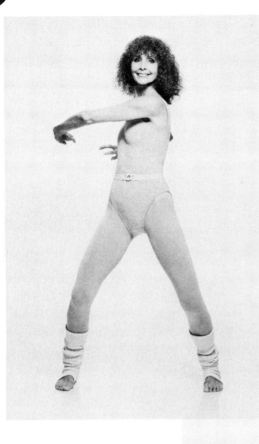

Bend your knees, feet parallel and slightly more than hip distance apart. Elbows are bent and arms just below shoulder level. Swing arms and shoulders to the right . . .

and swing to the left (one set). Alternate right and left for a total of 16 sets. Be sure knees remain bent and hips as stationary as possible. Don't let knees roll in. Breathe normally.

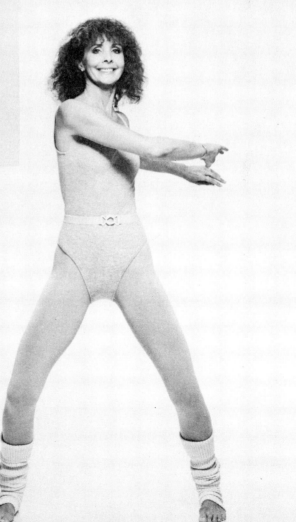

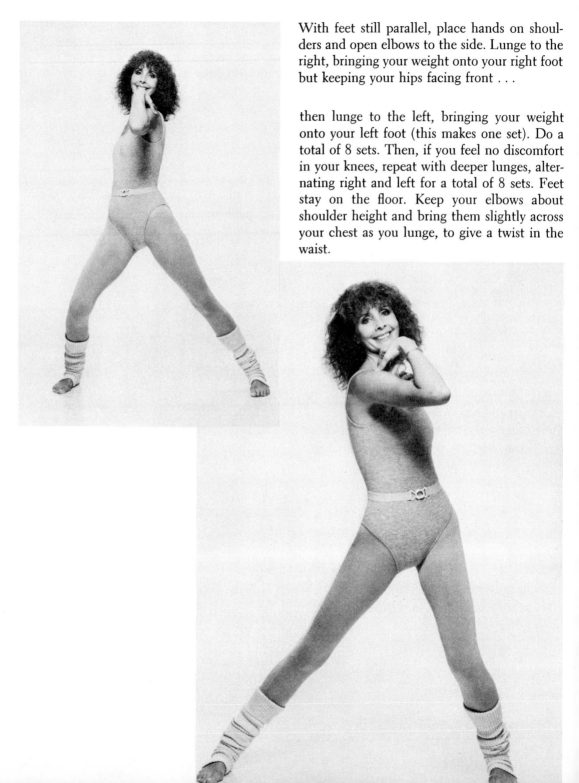

With feet still parallel, place hands on shoulders and open elbows to the side. Lunge to the right, bringing your weight onto your right foot but keeping your hips facing front . . .

then lunge to the left, bringing your weight onto your left foot (this makes one set). Do a total of 8 sets. Then, if you feel no discomfort in your knees, repeat with deeper lunges, alternating right and left for a total of 8 sets. Feet stay on the floor. Keep your elbows about shoulder height and bring them slightly across your chest as you lunge, to give a twist in the waist.

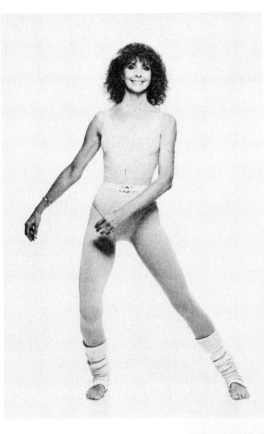

Bring your arms down, bend knees, and shift your weight to the right, then to the left (one set) . . .

. . . while gradually bringing feet together in 4 sets. (This will let you go right into the aerobics without stopping.)

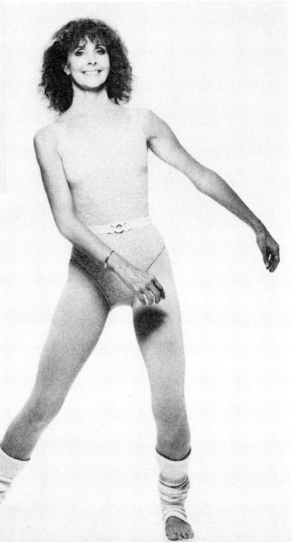

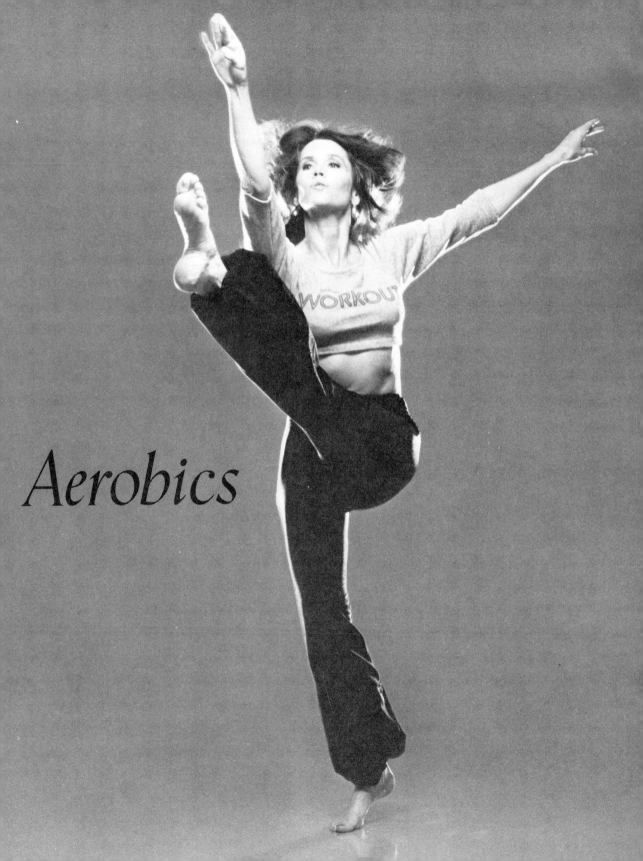

Aerobics

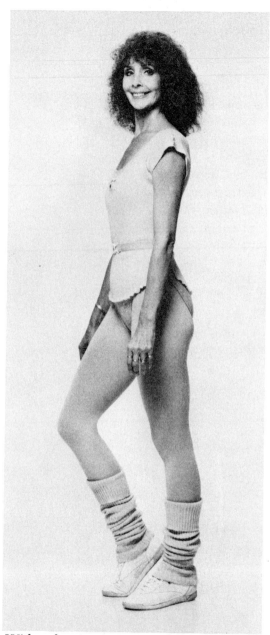

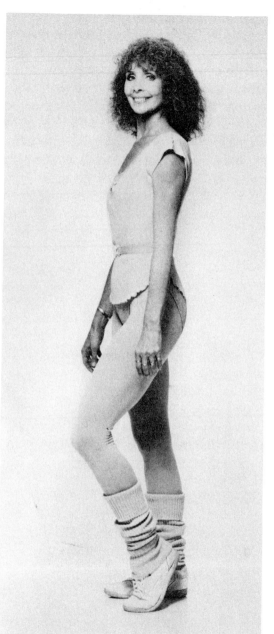

With a slow jogging tempo, lift right heel and press forward over your toes . . .

then repeat with the left foot. Continue these small heel presses for 5 minutes as you warm up the large muscles in your hips and thighs. Be sure to keep your spine lengthened, weight slightly forward, pubic bone lifted. The movement should be smooth and fluid, not jarring to your ankles.

Put on music that makes you want to move and dance. The tempo should be one you can comfortably skip and jog to.

Your eventual goal is to do 12 to 20 minutes of nonstop aerobic movement. Start very gradually with these small steps for 5 minutes, just lifting your heels off the floor. Then take small jogging steps for several minutes. When you are able to do this without panting or undue strain, increase your time, lifting your knees a little higher or adding other steps such as skipping, swinging your legs side to side, pretending to jump rope. As you improve your cardiovascular fitness, feel free to prance, Charleston, boogie, do can-can kicks . . . whatever gets you going. The more you vary the steps, the more you will dissipate the stress to your joints and shins. It will also help to lessen the impact if you move about over at least a 3- to 4-foot area as you step and jog. The more room you have to move about in, the better.

To maximize the burning of fat calories, keep your heart rate within the parameters of its training range. See page 246 for how to determine your ideal training heart rate during aerobic exercise. A rule of thumb is to maintain breathing that allows you to carry on a conversation.

Lifting your knees higher, kicking your legs up, bringing your arms overhead as you jog in place, all will raise your heart rate. If you become breathless take smaller steps, lifting only your heels for a while till your heart rate decreases.

MOST IMPORTANT, remember to:
- Breathe deeply throughout. It is counterproductive to push yourself so much that you are panting.
- Land on the balls of your feet and allow your heels to touch down.
- Pull up tall. Do not let yourself slouch.
- Land with bent knees.

You should never stop aerobic activity abruptly. Always allow time for a gradual decrease in your heart rate and a good stretch to lengthen your muscles and prevent soreness.

AEROBIC COOL-DOWN

At the start of this cool-down you should take your pulse to see if you have raised your heart rate to its safe training range (see page 246).

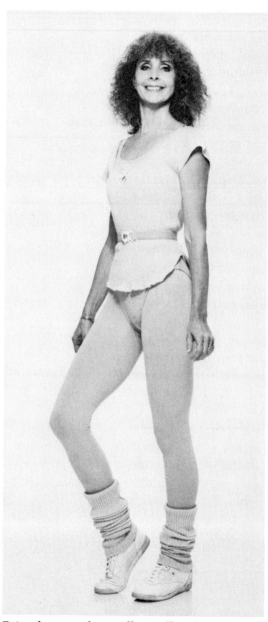 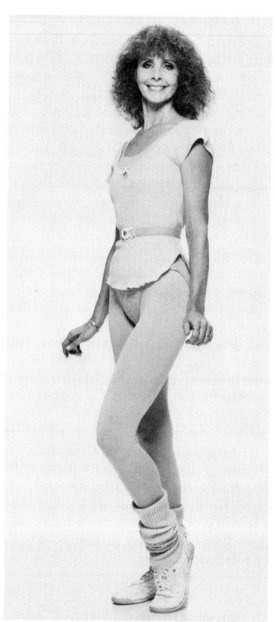

Bring feet together, pull up tall with your stomach in. Lift right heel and press over your toes . . . and repeat with left foot (one set). Do 32 sets, or until you are no longer breathless. Be sure not to sink into your hips. Stretch up and work through every part of your foot in a gentle, fluid motion, with your weight slightly forward and pubic bone lifted.

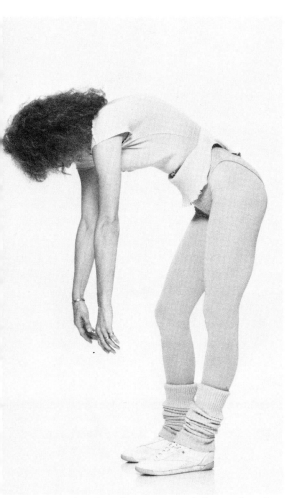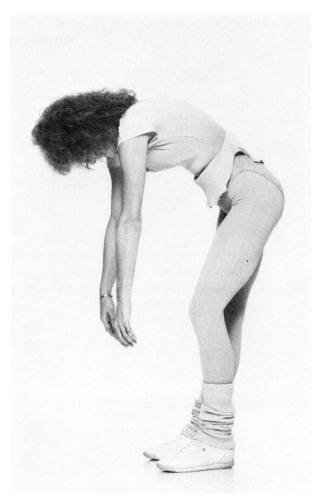

Let your head and torso round down, bending your right knee . . .

. . . then your left knee, in 6 sets. If you feel out of breath keep bending your knees and stay at this level with hands on thighs—don't lean all the way over.

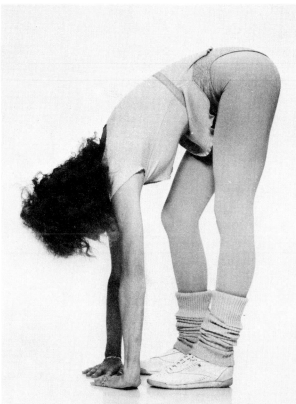

Letting your head and shoulders relax down even farther, bend the right knee and hold for 4 counts (hands may be on ankles, lower legs, or thighs) . . .

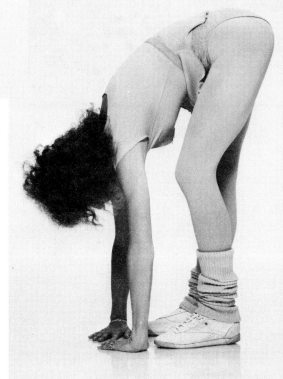

then bend the left knee and hold for 4 counts. Repeat to each side.

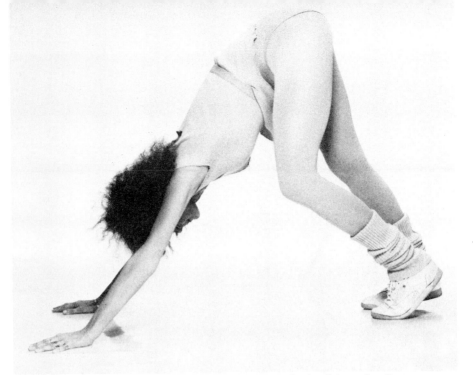

Walk hands out in front of you, pressing the right heel into the floor . . .

then press the left heel into the floor (one set). Repeat for 8 sets. Lift your hips to the ceiling while lengthening your spine. To prevent your back from arching, think of curling your pubic bone toward your navel.

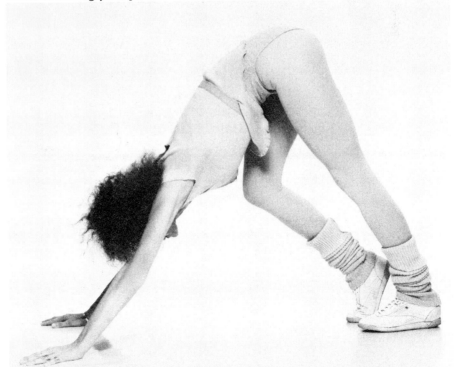

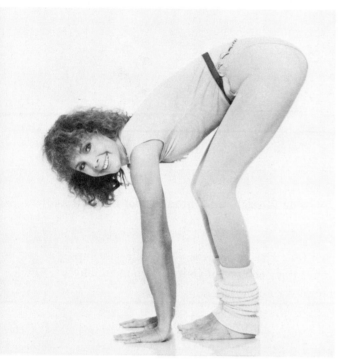

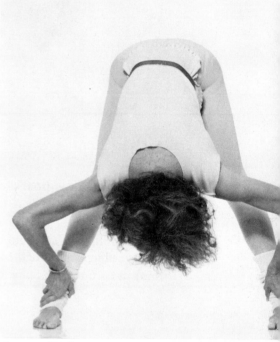

Keeping knees bent, walk feet toward your hands . . .

then walk feet out wider than hip distance apart, placing your hands on your lower leg or ankles.

We'll go right into the hamstring stretches.

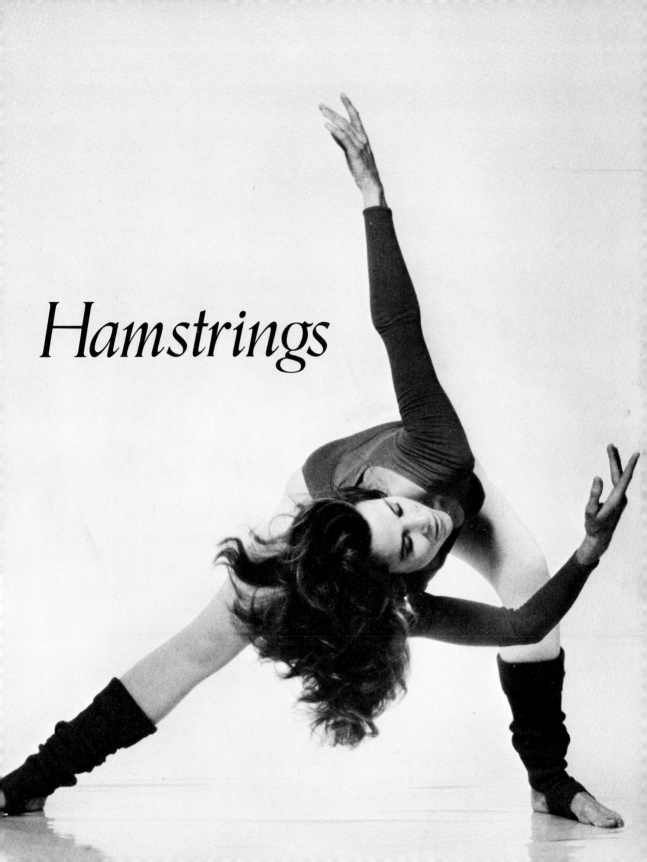

Hamstrings

1

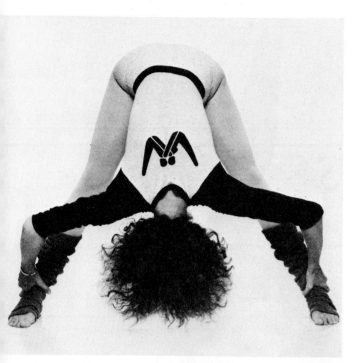

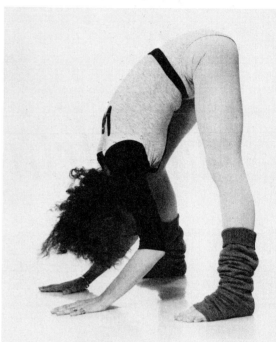

Standing with feet apart, bend over and place your hands on thighs, lower legs, or the floor in front of you. Feet should be parallel, *not turned out.*

Slightly bend your right knee . . .

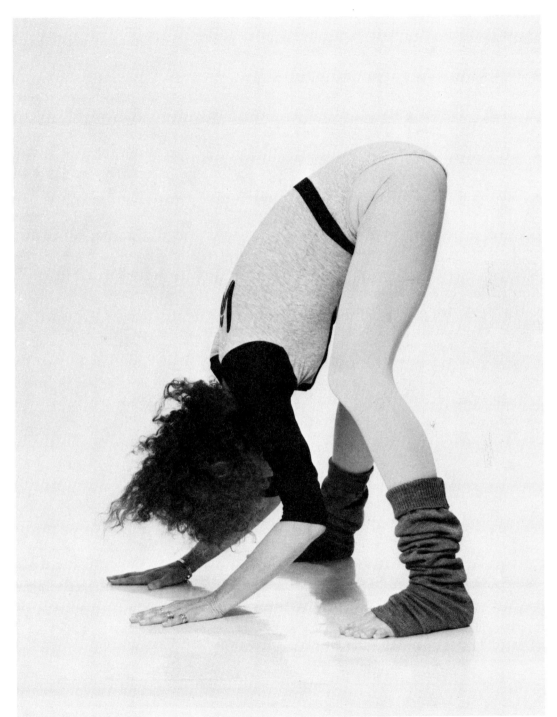

then slightly bend your left knee as you straighten the right (this is one set). Try to bend your knees without dropping your hips. Think of stretching and lengthening the back of your leg as you straighten it. This is a fluid, not jarring, movement. Keep the front of your thigh relaxed. Do 8 sets.

2

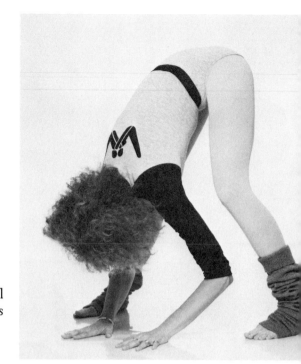

Being careful not to allow your knees to roll in, bend both knees without letting your hips drop . . .

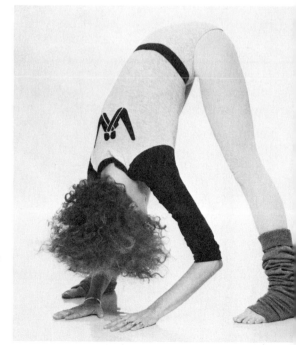

then straighten both knees. Do 8 sets. You do not need to put your hands on the floor. *Breathing:* Exhale as you straighten knees.

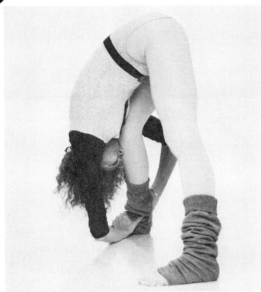

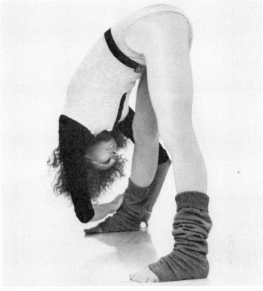

Still bending forward with hands on floor, lower leg, or thigh, face your right knee. Bend...

... then straighten your right knee, concentrating on lengthening the back of the leg. (This is a gentle movement. Don't let your knee snap back, and keep your feet flat on the floor at all times.) Do 8 sets. Bend your right knee again, slowly straighten it, and stretch over for 8 counts.

... then straighten your left knee. Do 8 sets. Bend your left knee again, slowly straighten it, and stretch over for 8 counts. *Breathing:* Exhale when you straighten your knee.

Now repeat on the left side. Bend . . .

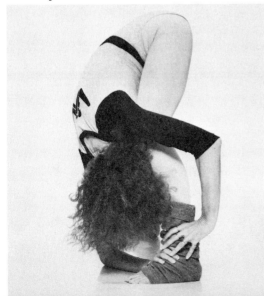

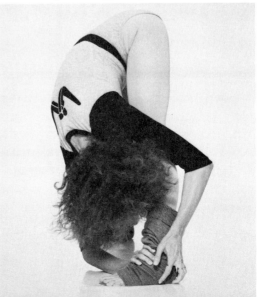

341

4

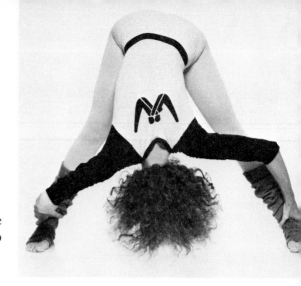

Bending forward, legs wide, feet parallel, place your hands on your lower legs. Move hips to the right . . .

. . . then to the left. Do 4 sets. You should feel a stretch in the inner thighs.

Stretch over center, holding for 8 counts. Be sure to keep your weight forward toward the balls of your feet. Breathe normally.

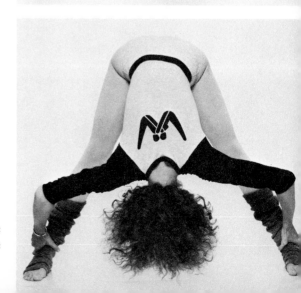

5

Keeping your knees bent, relax your arms and
slowly roll up, pulling in your abdominals, one
vertebra at a time . . .

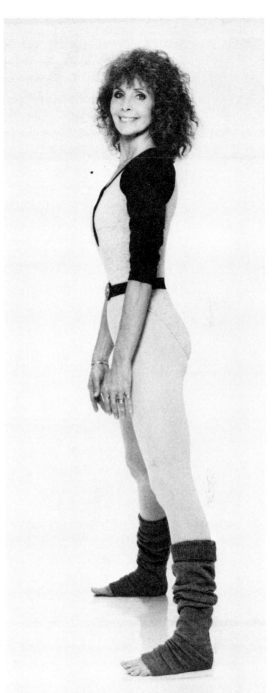

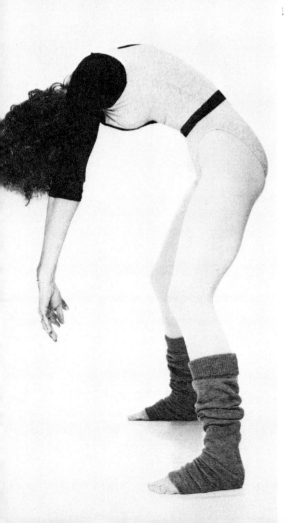

to an erect standing position, stomach pulled
in, pubic bone lifted, pulling up tall in the
waist, chest lifted. Breathe normally.

Floor Work

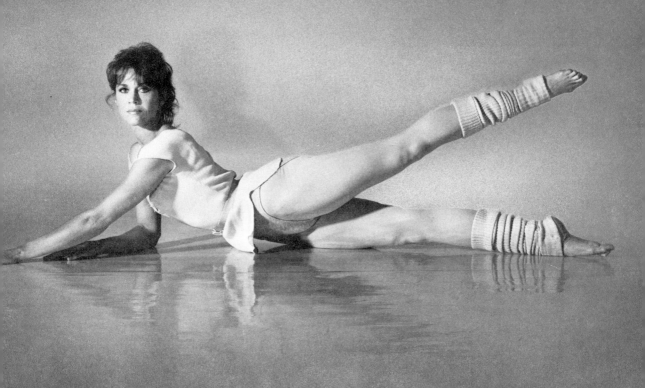

1

You should use a mat, folded blanket or towels to cushion your back and hips, and to keep dust and carpet fibers out of your hair and nose.

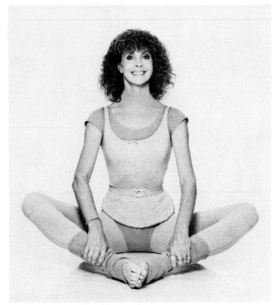

Starting position: Sit on the floor with soles of your feet together, hands on ankles, knees dropped gently open.

Lower your head. Pull in and tighten the muscles between your legs as if holding in a urination, for 2 counts. Release for 2 counts. (This makes one set.) Do 4 sets. Repeat the movement, doing 24 sets double time. Contract the muscles and hold in for 8 counts, then release.

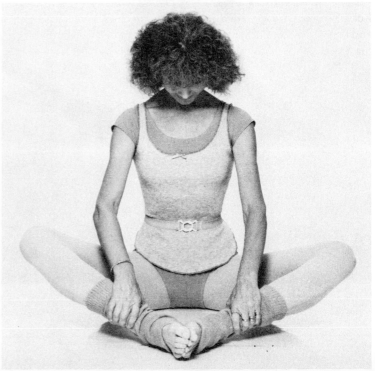

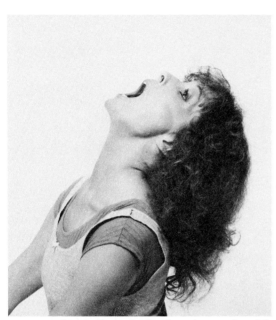

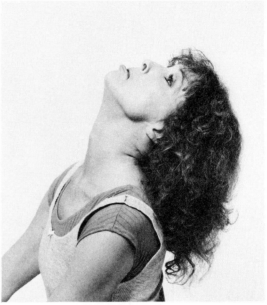

Let your head tilt as far back as is comfortable and open your mouth wide, stretching your jaw for 8 counts.

Then close your mouth. Cover your top lip with your bottom lip, stretching your chin for 8 counts. Then release. Bring head back to center. Breathe normally. If you start to feel dizzy with your head held in this position, please raise your head to center and go on to the next exercise.

3

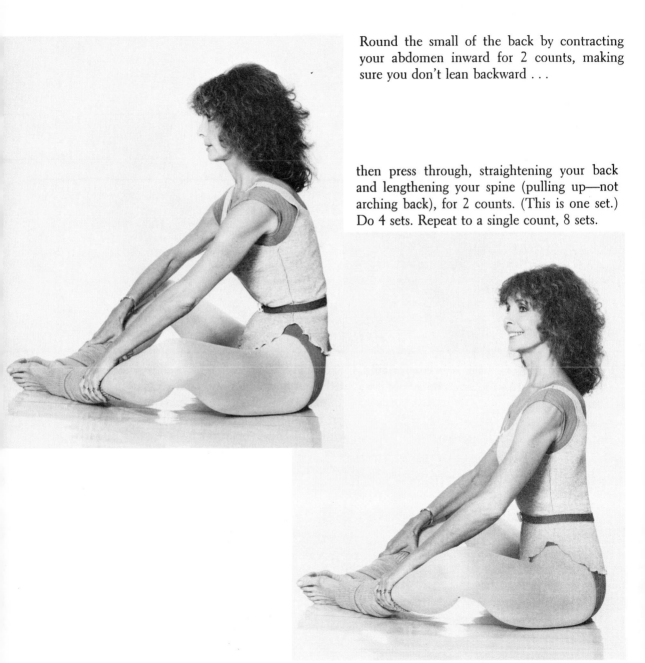

Round the small of the back by contracting your abdomen inward for 2 counts, making sure you don't lean backward . . .

then press through, straightening your back and lengthening your spine (pulling up—not arching back), for 2 counts. (This is one set.) Do 4 sets. Repeat to a single count, 8 sets.

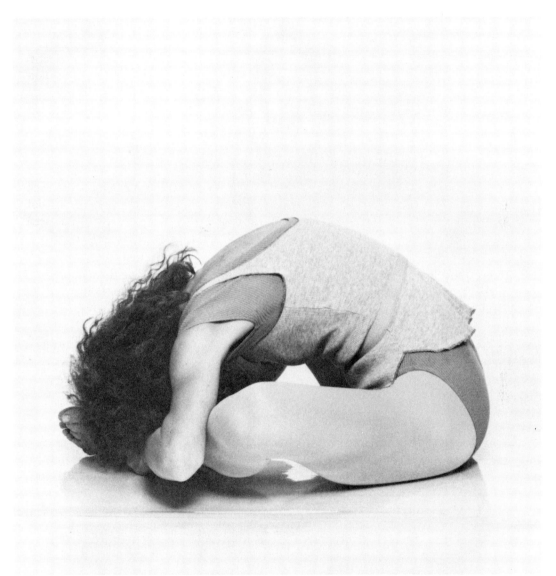

Let your head and torso round forward. Hold this position for 8 counts, trying to press your knees toward the floor with abdominals pulled in. Roll up. *Breathing:* Steady, normal.

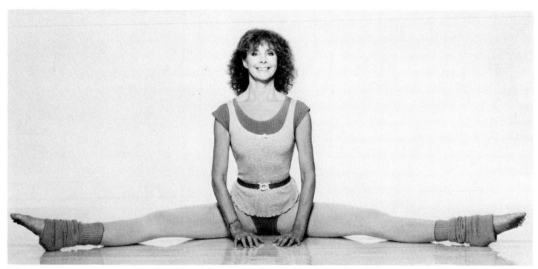

Still sitting on the floor, open your legs as wide as you can without straining the tendons in the inner thighs. You can do this stretch either with straight legs or bent knees. Point your toes. (Don't feel you must open your legs as wide as Shirlee does.)

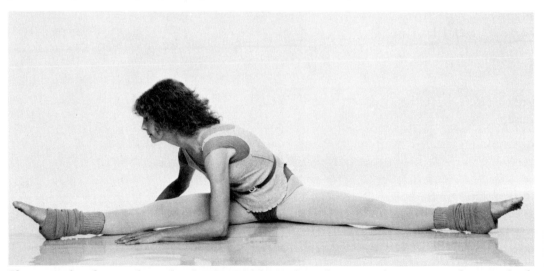

Place your hands on either side of your right leg and reach over with your torso, keeping both hips on the floor and left thigh turned out. Gently pulse for 8 counts.

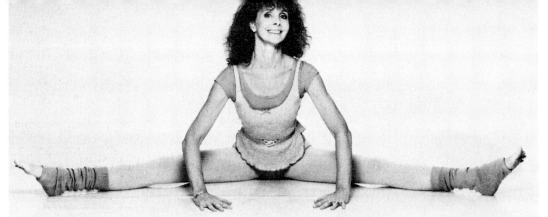

With your hands on the floor in front of you, stretch out of your hips and "walk" yourself around to the left leg in 4 counts.

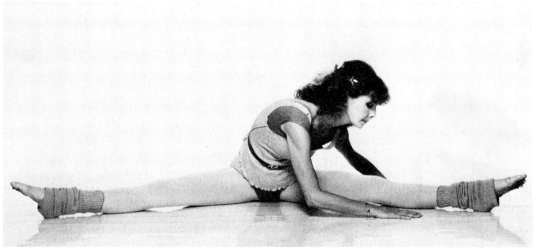

Stretch over your left leg, keeping both hips on the floor and turning your right thigh out. Pulse gently for 8 counts. "Walk" back to center in 2 counts.

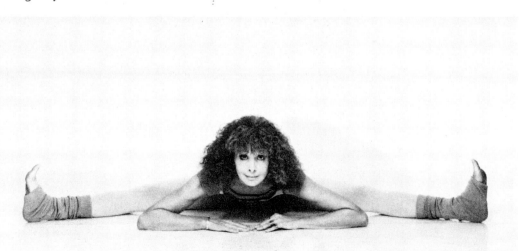

Flex your feet and stretch to the center, trying to lengthen your spine for 16 counts. Do not arch. Shake your legs out and bring them together. Breathe normally.

6

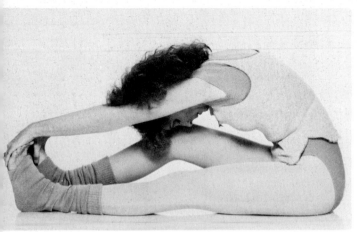

Slowly bring your legs together in front of you and round forward over them. Flex your feet, hold your toes or your lower legs, and bend the right knee . . .

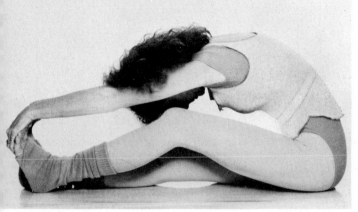

then bend the left knee (this makes one set). Do 8 sets.

Stretch forward over both legs, knees slightly bent, for 8 counts. Then roll up. Breathe normally.

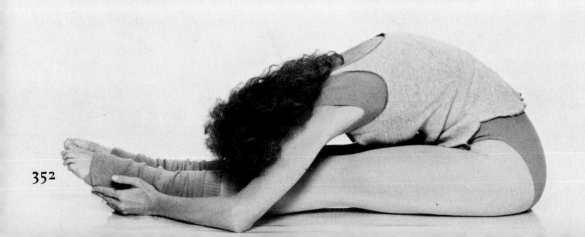

352

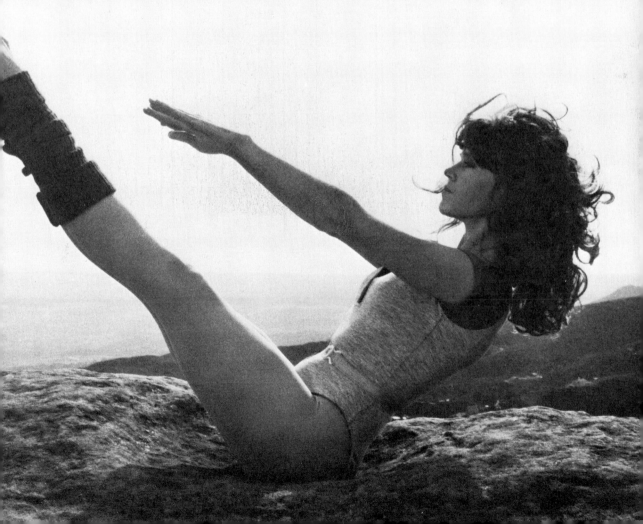

Abdominals

1

You may not be able to do all these stomach exercises at first, or as many repetitions as I've given. Feel free to do as much as you can and build up gradually.

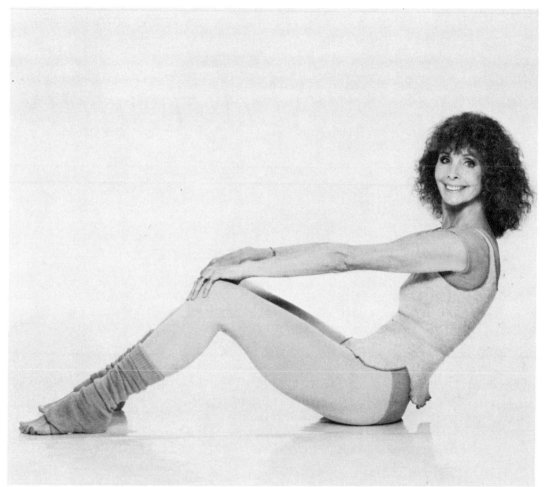

With knees bent and feet flat on the floor, hold on to your knees or thighs to help you roll down onto your back, one vertebra at a time.

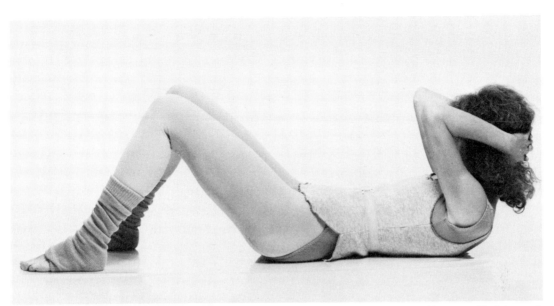

Keeping your feet on the floor, place your hands behind your head with elbows pulled in and lift your head off the floor. Don't attempt to pull your neck up with your hands—all the work should be done with the abdominals. Don't let your hips leave the floor.

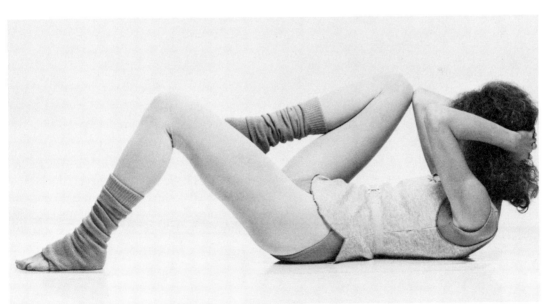

Curl your pubic bone up toward your navel and pull your right knee in toward your right elbow for 2 counts. Lower your leg for 2 counts. Repeat with your left leg to left elbow. (This makes one set.) Do 4 sets. Your head stays lifted throughout the exercise. *Breathing:* Exhale as knee comes in.

2

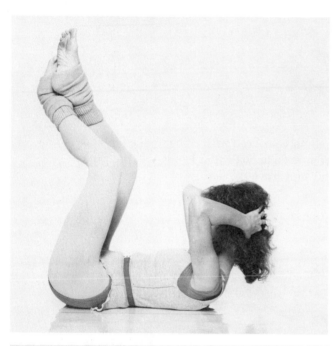

Keeping your head lifted, bend both knees in toward your chest, ankles crossed, hands behind your head with elbows alongside your ears.

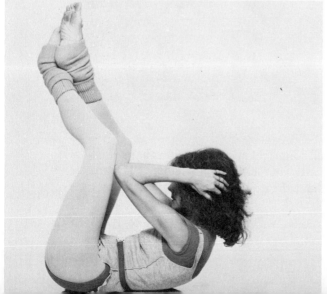

Reach to your knees with your upper body, releasing back a little after each reach, for 8 slow counts and 16 counts double time. Keep your chin to your chest. Use the abdominals to lift, not your arms. *Breathing:* Exhale as you lift.

Reach your right elbow to your left knee . . .

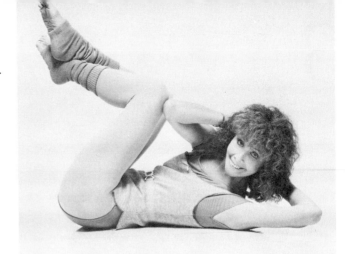

and reverse, reaching your left elbow to your right knee. Do 8 sets slowly, 16 double time. Really try to lift your whole chest and shoulder area—not just your elbows—making the muscle between your navel and pubic bone do all the work. *Breathing:* Exhale each time you reach your elbow to your knee when doing the 8 slow sets, inhaling as you change sides. Exhale every other time when doing the 16 sets double time.

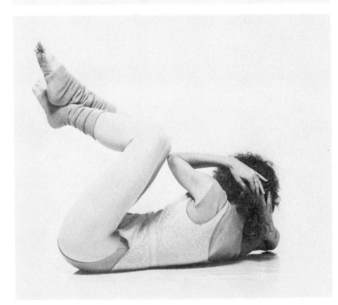

Reach both elbows toward your knees again for 8 counts double time. Exhale as you lift.

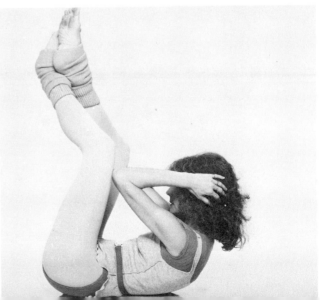

3

Release your head and abdominals and hug your knees tightly to your chest. If this position bothers your knees, clasp your thighs from behind your knees instead of on top.

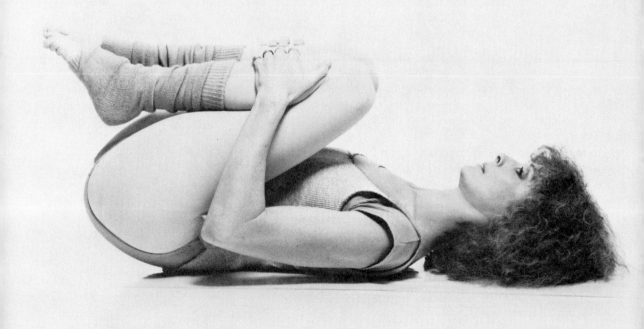

Place your feet on the floor. With left hand behind your head, lift your head and reach
through your legs with your right arm. Keep
your chin to your chest and exhale as you
reach, inhale as you release back a little, 16
times.

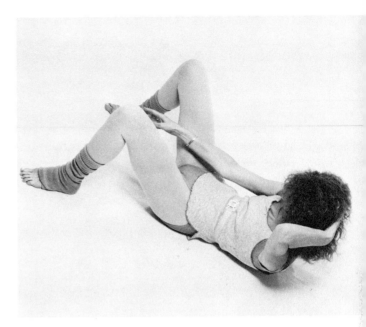

Rest your head and neck for a moment, then reverse arms and repeat 16 times. Be sure not to
put pressure on your neck with your hand. It is the abdominals that should be doing the lifting.

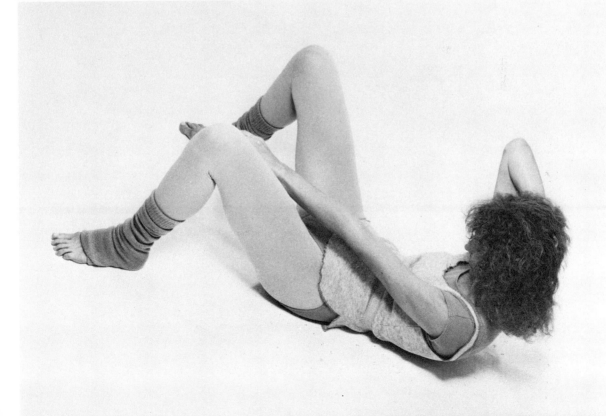

Release your head and abdominals and hug your knees tightly into your chest. If this position causes any discomfort, hold thighs from behind knees instead.

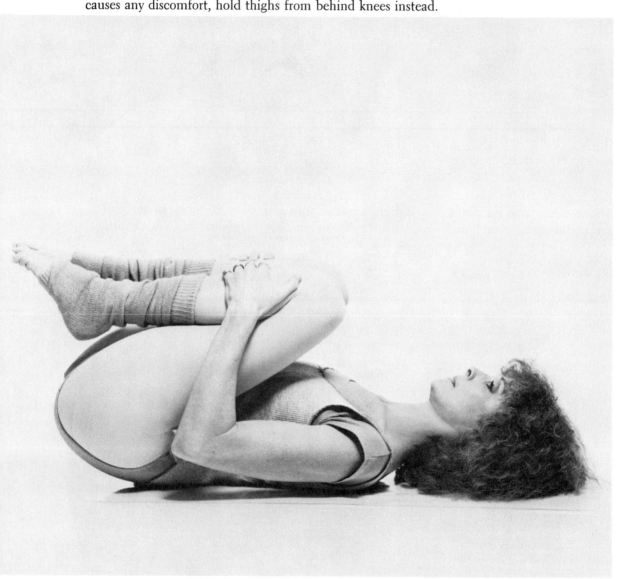

5 Put your feet on the floor and relax your legs. Take your legs to the right side and your arms to the left, and relax.

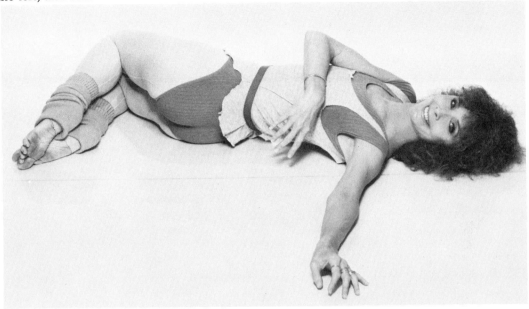

Reverse sides.

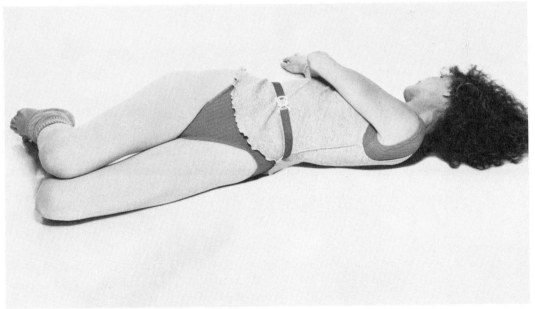

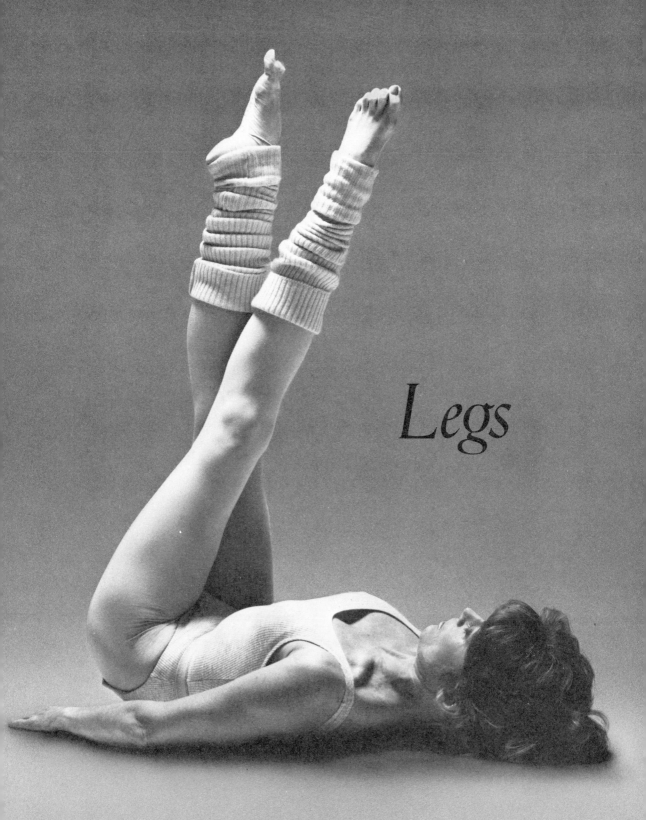

Legs

1

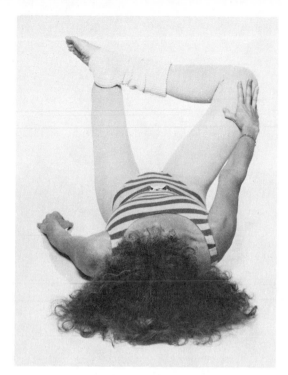

Lying on your back, head and shoulders on the floor, bend both knees. Place your right ankle against your left knee and press the right knee away from you, stretching the inner thigh, for 8 counts.

Repeat with left foot on right knee for 8 counts.

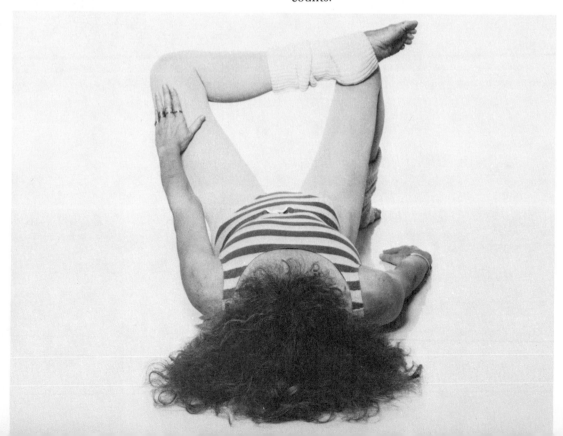

2

Extend your legs straight up, keeping your hips on the floor and your toes pointed.

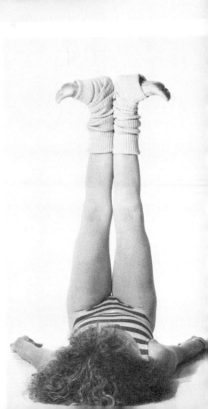

Rotate your legs out from hips, keeping your heels together, and exhale. Rotate legs back to parallel position. Inhale. Do 4 sets.

Keeping your legs straight up, flex your feet . . .

and rotate your legs out from your hips. Rotate them back in. Do 4 sets. Repeat the entire sequence, rotating with pointed toes for 8 sets double time and with flexed feet 8 sets double time.

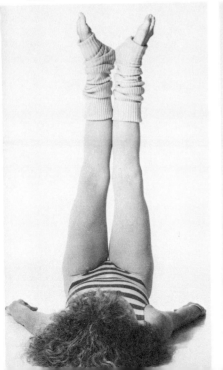

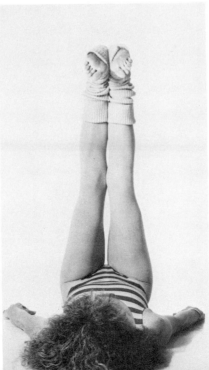

3

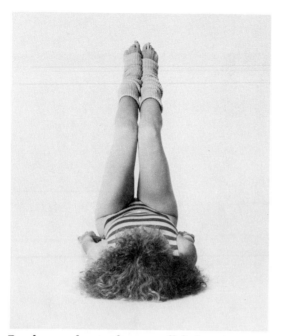

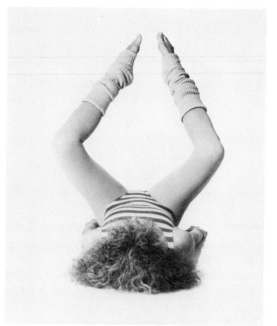

Bend your knees, legs parallel, keeping toes pointed and hips on the floor.

Open bent knees out to side, keeping hips on floor and feet together . . .

extend legs out to the side, still keeping hips on floor . . .

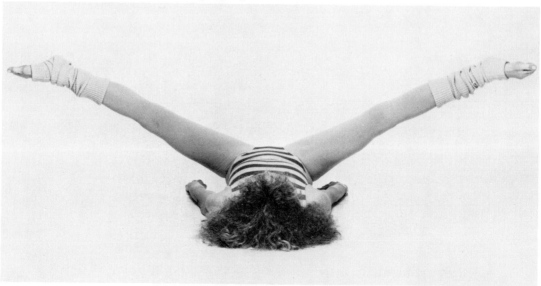

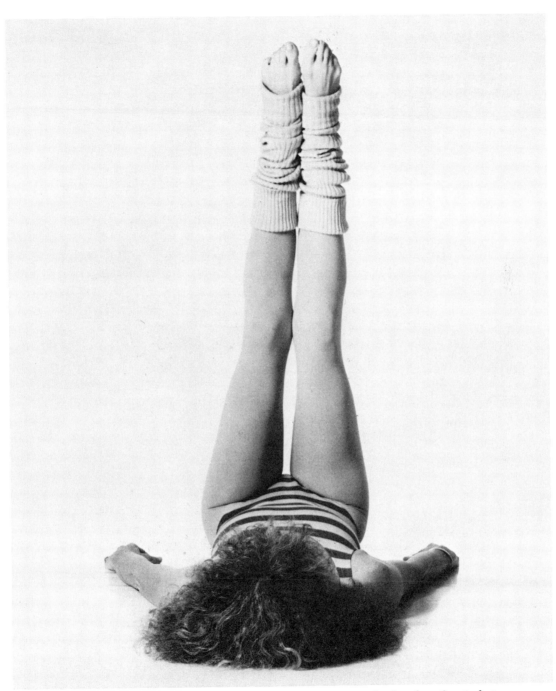

and bring straight legs together. Do the entire sequence once slowly, then 8 sets faster.

4

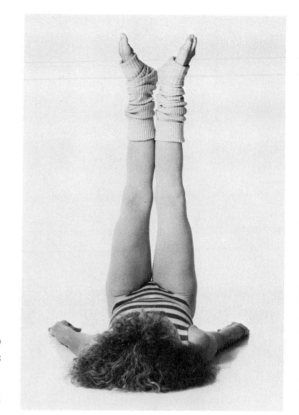

Starting with legs stretched perpendicular to body, turned out from the hip socket, toes pointed . . .

extend legs out to the side, keeping hips on floor, in 2 counts.

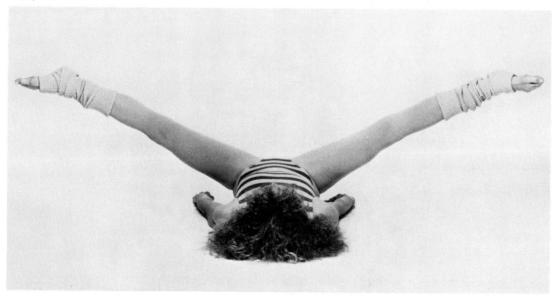

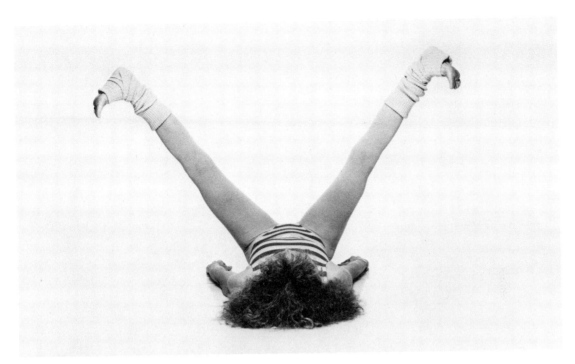

Flex your feet . . .

and bring legs together in 2 counts until heels touch. Point toes and repeat entire sequence once more. Then repeat sequence faster, opening legs only halfway, for 8 sets.

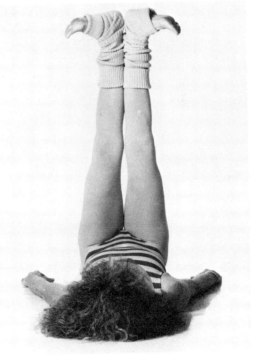

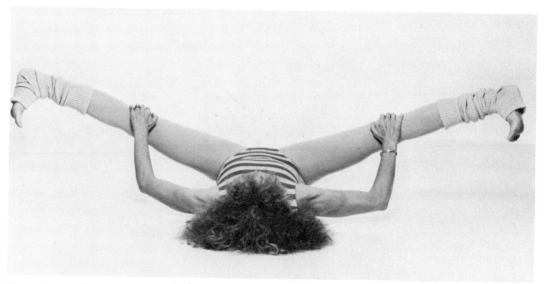

5

Extend your legs out to the side with flexed feet and place your hands on your inner knees. (Don't bounce legs toward the floor.)

Keeping your knees stationary, bring your heels halfway in for 4 counts and extend them out again in 4 counts. Do 2 sets. *Breathing:* Exhale as you extend heels.

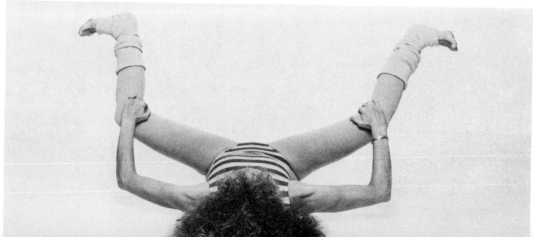

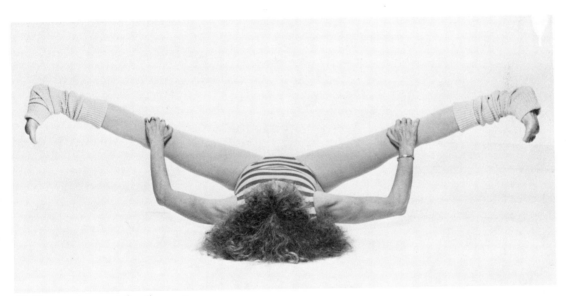

Hold your legs out for 5 counts.

6

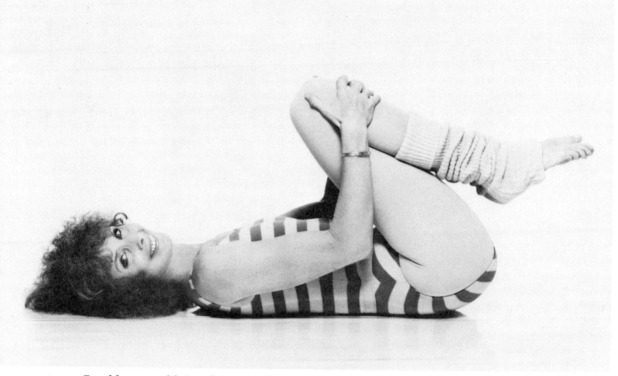

Bend knees and bring them together. Holding your knees, press them to your chest. If this position bothers your knees, clasp your thighs from behind your knees instead of on top.

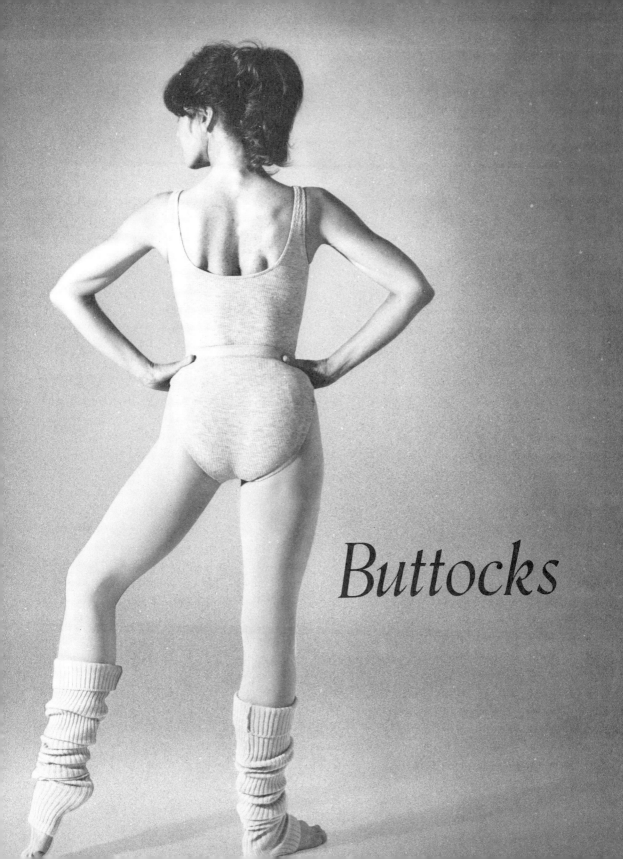

Buttocks

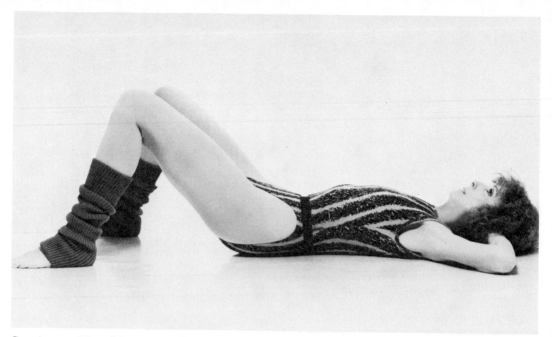

1

Starting position: Lie on your back, knees and feet parallel, feet flat on the floor a little more than hip distance apart, your hands behind your head, small of the back pressed toward the floor.

Curl your pubic bone up toward your navel and squeeze the buttocks muscles, letting hips come slightly off the floor, then relax, letting hips return to floor. Curl up and release 8 times, then repeat for 32 counts double time. It may help prevent your back from arching if you place both hands palms down beneath your lower back and make sure your lower back is touching the tops of your hands throughout the exercise.

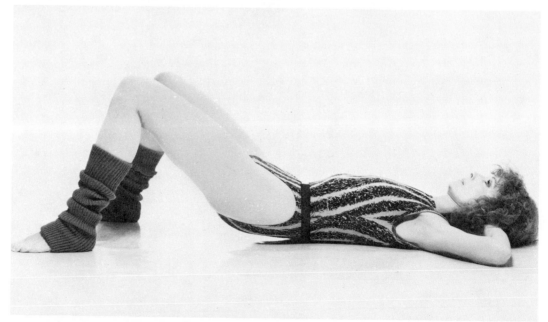

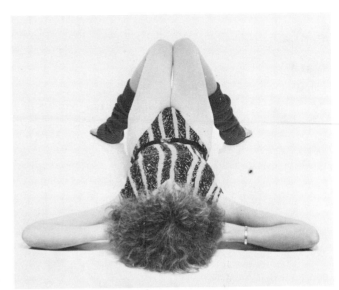

Move your feet slightly farther apart. With pelvis curled upward, hips slightly off the floor, squeeze the buttocks as you press knees together . . .

. . . then open them to the side, keeping hips stationary. Repeat opening and closing the knees as you keep the pubic bone lifted and buttocks squeezed tight for 16 sets.

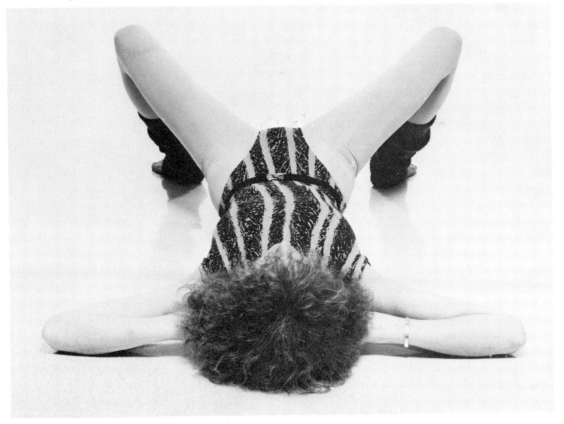

3

Adjust your knees and feet to a parallel position. Keeping your lower back pressed down, curl up then release your hips 8 times double time. Hold for 8 counts, then lower.

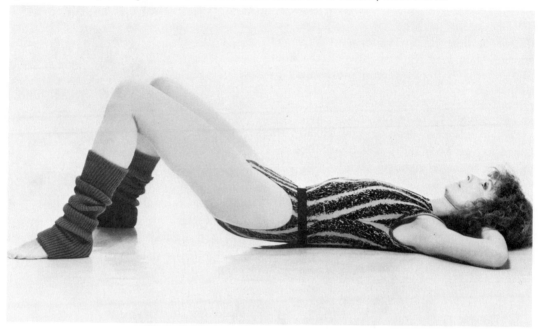

4

Place right ankle against your left knee and with your hands pull left knee to chest, stretching right hip for 8 counts. Repeat with other leg.

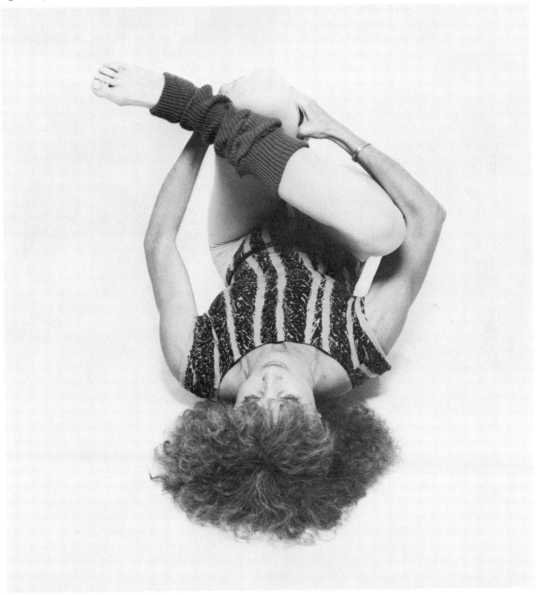

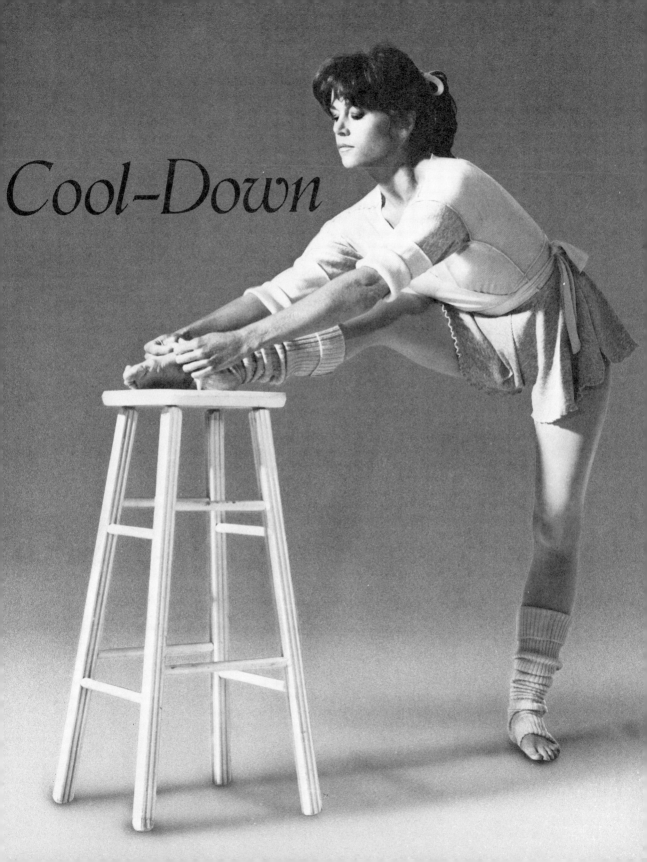

Cool-Down

1

Stretch your legs and your arms straight out on the floor, so you're in one long line. Clasp hands, flex feet and reach with your arms as you inhale. Hold.

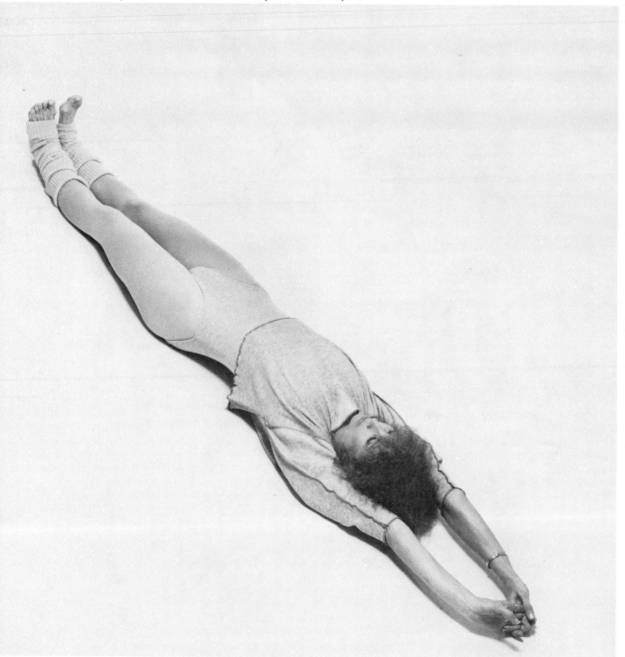

Release the stretch as you exhale. Do 2 times.

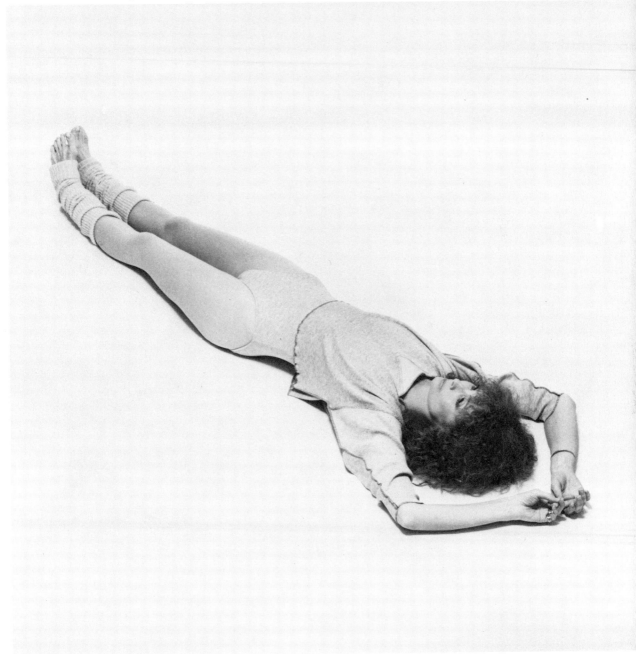

2

Bend both knees into chest . . .

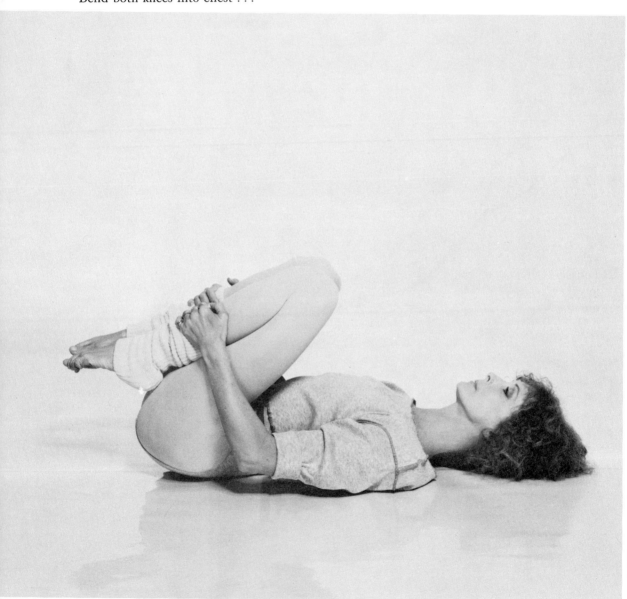

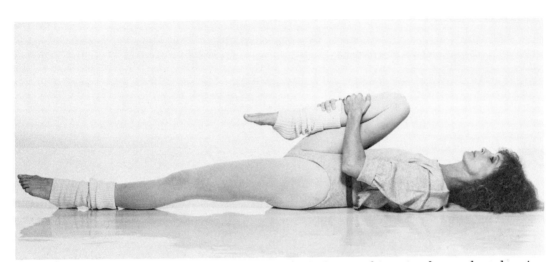

then clasp the right knee and extend the left leg. Stretch your chin toward your chest, keeping head on the floor to lengthen the spine, and keep the small of your back pressed into the floor. Clasp your thigh from the back of the knee instead of from above if this position causes any discomfort.

Then reverse.

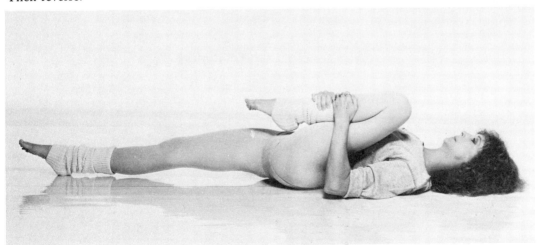

3

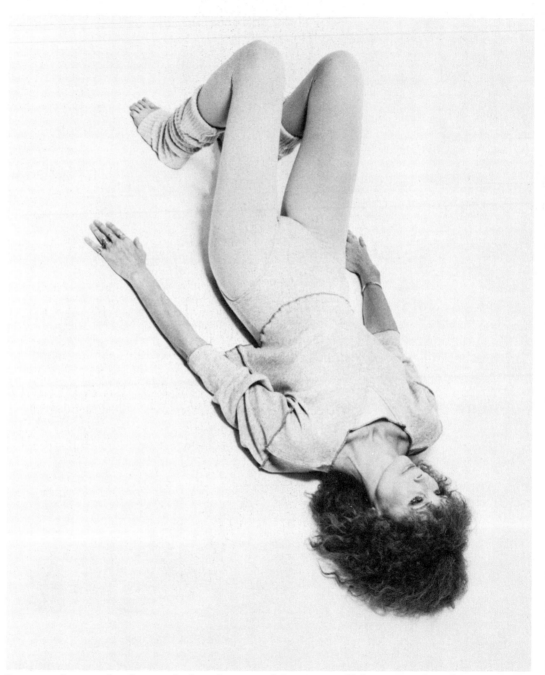

Put your feet on the floor and place knees and feet in parallel position, hip distance apart. Bring your arms to your sides and press the small of the back into the floor.

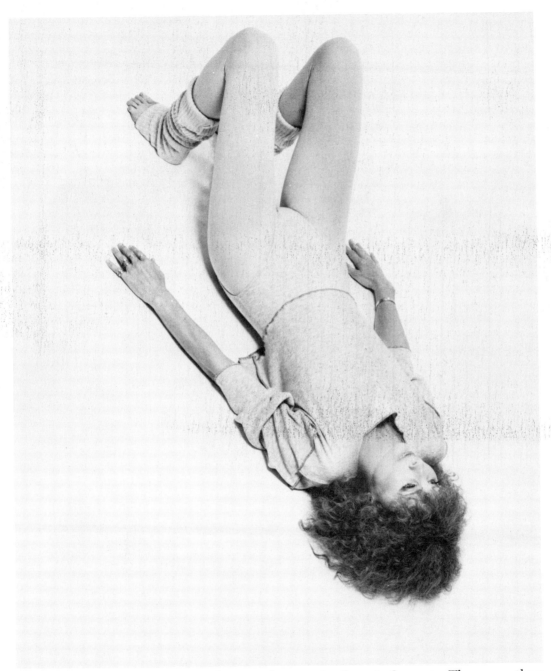

Shrug both shoulders to your ears, keeping them on the floor, in 2 counts. Then press them back to normal position in 2 counts. Do 2 sets.

Turn head to the right in 2 counts . . .

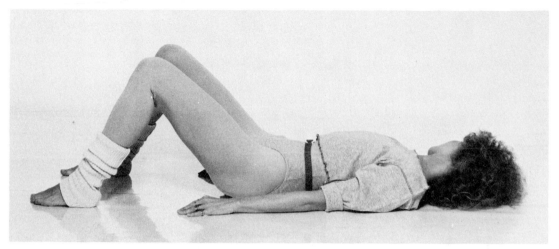

then back to center in 2 counts . . .

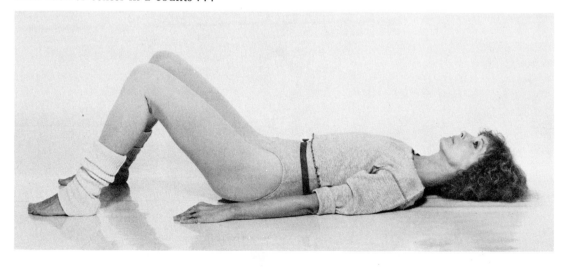

then to the left in 2 counts . . .

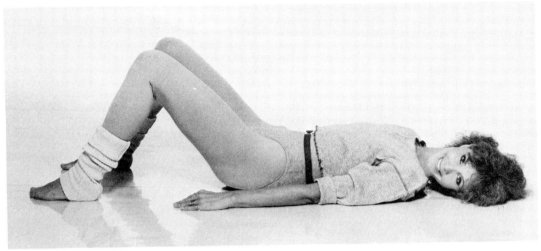

and back to center in 2 counts. Take a deep breath and as you exhale try to lengthen your spine along the floor. Repeat one more time.

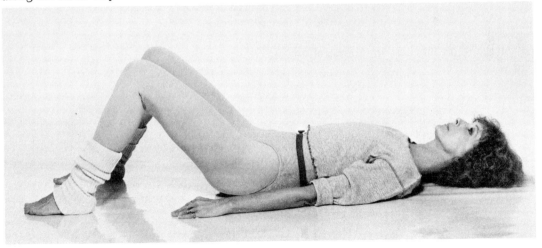

5

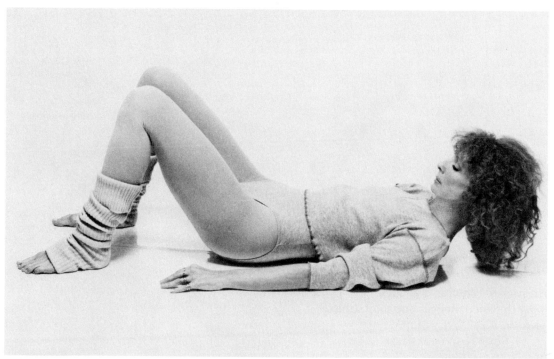

Bring your chin to your chest and roll up slowly
toward your knees.

Place your right leg in front of your left leg and
come up onto your feet.

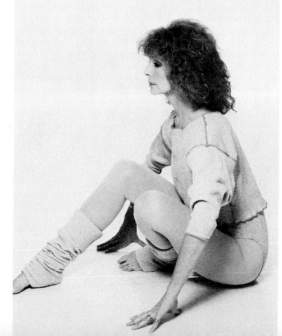

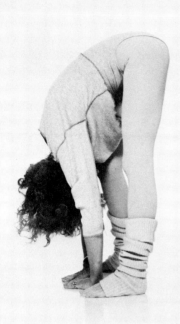

Stretching over your legs, bend the right knee and hold for 4 counts, feeling the back of your left leg lengthening . . .

then bend the left knee and hold for 4 counts. Concentrate on stretching the back of your right leg. You should place your hands on your lower legs or thighs if it is difficult to reach the floor.

Bend both knees, pull in your abdominals, and roll up to a standing position, one vertebra at a time.

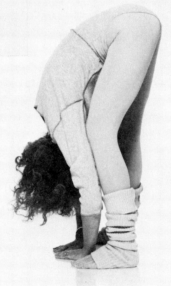

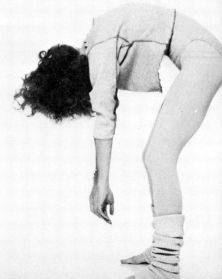

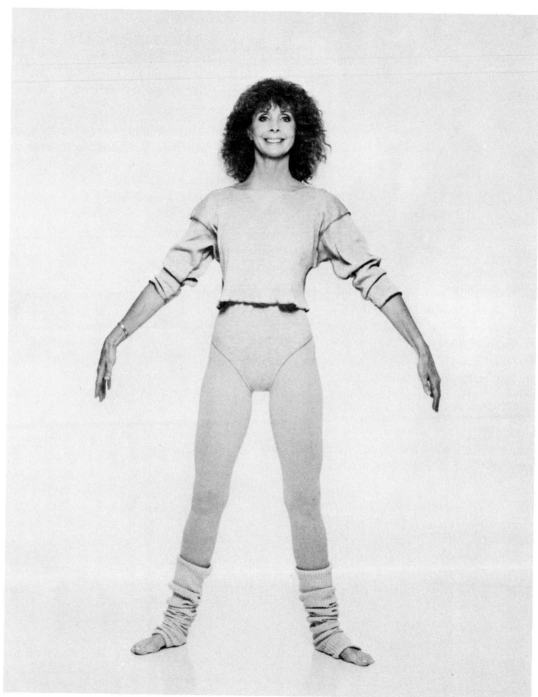

Place feet, slightly turned out, a little more than hip distance apart. Inhale while lifting arms above head, palms down.

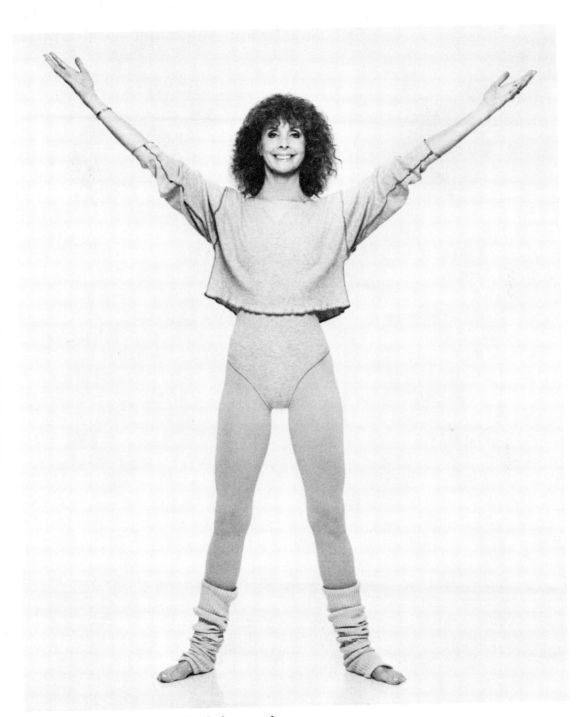

Exhale while bringing arms back down, palms up.

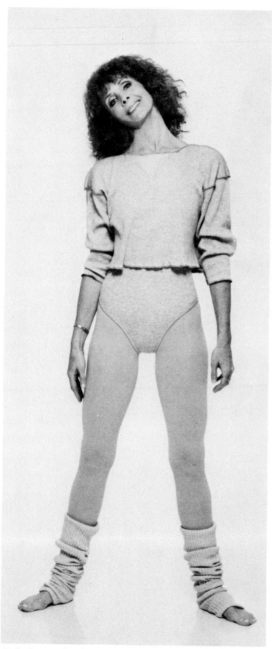 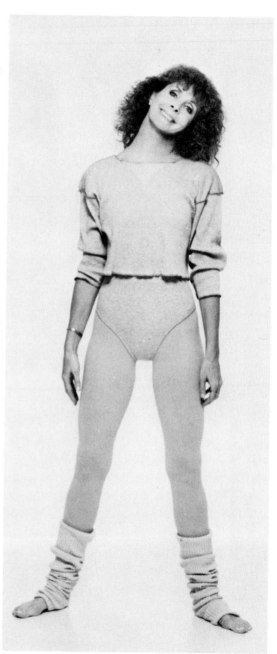

Inhale. Exhale as you take your head to the   then repeat to the left.
right, ear to shoulder, and stretch. Inhale . . .

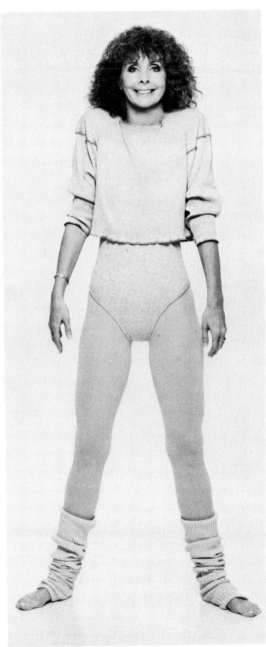

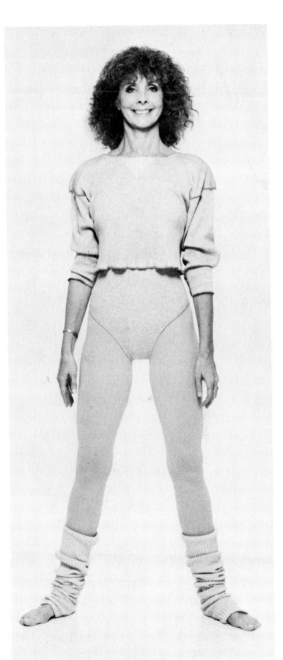

Inhale while lifting shoulders up . . .

exhale while pressing shoulders down. Do this 2 times. As you lower your shoulders think of lengthening your spine and growing taller.

Good work!

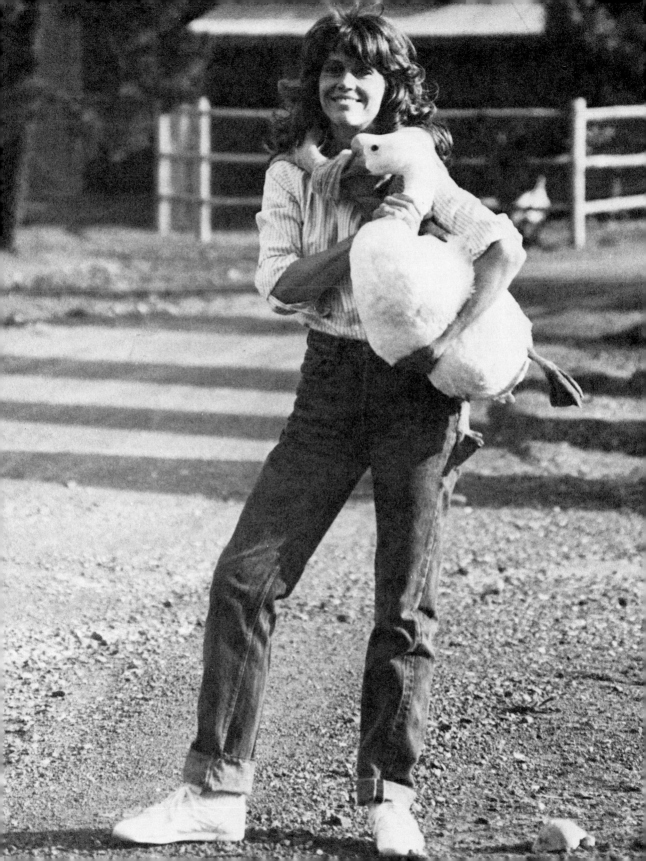

PART SIX

Completing the Picture

Me with Newton, our goose, at Laurel Springs.

CHAPTER **15**

PLANNED PATIENTHOOD

THIS BOOK IS PRIMARILY ABOUT taking responsibility for your own health and fitness during midlife and beyond. Regular exercise and good nutrition are the cornerstones of a self-help approach. But there is one final key ingredient that must be addressed: developing a *partnership* of trust with a physician. I stress partnership because we want to avoid giving ourselves blindly over to anyone's care. We have to equip ourselves with enough information so that we can have an informed dialogue with the physician we choose. The following guidelines will help you move in this direction:

1.   **Build an ongoing relationship with a primary-care physician.**
     Each of us should have a knowledgeable, personable doctor to whom we can turn for our overall health care needs. You don't want to wait until there's an emergency, then search hurriedly for a doctor whom you don't know and who doesn't know you. Choosing your regular primary-care physician takes time and is best done when you are well. This will give you a chance to become acquainted with each other before a medical need arises.
     Primary-care physicians for women are frequently gynecologists with a knowledge of general medicine. Your doctor can also be an internist or a general practitioner with a sound knowledge of gynecology. Ask friends, neighbors, or other doctors you may know if they have someone to recommend. If a doctor has a good reputation, she or he will be more apt to be someone you'll want to stay with.
     Here are the most important qualities to look for as you search for and interview health care professionals:

- Experience and ease working with women in their middle years
- The perspective that the processes of aging and menopause are normal
- Good ability to communicate—an openness to your questions and concerns, willingness to provide complete information about the state of your health, full explanations of any recommended treatment and the alternatives, and willingness to give you access to your records
- The consistent practice of keeping up-to-date on the latest medical information
- A philosophy of prevention and the understanding that health depends on many interacting factors
- A conservatism when it comes to prescribing tests, drugs, and surgery
- Reasonable availability
- Confidentiality
- A sense of mutual regard and friendliness
- The presence of a competent and supportive staff (Often, the morale of the staff can tell you a great deal about the nature of the physician or group of physicians they work for.)

2. Keep written records of your health.

If you don't already do so, I suggest you begin to keep a personal file or ongoing notebook of your physical health. I've found the longer one's medical history gets, the harder it is to remember everything and the more important the specifics seem to become. A brief, to-the-point journal will keep all the information you need at your fingertips. If it's convenient, you can even bring the notebook with you on doctor visits, along with a list of any questions you might want to ask or copies of X rays from your file that may be pertinent. Here's what I recommend including:

- The names and addresses of doctors you've visited, along with the dates and purposes of the visits
- Your notes about the outcome of these visits, including any medication prescribed
- Your experience with the medication and whether there were any negative side effects or allergies

- Any surgery performed, as well as the name and address of the hospital and surgeon
- Currrent or past occupational hazards
- The health history of your immediate family—your parents, sisters, and brothers
- The chart of your menstrual patterns and any signs of menopause
- Anything else regarding your physical health you'd like to remind yourself about

If you want a copy of your official medical records either from a hospital or a private physician, you should know that every state regulates patient access differently. As of 1980, only 25 states had a law on the books allowing direct access to hospital records, and only 15 states to private physicians' records. And even these regulations vary. Some permit copying the whole file, some just reading it. Some specify the right to receive only a summary of the file. In the best of circumstances, a physician may allow patients access to their records even when not legally bound to do so by state regulations. But whatever the case, *every* state requires that your medical record be forwarded to another physician or to an attorney upon your written request and authorization.

3.   Know the special health concerns of women in midlife.
Menopause, a healthy aspect of women's aging, has already been discussed at length. In the remaining pages of this chapter I want to outline the basics of two other of the most important health issues for midlife women—the surgical operation of hysterectomy and the chronic disease of breast cancer. These are *not* normal aspects of the aging process. Both tend, however, to be increasingly prevalent as women grow older. For that reason, I believe it essential to find out what we need to know in order to minimize our risk of experiencing either.

HYSTERECTOMY

Hysterectomy is the most common major operation in the United States. In fact, our country has the highest hysterectomy rate in the world and the numbers continue to rise. If this continues, *more than*

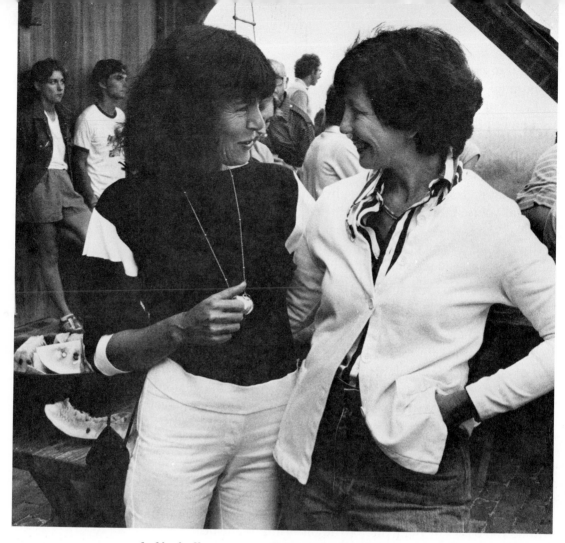

half of all women will have had a hysterectomy by age 65—and many needlessly. An estimated 40 percent of all hysterectomies are believed to be unnecessary! In addition, there is a high rate of complications, a long recovery period, and the operation is expensive. For all of these reasons, I think we need to be fortified with facts should such surgery ever be recommended to us.

One of the most important decisions involved in having a hysterectomy regards the extent of the operation. A hysterectomy is the surgical removal of the uterus, but the procedure frequently means more than that. If "partial," the surgery will remove the uterus only and exclude the cervix or uterine opening. If "simple," it will remove the cervix as well. A "total" or "complete" hysterectomy will include the uterus and the cervix along with the ovaries and fallopian tubes. (The removal of one or both ovaries is often referred to as an oophorectomy.)

We have to be absolutely certain what the physician is suggesting and why. I know of instances where women have had their ovaries removed without realizing it in advance, for example. And now that we know the ovaries continue to play a role in hormone production after menopause, their removal should never be routine.

The removal of any part of our reproductive organs should *only* be done in response to the threat of a major disease—after all other medical alternatives have been explored. A hysterectomy should *not* be done for purposes of sterilization, for instance. There are other methods available—such as tubal ligation—and they are much safer, simpler, less expensive, and don't have the possible aftereffects of a hysterectomy. Nor should a hysterectomy necessarily be done for a prolapsed or "fallen" uterus (this can be a matter of a simple surgical repair) or for small fibroid growths (these usually shrink on their own following menopause). Lastly, a hysterectomy should not be done for reasons of prevention when there is no indication of disease present. The ovaries, for instance, have sometimes been removed just as a precaution against ovarian cancer, a highly fatal but relatively uncommon cancer among women.

The following conditions are valid reasons to consider hysterectomy:

- Cancer of the cervix, uterus, ovaries, tubes, or vagina
- Extreme endometriosis that is unresponsive to other treatments (this is the appearance of uterine lining tissue outside the uterus)
- An excessive number of *large* benign fibroids which may be pressing on the bladder or other organs
- Excessive and prolonged bleeding that doesn't respond to a D&C or other medical treatment
- *Chronic* disease or infection in the tubes or ovaries.

The Second Opinion

Unless the surgery is an emergency, ALWAYS seek a second opinion. Usually hysterectomies are elective non-emergency surgery and you will have enough time to make the best decision and to avoid the experience of an unnecessary operation. Don't be shy about getting a second opinion. This is a long and honored practice in the medical profession and should be routine for anyone facing elective surgery—particularly in the area of gynecology, where the first doctor's opinion is often reversed.

You want the second opinion to be *independent* and you can go about obtaining it in several ways. You can ask your physician to refer you to another surgeon not connected to her or his own practice. You can also find another surgeon on your own by asking friends for recommendations or by calling the Second Surgical Opinion Hot Line (800-638-6833). This is a national toll-free number that will provide you with local contacts and with a list of questions to ask the surgeon. Whomever you finally select, let this surgeon know you are seeking her or his opinion but that she or he will not do the surgery if indeed it is necessary. You can ask your physician to brief the other—at least to send on a copy of your records. Or you may decide you want to go to a second physician with no information having been exchanged. If the first doctor seems uncooperative about your seeking a second opinion, that's a clue to go elsewhere.

If the second opinion doesn't agree with the first, or if you're still not convinced the operation needs to be done, then seek a third opinion. Your insurance will usually cover the cost.

BREAST CANCER

Over the last few years, I've noticed more of my friends going to the doctor because of a lump in their breast. Most are relieved to find the growth is benign. Some have to face the frightening and painful reality that they have a malignancy. All of us need to learn as much as we can about these phenomena because the plain fact is one out of eleven women will experience breast cancer—normally but not always after age thirty-five. Breast cancer remains the leading cause of death for midlife women until age fifty-five, at which time it trades place with heart disease. But there are things we can do that can make a difference.

Like all cancers, breast cancer is a disease of the cells. There are actually about fifteen different types of breast cancer. For example,

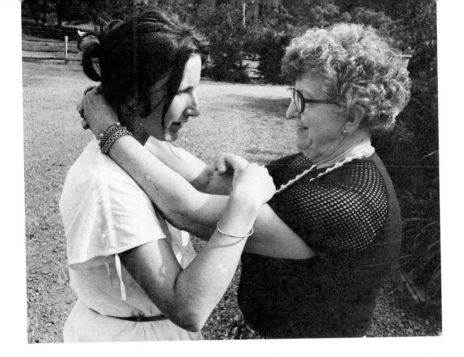

some tumors grow and eventually invade other tissues outside of the breast, while others grow but stop before spreading. The bad news about every kind of breast cancer is that we still haven't found the cause or the cure and the overall mortality figures have been more or less constant over the last fifty years. And in spite of the fact that breast cancer is the *leading* cause of cancer death for all women and a special danger to midlife women, only *four percent* of the national cancer research budget is spent on breast cancer! We have to see that this is changed. The good news is that a great deal of progress is being made. Treatment of breast cancer today is often less radical than in the past and, if the tumor is discovered early, the chances for a longer survival are much better.

Being Prepared

Let me walk you through what I've learned about what to do if you think you've detected a sign of potential cancer in one of your breasts. These signs might be any of the following:

- A lump or thickening in the breast
- A discharge from the nipple
- A scaliness of the skin, especially around the nipple

- A change in color or texture
- A dimpling or puckering
- A change in shape
- Any change from your normal patterns not related to the menstrual cycle

The first thing to remember should you notice one or more of these changes is that 85 percent of the lumps discovered turn out to be benign or nonmalignant. Such breast lumps, in fact, are more common than we tend to think. Knowing this, I hope, will help you to be less fearful and to see a doctor without delay if you notice anything unusual about your breasts. This is the immediate step to take. You will probably want to go to your primary care physician or gynecologist first. You might also want instead to seek out a doctor specifically trained or interested in the detection and diagnosis of breast disease. (This should *always* be done before any breast surgery.) You can find such a specialist through your primary-care physician or gynecologist, from friends or a local medical school, or by calling the national toll-free Cancer Hot Line (800-4-CANCER) or your local American Cancer Society.

The diagnosis should proceed in a series of steps. (In fact, if the doctor you select doesn't follow these, you should ask why.)

The physician will begin with a manual breast exam and two key tests: a *mammography*, which is an X ray of the breast, and a *needle aspiration* of the breast lump. The insertion of a fine needle will generally yield fluid if the lump is merely a benign cyst and this fluid will then be analyzed. (This is not painful.) The mammography will detect, with 85 percent accuracy, tumors too small to feel. Other less accurate breast "pictures" may also be taken and used for later follow-up testing. Thermography uses infrared scanners to detect abnormalities; it's best for confirmations and watching changes in the breast over time. Ultrasonography uses sound waves for detecting breast patterns but is best for finding cysts and not for distinguishing between malignant and benign breast lumps, as a mammogram can.

If the needle aspiration doesn't yield fluid or if the lab analysis and breast X ray don't give you an absolutely clean bill of health, the physician will recommend a *surgical biopsy* which usually involves removing the whole mass for lab analysis. In years past, women were asked to sign a form which authorized the surgeon to remove the entire breast at the same time if a quick examination of the tissue showed it to be malignant. *This "one-step procedure" is no longer recommended.* A short delay between the biopsy and whatever breast surgery may need to follow is now the preferred route should breast cancer be diagnosed. Such a time lapse gives us a chance to examine our options and decide with our physician upon the best course of treatment. It gives the lab a chance to study the tissue more carefully and the doctor the ability to determine more precisely the extent and type of the cancer.

Options

The most important thing to know about your surgical options is that you won't necessarily have to lose your breast. The old disfiguring "radical mastectomy" is on its way out. This procedure, sometimes called the Halsted after the physician who initiated it, removed not only the entire breast but also the chest muscles underneath and the lymph system extending throughout the chest and under the arm.

The most common treatment today is the "total mastectomy" (what used to be called the "modified radical mastectomy"). This surgery removes the breast and the lymph nodes under the arm but leaves the chest muscles in place. It has been shown to have the same survival rate as the more severe surgery and reconstruction of the breast is possible afterward if you want it. We now know that taking *more* is not necessarily better.

Another alternative, relatively new and increasingly chosen, spares all or most of the breast and may have equally good survival rates. Called a "lumpectomy," this procedure removes the lump itself, the tissue immediately surrounding it, and often some of the lymph nodes under the arm to determine whether the cancer has spread. The surgery is followed by treatments of radiation and later, if the cancer has moved beyond the breast, by chemotherapy or anticancer drugs. As I write, studies are being done to compare results of the total mastectomy and the lumpectomy, with *and* without radiation.

The size of the lump is a critical factor in deciding whether or not a woman can be a candidate for lumpectomy, so early detection again is crucial. A lump smaller than an inch in diameter is safest (Stage I breast cancer). A lump smaller than two inches, with or without evidence the cancer has spread, *may* qualify (Stage II). Fortunately, the vast majority of cancerous breast growths are caught before progressing beyond these stages, about half no further than Stage I.*

Before breast surgery, there are several other important steps to take. (1) Decide whether you may later want to have your breast rebuilt so the surgeon can make any necessary surgical variations in anticipation of the later reconstruction. (Should you not decide until afterward, however, such plastic surgery is still a possibility.) (2) Make advance arrangements to have your breast tissue tested immediately after removal for its responsiveness to estrogen and progesterone. One third of all breast cancers are strongly hormone-dependent, which means they are fostered by the body's own hormones. One third are not and the other third fall somewhere in between. The estrogen receptor assay (ERA) is now routine, but the progesterone receptor assay (PRA) is fairly new and you should be sure preparations are made for both of these tests. The results should be kept permanently in your records. They tell the physician whether manipulating your hormone balance can make a difference in follow-up treatment and in preventing a recurrence. (3) Plan an exercise program in advance. Discuss this with your physician or a physical therapist. Or seek out an already established program in your area such as Reach for Recovery, offered by the American Cancer Society, ENCORE by the YWCA, or services offered by many Jewish Community Centers. Thorough upper body exercise, offered by these programs and by the Prime Time Workout as well, is a crucial part of the recovery from breast surgery.

Prevention

Like most chronic disease, breast cancer is not thought to have any one cause. Our first clues for prevention are the known *risk factors:*

* If breast cancer is found early at Stage I, there is now an 87 percent chance of survival beyond five years, and 70 percent beyond ten years. If treated at Stage II, the figures are 70 percent and 50 percent. If discovered beyond that, there is a 47 percent five-year survival rate.

- Previous personal history of breast cancer
- Family history of breast cancer, on either side of the family, but especially in a mother or sister, especially if their cancer developed before the age of forty, and more so if it occurred in both breasts
- Being over the age of forty
- A long reproductive life—due to early menstruation (before twelve), late menopause (after fifty), or both
- No pregnancies
- Giving birth for first time after age thirty-five
- Not having nursed one's children
- Late or no sexual activity
- Excessive exposure to radiation
- Prior personal history of other cancer
- Prior personal history of benign tumors, for example, fibrocystic breast condition
- Unusual obesity or height
- European Jewish ancestry, non-Jews of northern European background, and affluent black women
- Living in urban industrialized areas of the northeastern United States

Unfortunately, even these risk factors are somewhat uncertain, so until more is known, *all of us* have to proceed as if we're at risk and, hence, need to integrate into our daily lives certain precautions that I'll now summarize for you.

1. Monthly Breast Self-Exam

You've already seen the importance of early detection. Breast self-examination is probably the most important part of that. *Ninety percent* of all breast lumps are found by women themselves or by their lovers—not by the physician. The biggest problem with self-exam, though, is that most of us tend to avoid it because it means looking for something we don't want to find. What we have to remember is that the vast majority of all lumps are benign. So we need to become familiar with our own breasts, develop the habit of observing them for any changes, and gain the confidence that we'll be able to recognize early anything that might be amiss. Your physician can teach you how to examine your breasts and can explain very graphically the feel of a breast lump. See also the chart on page 408.

How to Examine Your Breasts

With practice, these three simple steps will become second nature. Follow them *once every month.* Before menopause, the best time to check your breasts is about a week after your period, when breasts are usually not tender or swollen. After menopause or total hysterectomy, make the first day of the month your regular time.

1 IN THE SHOWER:

Examine your breasts during bath or shower; hands glide easily over wet skin. Fingers flat, move gently over every part of each breast. Use right hand to examine left breast, left hand for right breast. Check for any lump, hard knot or thickening.

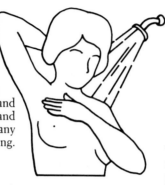

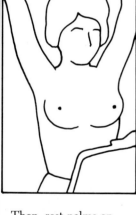

2 BEFORE A MIRROR:

Inspect your breasts with arms at your sides. Next, raise your arms high overhead. Look for any changes in contour of each breast, a swelling, dimpling of skin or changes in the nipple.

Then, rest palms on hips and press down firmly to flex your chest muscles. Left and right breast will not exactly match on most women.

Regular inspection shows what is normal for you and will give you confidence in your examination.

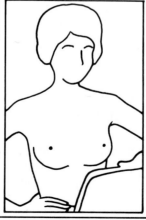

3 LYING DOWN:

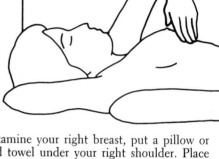

To examine your right breast, put a pillow or folded towel under your right shoulder. Place right hand behind your head—this distributes breast tissue more evenly on the chest. With left hand, fingers flat, press gently in small circular motions around an imaginary clock face. Begin at outermost top of your right breast for 12 o'clock, then move to 1 o'clock, and so on around the circle back to 12. A ridge of firm tissue in the lower curve of each breast is normal. Then move in an inch, toward the nipple; keep circling to examine *every part of your breast,* including nipple. This requires at least three more circles. Now, using your right hand, slowly repeat procedure on your left breast with a pillow under your left shoulder and left hand behind head. Notice how your breast structure feels.

Finally, squeeze the nipple of each breast gently between thumb and index finger. Any discharge, clear or bloody, should be reported to your doctor immediately.

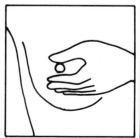

2. Periodic Checks by Your Physician

Breast examination by your doctor is important too, even though you still know your own breasts best. You and your physician should decide how often you need to see her or him, depending on your level of risk. The American Cancer Society recommends a physician's breast exam every three years between the ages of twenty and forty, and every year after that.

3. The Mammogram

Having a mammogram done to *diagnose* a suspicious breast lump is crucial. Having a mammography to *screen* seemingly healthy breasts for cancer is another matter and a step we need to consider carefully. The benefit is that a mammogram can detect cancer growths even *before* you can feel them. The danger is that the radiation involved is also a risk factor for breast cancer. Fortunately, new equipment which X-rays breasts at very low doses of radiation is now available.

The National Cancer Institute recommends that women in the following categories discuss with their physicians having *routine* mammograms:

- All women over the age of fifty
- Women over forty whose mothers or sisters have had breast cancer
- Women over thirty-five who have had breast cancer before

The American Cancer Society (ACS) goes a bit further and recommends that between the ages of thirty-five and forty *every* woman have a *baseline* mammogram to keep in her permanent records. This gives a standard by which to compare later tests. The ACS also suggests discussing with our physicians the possibility of having a number of follow-up mammograms in our forties. They recommend an *annual* mammogram for everyone after age fifty.

Whatever you decide with your physician, always make sure the latest low-dosage equipment is being used.* If you need to have X

---

* 1983 American College of Radiology mammography guidelines recommend the dosage not be higher than one rad (radiation absorbed dosage) for a two-view examination of each breast (or four pictures total). The latest equipment falls within these boundaries.

rays for any other reason, always make sure your breasts are protectively shielded.

4. Proper Diet and Regular Exercise

Diet is now thought to be a *major* factor in the development of breast cancer—particularly a *high-fat diet*. The highest rates of cancer appear in countries like ours where intake of fat is the highest. Conversely, countries with low-fat diets have little or no breast cancer at all. American women, for example, consume over three times the fat that Japanese women do—for whom breast cancer is almost nonexistent. When Japanese women migrate to the West and begin to eat a Western diet, they are known to become suddenly vulnerable to breast cancer. The hypothesis is that fat in the diet may indirectly intensify an estrogenic environment that can foster some kinds of breast cancer.

To reduce the incidence of all cancers, the following dietary guidelines are important:

- Eat less saturated *and* unsaturated fat.
- Eat more complex carbohydrates.
- Eat plenty of foods high in vitamin C and vitamin A (or beta-carotene, the vitamin A precursor found in dark green and deep yellow vegetables like carrots).
- Make sure you eat lots of vegetables such as broccoli, cabbage, cauliflower, brussels sprouts, and spinach, which appear to have a particularly potent detoxifying effect.
- Avoid processed foods and their additives.
- Maintain your normal weight and lose excess fat if necessary.
- Drink alcohol in moderation, if at all.
- Do not smoke.

The role of the immune system in protecting against cancer is imperfectly understood, but proper diet and regular exercise will help to keep your immune system functioning at its best.

5. Alleviating Benign Breast Conditions

About one in five women has some kind of benign or fibrocystic breast condition. This is characterized by cysts or solid fibrous growths that cause a tenderness and swelling similar to but independent of the swelling or lumps we often have before and during menstruation. We aren't sure of a direct connection with breast cancer, but at the moment benign breast disease appears to be a *possible* risk factor. Doctors have had some success in alleviating this condition when women eliminate caffeine altogether and take up to 600 I.U. of vitamin E daily (see p. 214 of "Eating for the Long Run"). If you have a fibrocystic breast condition, I suggest you talk to your doctor about these dietary suggestions. The fewer breast lumps you have the more accurate your self-exams will be and the better your peace of mind.

6.   Caution for Estrogen Therapy

Because some cancers are hormone-dependent, estrogen therapy for menopause may be a risk factor for breast cancer. If you have decided to take estrogen, be sure its effects are balanced by taking progesterone at certain prescribed times. Unfortunately, we don't yet know the long-range effects of progesterone therapy itself.

DO YOU SMOKE?

- Smoking is the largest single cause of premature death and ill health for women and men in America.
- Women are starting to smoke at an earlier age. Fewer teenage boys are starting but the proportion of girls is increasing and the younger you begin, the more likely you are to become a regular smoker.
- More women are becoming heavy smokers. American women are the heaviest smokers of all the women in the world—*especially American women between the ages of 35 and 44.*
- A woman who smokes runs eight to twelves times the risk of dying from lung cancer, three times the risk from a stroke, and twice the risk of dying from a heart attack, emphysema, or chronic bronchitis.

I address this section to the 30 percent of American women who smoke. Most of you *want* to quit. That's not the problem. Nor is weakness of character the reason it's so difficult to do so. To stop smoking is thought to be as difficult, if not more so, than quitting an alcohol habit. It's also known that kicking cigarettes has been harder for women than for men—though both sexes are making real progress in the antismoking battle. There are more ex-smokers than ever before. For those of you still smoking, to help you beat this beast I want to add a little to what I said early on in the book about its fast aging effects.

In the last few decades, women's health has improved in every area with one striking exception—lung cancer. In fact, by the time you read this, lung cancer may have taken the lead over breast cancer as the primary cause of cancer death in women—it already has in California and Washington! And it is already the leading cancer killer for men. We're catching up fast, largely because women now smoke as much as men do. Women began smoking in large numbers around the time of the Second World War and we'll be seeing the effects of this legacy for many years.

The devastating thing about lung cancer, which usually shows up during midlife, is that only about five to ten percent of those who have it are cured. Lung cancer is far more lethal and difficult to detect early than is breast cancer. So even though today fewer women

Chatting after Prime Time class with Hazel Washburn, who has successfully beaten the smoking habit.

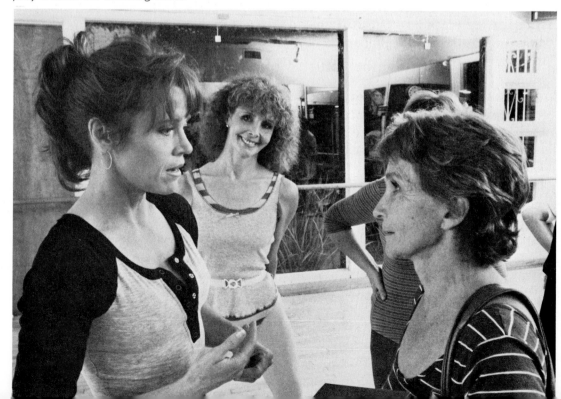

develop lung cancer than breast cancer, the risk of death is greater because lung cancer is the toughest cancer to defeat. But on the positive side, it may be the easiest to *prevent*. In most cases we just need to stop smoking.

What keeps us smoking? Habit. Stress. Other members of the family who smoke. The nicotine that's possibly addicting physically. And especially the tobacco industry, for whom women are a major target.

Cigarette ads make up 10 to 16 percent of all ads in women's magazines.* From the beginning, cigarette advertising has promised to all women who smoke a passport to slimness—"Reach for a Lucky instead of a sweet." Now, it's jumped on the feminist bandwagon and the "independent career woman" is considered advertising's most lucrative market for cigarettes—"You've come a long way, baby." Cigarettes are to bring not only "lightness" but liberation, and the poise, sexiness, energy, and self-assurance to make us successful in work and in love. Virginia Slims have now made it into the ranks of the Marlboro Man—an equal-opportunity tragedy, I'd say. Let's say No to the things that keep us smoking.

Switching to low-tar and low-nicotine cigarettes *can* reduce the risk of lung cancer and heart disease to some degree—but only if you don't inhale more often or deeper and only if you don't increase the number of cigarettes, which smokers usually tend to do when they switch to low-yield cigarettes. Smoking "lights" is *not* a viable alternative to giving up smoking completely. They still contain the harmful Toxic Three: tars, nicotine and carbon monoxide. What's more, additives are now used to replace the flavor lost by the less powerful tobacco. These additives may be *increasing* the danger of smoking rather than reducing it. And no one but the tobacco companies knows what these additives are.

In short, there is no safe cigarette.

I'm not a smoker, but I have worked with many women who have quit smoking and taken up instead a program to improve their overall fitness. From all that I have seen and heard, my best advice is to begin by deciding how you personally want to go about giving up

---

* A growing number of magazines now refuse these ads as a matter of policy. Among those to be applauded are *Good Housekeeping, Seventeen, Mother Jones, Prevention,* and *National Geographic.*

smoking. The kind of healthy diet and exercise program I've talked about can be a tremendous help as it will reduce the initial stress of stopping smoking, and it will increase your resistance to starting again. There are also many good resources available, some free of charge which I've listed in the Resource Guide. But remember, smoking is one of the hardest things to give up. Don't expect it to be easy. You might be at war with the desire to smoke for the better part of a year. So you have to be prepared to give it all you can and put up a good fight.

ESTING, TESTING

The following is a basic list of routine examinations recommended by health practitioners and organizations. By suggesting these, I don't mean to replace the need for you decide with your primary-care physician what regular sting is best for you. A good physician will help you to stay on top of all this. But it's always good for us to have an overview too, especially if you have not yet found a physician in whom you have great confidence. This schedule of check-ups is not a rigid one. Never wait before consulting your doctor if you experience any unusual symptoms.

EARLY

ental exam
Every six months is even better. By age sixty, 45 percent of Americans now lose their teeth—not because of aging or cavities, but largely because of periodontal disease caused by poor dental care. Bacterial deposits called plaque accumulate under the gum line. The supporting bones recede to protect themselves from infection and as a result teeth fall out. Thorough flossing and brushing with the least abrasive toothpaste you can find are essential—every day—to prevent periodontal disease, as are regular visits to the dentist for a check-up and a cleaning. Dental X rays every two years are also a good idea.

ynecological xam
After age forty, this should include an annual *Pap smear* as a check for cervical cancer. Sexually active women with several partners should have Paps twice a year. Before forty, a Pap smear is recommended every three years if you have had two consecutive years of healthy results (unless you are at special risk). This would also be a convenient time to include a breast exam.

Rectal exam
After age forty, this exam is important to screen for colorectal cancer, the third leading cause of cancer death in midlife women.

After age fifty, this should include an annual stool test and possibly a deeper rectal exam.

General physical
The following are best done yearly:

Blood pressure check

A complete blood panel that includes the measurement of blood fats and a check for anemia

Urinalysis that includes a measurement of sugar, protein, and calcium

EVERY TWO YEARS

Glaucoma test
There's an increasing susceptibility to glaucoma with age. This eye disease is characterized by a hardening of the eye and excessively high pressure within the eyeball that can damage the optic nerve and cause blindness. After age forty, an eye exam that includes a test for glaucoma is recommended every two years. See an ophthalmologist for this test.

TO BE DECIDED WITH YOUR PHYSICIAN

Baseline mammogram and follow-up mammogram screenings

Baseline bone measurement for osteoporosis (equipment permitting)

Regularity of breast exam by physician

Regularity of gynecological visits and testing if currently on estrogen therapy

THE COMPLETE PHYSICAL EXAMINATION

A good rule of thumb for how often to have a complete physical examination, one that looks at *everything* including most of the above tests, is the following: three in your thirties, four in your forties, five in your fifties, and annually beginning in your sixties.

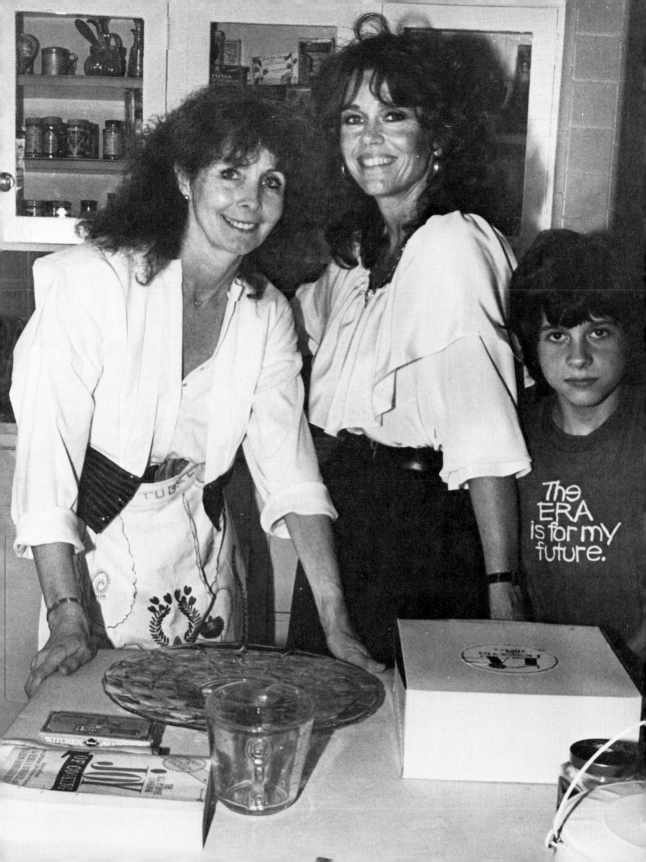

CHAPTER 16

CONCLUSION: A VIEW FROM THE BRIDGE

SO. A YEAR HAS PASSED since we began our writing. We've traveled further and covered far more ground than I expected when we began. Mignon has become what is probably the world's youngest expert on midlife. Together we have vicariously experienced every symptom we've written about. Every ache. Every pain.

For me personally, the writing of this book has been extremely important. Having delved to the very heart of the midlife experience, explored its every facet, I feel less frightened about getting older, better prepared for what is to come, ready to make the most of this time in my life. I hope this is true for you as well.

I feel more strongly than ever that we owe it to our children—our girls *and* boys—to build a new image of women that is not based on age and that includes a vision of mature beauty, mature sexuality, and the potential for a fully powerful role late into life. Otherwise, there is nothing to tempt the young ones to prepare for their futures—or ourselves for that matter. If we continue to believe that all we have to offer are a youthful face and body and an ability to bear children, growing older will remain the terrifying "ordeal of the imagination" it was for those who came before us. We will be left extraordinarily vulnerable as we age. We will be cut off from the fulfillment that comes from developing every aspect of our lives.

It is women who must explode the myth that womanliness ends in middle age, women alone who must redefine femininity. We have a unique perspective to offer the young, the rare vantage point of

Shirlee, me, and Troy getting ready to celebrate what was to be Dad's last birthday.

standing between generations, between old and new values, between old and new frontiers—a view from the bridge.

We are the pioneers—a first generation of consciously, admittedly midlife women, charting a positive new trail for ourselves and our daughters through a previously misunderstood and ignored part of life. It's up to us. We are women coming of age.

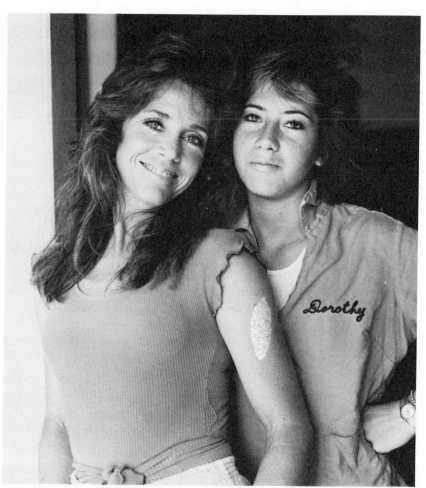

Vanessa and me at the beginning of the summer, 1984.

RESOURCE GUIDE

WORKOUT RESOURCES

1. The Prime Time Workout
- *Jane Fonda's Prime Time Workout Record* (Album)
- *Jane Fonda's Prime Time Workout* (Audio cassette)
- *Jane Fonda's Prime Time Workout* (Video cassette, Beta and VHS)

To complement the Prime Time Workout exercises introduced in this book, I've designed an album, audio cassette, and video. Each offers a 45-minute program designed especially for women and men in midlife and also for those who want a comprehensive exercise program but find the Beginners' and Advanced Workout from my first book too difficult. Prime Time is also excellent for anyone who does the regular Workout but simply wants a change of pace. With its emphasis on flexibility and proper form, Prime Time is especially good for those who haven't been exercising, who may be overweight, or who are suffering from back problems, arthritis, or injuries due to overuse.

2. The Original Workout
- *Jane Fonda's Workout Book*
My first book on health and fitness. Along with the basics of good nutrition and exercise, I present the complete Beginners' Workout and Advanced Workout, based on the program offered at the Workout studios. Available in both hard and soft cover.
- *Jane Fonda Workout Record* (Album)
- *Jane Fonda's Workout* (Audio cassette)
- *Jane Fonda's Workout* (Video cassette, Beta and VHS)
These are based on the Workout program introduced in my first book. All three are designed to give a thorough workout to the beginning and also the advanced exerciser. The Beginners' Workout on the album and audio cassette takes 25 minutes; on the video, 30 minutes. The Advanced Workout on the album and audio cassette takes 50 minutes; on the video, 55 minutes.

3. The Challenge Workout
- *The Jane Fonda Workout Challenge* (Video cassette, Beta and VHS)
For experienced exercisers, a vigorous 90-minute video cassette class. The Challenge is designed to build strength, to develop flexibility, and to increase endurance. Excellent for those who have been doing the Advanced Workout and feel ready to move on to a more strenuous class with 20 minutes of choreographed, highly energetic aerobics.

4. The New and Improved Workout (available Spring, 1985)
- *Jane Fonda Workout Record—New and Improved* (Album)
- *Jane Fonda Workout—New and Improved* (Audio cassette)
- *Jane Fonda Workout—New and Improved* (Video cassette, Beta and VHS)
A newly updated album, audio cassette, and video of the original Workout, Beginners' and Advanced, including an extended aerobics section. Special emphasis is given to exercising safely and with proper form. Both the album and audio cassette come complete with a manual of diagrams and instructions that make the exercises easy to follow. The Beginners' Workout on the album and audio cassette takes 30 minutes; on the video, 35 minutes. The Advanced Workout on the album and audio cassette takes 50 minutes; on the video, 55 minutes.

5. **The Stretch and Strengthen Workout** (available Fall 1985)
- *Jane Fonda's Stretch and Strengthen Workout* (Video cassette, Beta and VHS)
  A program that concentrates on deep stretching and deep muscle toning. Excellent for developing greater flexibility and strength. Ideal for alternating with the other Workout programs.

6. **The Pregnancy, Birth, and Recovery Workout**
- *Jane Fonda's Workout Book for Pregnancy, Birth, and Recovery* by Femmy DeLyser
  Beautifully written, this book presents the unique program created by Femmy DeLyser to guide women safely through the rapid physical changes involved in becoming a mother. It covers the entire year from conception to recovery and nursing, includes birthing skills and baby massage, and presents the special exercise program given at the Workout studios for expectant and new mothers. Available in hard cover.
- *Jane Fonda's Workout Record for Pregnancy, Birth, and Recovery* (Album)
- *Jane Fonda's Workout for Pregnancy, Birth, and Recovery* (Audio cassette)
- *Jane Fonda's Workout for Pregnancy, Birth, and Recovery* (Video Cassette, Beta and VHS)
  Based on Femmy's book, each of these—the album, audio cassette, and video—offers a complete 90-minute program led by Femmy DeLyser and myself.

WHERE TO FIND WORKOUT RESOURCES
The Workout books, albums, audio cassettes and videos are available locally at all regular outlets. You may also order by mail. Write to:
The Workout, Inc.
P.O. Box 2957
Beverly Hills, CA 90213

LOOKING TO THE FUTURE: YOUR FISCAL FITNESS

Health is more than a medical question. It's an economic one as well. Our financial circumstances affect both our physical and our mental well-being. They determine where we live, how we live, whether we live with a sense of security and balance or a sense of anxiety and stress, and, of course, whether we can even afford health care when we need it. Yet, all too often the economic side of our health is the one for which we are the least prepared. It is also the arena in which women come up against the toughest realities.

Most of us who've been married will survive our marriages by many years. No matter what our marital status, however, each of us needs to be able to support ourselves in midlife and beyond. We have to plan for the second half of our lives as consciously and as enthusiastically as possible, putting as much attention into shaping up financially as we do into shaping up physically. In addition, we need to work toward having a lasting network of friends, family, and community to sustain us. The more solid the fiscal and social foundation we build in midlife, the more security we will have as we grow older.

The following organizations and publications are excellent resources to which you can turn for more information and assistance in these aspects of midlife well-being: employment, social security, pensions, health insurance, and the changes to public policy that need to be made in order to correct the inequities that now exist for women in each of these areas.

Older Women's League (OWL)
1325 G. St, N.W.
Lower Level B
Washington, DC 20005

An effective national membership organization with over 70 local chapters in the forefront on issues concerning midlife and older women. The importance of physical fitness is emphasized too; an increasing number of chapters have begun walking clubs. Membership dues of $5.00 a year include 10 issues of the *OWL Observer* newspaper, a reliable update on national policy issues. Write for a list of OWL's excellent publications and series of *Gray Papers*.

National Organization for Women (NOW)
425 13th St, N.W.
Washington, DC 20004

A strong national membership organization with local chapters across the country and specific task forces on issues concerning midlife and older women. NOW has been the lead organization working for the passage of the Equal Rights Amendment (ERA) and legislation for women's economic rights. It also works actively to elect progressive women candidates and to support those male candidates and elected officials who stand up for women's equal rights. Membership dues of $25.00 a year include a subscription to the monthly *NOW Times*.

Displaced Homemakers Network
1010 Vermont Ave. N.W., #817
Washington, DC 20005

Purpose is to foster the development of displaced-homemaker programs throughout the country and to advocate on their behalf. Millions of midlife women today are displaced homemakers, usually between the ages of thirty-five and sixty-five. They are women often still responsible for dependent children, who have worked in the home providing unpaid household service to family members and therefore been dependent on the income of their husbands, but who have lost this source of support through death, divorce, separation, or disability. These women have or will have difficulty in finding a job. Contact the national Network office for the location of the program nearest you. For a donation of $5.00–$15.00, depending on your means, you will receive six issues a year of *Network News*. You might also want to order the Network's excellent book *Displaced Homemakers* by Laurie Shields ($6.00, by mail or in bookstores).

9to5
National Association of Working Women
1224 Huron Road
Cleveland, OH 44115

Most midlife women work outside the home, and most of those who do are office workers. 9to5 is a national membership organization of office workers with over 20 chapters across the country and with members in nearly every state. It has won many victories for the rights and respect of office workers and has also cofounded a national union for office workers, District 925, affiliated with the Service Employees International Union (SEIU). An organization such as 9to5 is essential when more midlife women than ever before, trying to find jobs or to hold on to jobs, encounter the double whammy of sex and age discrimination. There is also evidence that the increasing number of women who operate video display terminals (VDTs) are being exposed to serious health hazards. In addition, the heavy, speeded up, monotonous work load of office work lacking challenge or decision-making authority is very stressful. If you are an office worker and get a headache every day, don't call a psychiatrist, call an organizer. You might also want to read 9to5's excellent book *9to5: The Working Woman's Guide to Office Survival* by Ellen Cassedy and Karen Nussbaum ($6.00 by mail or in bookstores).

Gray Panthers
3635 Chestnut Street
Philadelphia, PA 19104

An effective national membership organization with local chapters whose far-reaching concern with the aging issues of our country takes into account the needs of future generations as well. The membership is intergenerational although the majority are in midlife and their later years. A donation of $12.00 a year will bring you six issues of *Gray Panther Network*, the organization's national newspaper.

Women's Equity Action League (WEAL)
805 15th St, N.W., #822
Washington, DC 20005

WEAL's purpose is to secure legal, educational, and economic rights for all women by monitoring the implementation and enforcement of equal-opportunity laws, including those related to social security and pensions. Publishes the excellent *WEAL Washington Report* six times a year, which follows national legislation specifically affecting women. This is included in the $30.00 yearly membership fee ($15.00 for those with limited resources). WEAL also offers "Women Growing Older," a set of excellent fact sheets on policy issues affecting midlife and older women ($2.50).

RECOMMENDED READING:

"A Guide to Understanding Your Pension Plan" ($2.50)
"Your Pension Rights at Divorce" ($2.00)
Write to:
Pension Rights Center
1346 Connecticut Ave, N.W.
Washington, DC 20036

Provides excellent educational information to individuals and organization about pension and social security issues.

"Directory of Services for the Widowed in the United States and Canada" (free)
"Widowed Persons Service Bibliography" (free)
Write to:
National Retired Teachers Association/American Association of Retired Persons (NTRA/AARP)
1909 K St, N.W.
Washington, DC 20049

Large national membership organization for persons over age fifty. Publishes very useful preretirement and retirement booklets. Also, its Widowed Persons Service offers programs in many communities across the country listed in the directory above. Membership dues of $5.00 a year include a subscription to six issues of the magazine *Modern Maturity* and the monthly *AARP News Bulletin*.

"On Being Alone" (free)
Write to:
Widowed Persons Service
NRTA/AARP
Box 199
Long Beach, CA 90801

A very helpful 15-page publication for the widowed.

"A Woman's Guide to Social Security" (free)

Call or write your local Social Security Office (found in the phone book under U.S. Government) and ask them to mail you a copy of this helpful booklet published by the U.S. Department of Health and Human Services. Ask them for any other useful publications they may have. You may also obtain a record of your personal lifetime social security earnings to date by asking them to mail you a "Request for Social Security Statement of Earnings."

THE GROWING FORCE OF OUR VOTE

There's a large poster that catches my eye every time I visit my husband's Assembly District office here in Santa Monica. In bold black and white are the following simple words: "Two out of three adults in poverty are women. What if we were all to go to the polls?"

This message states a harsh reality. It also shows us the most basic of steps we can take toward economic equity for women—exercising our right to vote! The vote is one way every woman can and must participate in the political process—from age eighteen onward. In the 1980 election, more women voted than ever before and, for the first time, in numbers slightly higher than men. And, not surprisingly, as a group we appear to vote differently from men on both candidates and issues.

As midlife women, our vote can play a special role in shaping policy and in ensuring women's full place in the arena of political power. In this society, because the squeeze of inequality intensifies as women grow older, we are in the best position to fight for change. We're like the "point

men" of aging. We come upon its dangers first. Accordingly, no one knows what needs doing quite as well as we do and, fortunately, as Gray Panther Founder Maggie Kuhn says, "we will outlive much of our opposition." Historically, this is the first time our numbers have been so great that public policy will have to move, however slowly, in our direction. Possessing this political strength, let's be sure to use it, letting no election go by, national or local, without our voices being heard. Please be sure you're registered.

To register to vote:

Call your state or county Registrar of Voters or Elections Office for information on how to register. Every state has different guidelines. You can also contact your local chapter of the nonpartisan League of Women Voters. The voter registration form is often brief and easy to fill out. In some states you can readily find registration forms in libraries, city halls, fire stations, and post offices.

GENERAL RESOURCES

Women in Midlife

FURTHER READING:
Growing Older, Getting Better:
A Handbook for Women in the Second Half of Life
Jane Porcino (Addison-Wesley, 1983)

An excellent sourcebook on the personal, social, and financial aspects of being a woman in midlife.

Hot Flash
A Newsletter for Midlife and Older Women
School of Allied Health Professionals
State University of New York
Stony Brook, NY 11794

Edited by Jane Porcino, Ph.D., the author of *Growing Older, Getting Better*, this is a very readable, concise quarterly update on a broad range of topics of concern to midlife and older women, from physical to fiscal fitness, reviewing the latest publications, books, and research with an action agenda on national legislation. Subscription is $10.00 a year/4 issues.

The Process of Aging

FURTHER READING:
Vitality and Aging
James F. Fries and Lawrence M. Crapo (W. H. Freeman, 1981)

One of the best general books on aging I have found, with a strong belief in people's ability to prevent chronic disease and to live long active lives through a program of good nutrition and regular exercise.

The Skin

PRODUCTS:
Caswell-Massey Company, Ltd.
Mail Order Division
111 Eighth Avenue
New York, NY 10011
(212) 691-4090

For a catalogue of Caswell-Massey's wonderful cu-

cumber products, soaps, and other cosmetic items, send $1.00 to the above address. Their retail store is located at 518 Lexington Avenue, New York City.

SERVICES:
American Society of Plastic and Reconstructive Surgeons
233 N. Michigan Avenue, #1900
Chicago, IL 60601
Special referral number: (312) 856-1834

Write or call for the names of board certified plastic surgeons in your area who specialize in general plastic surgery of the *entire body*, including cosmetic surgery of the face.

American Academy of Facial Plastic and Reconstructive Surgery
1101 Vermont Avenue NW, #304
Washington, DC 20005
(202) 842-4500

Write or call for the names of board certified plastic surgeons in your area who are specialists for the *head and neck only*, which includes cosmetic surgery of the face.

Middle-Age Spread

FURTHER READING:
Fit or Fat?
Covert Bailey (Houghton Mifflin, 1977)

A lean little book that offers the most compelling and clear explanation of the relationship between muscle, metabolism, exercise, and maintaining your ideal weight.

Body Mechanics

FURTHER READING:
Arthritis: A Comprehensive Guide
James F. Fries, M.D. (Addison-Wesley, 1979)

The Arthritis Helpbook
Kate Loring, R.N., Dr. PH, and James F. Fries, M.D. (Addison-Wesley, 1980)

Self-Help Manual for Patients with Arthritis
Arthritis Foundation
National Office
3400 Peachtree Road, N.E.
Atlanta, GA 30326

Additional free literature is also available by writing to the Arthritis Foundation, a highly respected voluntary organization with local chapters across the country.

Oh, My Aching Back
Leon Root, M.D. and Thomas Kiernan (New American Library/Signet, 1973)

Stand Tall! The Informed Woman's Guide to Preventing Osteoporosis
Morris Notelovitz, M.D. and Marsha Ware (Triad Publishing Co., 1982)

Is There Life After Menopause?

FURTHER READING:
Hot Flash
A Newsletter for Midlife and Older Women
(See address and description above.)

Midlife Wellness: A Journal for the Middle Years
Center for Climacteric Studies
University of Florida
901 NW 8th Avenue, Suite B-5
Gainesville, FL 32601

Edited by Morris Notelovitz, M.D., the author of *Stand Tall!*, this is a national medical journal for the public that focuses on wellness in the midlife years. A good resource for current documented information on the menopause and other health concerns of the climacteric. Subscription is $12.00 a year/4 issues.

Menopause, Naturally: Preparing for the Second Half of Life
Sadja M. Greenwood, M.D.
(Volcano Press, 1984)

Offers reliable medical information about menopause, with a strong emphasis on the importance of good nutrition and regular exercise. Write Volcano Press, 330 Ellis Street, San Francisco, CA 94102, to order a copy of the book and to be placed on a mailing list for an annual update, the *PMZ Newsletter.*

SERVICES:
Association for Voluntary Sterilization
122 E. 42nd St.
New York, NY 10168
(212) 573-8322

Contact this organization for more information on sterilization and for guidance in locating qualified physicians and clinics.

Eating for the Long Run

FURTHER READING:
Diet for a Small Planet
Frances Moore Lappé
10th Anniversary Edition (Ballantine, 1982)

Tufts University Diet and Nutrition Letter
Subscription information: PO Box 2465
Boulder, CO 80322

The Human Nutrition Research Center at Tufts University is in the forefront of research on nutrition and aging. Its monthly newsletter offers excellent, up-to-date information for the general public. Subscription is $24.00 a year.

Nutrition Action
Center for Science in the Public Interest (CSPI)
1501 16th St., N.W.
Washington, D.C. 20009
(202) 332-9110

CSPI is a nonprofit, consumer advocacy organization that investigates and seeks solutions to problems related to nutrition and food policy. Its very informative membership newsletter is published 10 times a year. Membership is $20.00 a year/$12.00 for students and senior citizens. CSPI also offers a wide range of products, such as colorful nutritional posters, recommended books, and even fun-to-use software, adaptable to most personal computers, which teaches basic principles of good nutrition, analyzes your eating and shopping habits, and provides a data base distinguishing safe from dangerous food additives.

Hitting our Stride

FURTHER READING:
Women's Running (Anderson World, 1976), and *Running Free* (Putnam, 1980)
Joan Ullyot, M.D.

If you include running or walking in your exercise

program, you'll find both of these books inspirational and informed guides. They are written for women by a physician, self-described as a "cream puff" in her prerunning years, who describes her own physical transformation through aerobic exercise.

Women and Sports
Janice Kaplan (Viking, 1979)

A hard-to-put-down book that talks about the importance of physical expression to the development of a woman's strength in every area of her life. The author makes a convincing and well-written case for the necessity of exercise and sports in our early girlhood, while also emphasizing that it's never too late to start.

Planned Patienthood

Hysterectomy
SERVICES:
HERS
Hysterectomy Educational Resources
501 Woodbrook Lane
Philadelphia, PA 19119
(215) 247-6232

Provides comprehensive information on hysterectomy and coping with its aftereffects for women to whom hysterectomy has been recommended and for those who have already had a hysterectomy. HERS also issues an excellent quarterly newsletter for $10.00 a year.

FURTHER READING:
Coping with a Hysterectomy
Susanne Morgan (Doubleday, 1982)

Breast Cancer
SERVICES:
CANCER HOT LINE
(800) 4-CANCER
Toll-free
Alaska (800) 638-6070, New York City (212) 794-7982, Washington, DC and suburbs of Maryland and Virginia (202) 636-5700, and Oahu (808) 524-1234 (neighboring islands call collect).

Sponsored by the National Cancer Institute, this Hot Line will connect you to any one of 27 different regions of the Cancer Information Service of-

fering up-to-date facts about all types of cancer. Spanish-speaking staff members are available to callers in California, Florida, Georgia, Illinois, Texas, northern New Jersey and New York City.

National Cancer Institute
Office of Cancer Communications
Building 31, Room 101A18
9000 Rockville Pike
Bethesda, MD 20205
(800) 638-6694

The National Cancer Institute has many excellent, very readable publications on breast cancer as well as other cancers. Call their toll-free number or write to request their list of materials. I recommend the following free resources:

"The Breast Cancer Digest"
A beautifully illustrated and well-written guide to medical care, emotional support, educational programs and resources for breast cancer (165-page softcover).

"If You've Thought About Breast Cancer . . ."
Rose Kushner, author of *Alternatives* (formerly *Why Me?*).
A regularly updated guide full of information, written by a woman who has personally experienced breast cancer (28-page booklet).

SERVICES:
American Cancer Society (ACS)
777 Third Avenue
New York, NY 10017

A national voluntary organization with local chapters across the country, offering many free and useful publications on breast cancer as well as other cancers. The ACS also offers the "Reach to Recovery" program for women who have had breast surgery. Write for their list of free materials.

ENCORE Program
YWCA
726 Broadway
New York, NY 10003

An excellent, affordable 10-week program of pool and floor exercises for women who have had breast surgery. The ENCORE program also offers time to talk with other women who have had mastectomies. Call your local YWCA or contact the national headquarters above to determine whether ENCORE is offered in your area.

American Society of Plastic and Reconstructive Surgeons
(See address above.)

Write or call for information on board-certified plastic surgeons in your area who do breast reconstruction.

FURTHER READING:
Alternatives: New Developments in the War on Breast Cancer (formerly *Why Me? What Every Woman Should Know About Breast Cancer to Save Her Life,* rewritten for the 1980's)
Rose Kushner, 1984

For a copy of the book, write The Kensington Press, c/o P.B.S., P.O. Box 643, Cambridge, MA 02139.

Smoking
American Lung Association
1740 Broadway
New York, NY 10019

National office with local chapters that offers valuable literature free-of-charge on how to quit smoking.

Office of Smoking and Health
Room 116, Parklawn Building
5600 Fishers Lane
Rockville, MD 20857

Write for list of free publications on smoking, its dangers, and suggestions for how to give it up.

General Health Concerns
SERVICES:
SECOND SURGICAL OPINION HOT LINE
(800) 638-6833
Toll-Free

This Hot Line will put you in touch with a phone number in your local area to call for a list of qualified physicians for second opinions. Also has information on questions to ask the physician.

Alcoholics Anonymous (AA)
P.O. Box 459
Grand Central Station
New York, NY 10017

One of the most highly respected and successful programs for fighting alcoholism and other addictions. (No dues or fees.)

Pills Anonymous
P.O. Box 473
Ansonia Station
New York, NY 10023

A self-help, self-supporting program modeled on AA, for those who wish to stop taking pills or other mood-altering chemicals. (No dues or fees.)

FURTHER READING:
Our Bodies, Ourselves
Boston Women's Health Collective, Third Edition (Simon and Schuster, 1984)

The latest edition of this excellent self-health book offers a considerably expanded section called "Growing Older" that discusses women's aging in general and menopause in particular.

The Complete Book of Women's Health
Gail Hongladarom, Ruth McCorkle, and Nancy Fugate Woods (Prentice-Hall, 1982)

A very readable reference book whose purpose is to assist women in becoming more responsible for their wellness. A wide range of medical topics is covered in addition to health issues such as smoking, alcohol, over- and under-nutrition, and environmental toxins.

NOTES

Page 17
Longest running study on aging in U.S.: The Baltimore Longitudinal Study of the National Institute on Aging.

Page 17
"Women have been badly neglected . . ." Robert N. Butler, M.D., Former Director, National Institute on Aging.

Page 19
"We who are older have nothing to lose! . . ." Maggie Kuhn, Founder, Gray Panthers, "Advocacy in This New Age," *Aging*, August 1979.

Page 25
Ten-year study of prime time and children's weekend television: "Women and Minorities on TV, 1969–1978," George Gerbner and Nancy Signorielli, Research Report by the University of Pennsylvania Annenberg School of Communications, released in collaboration with the Screen Actor's Guild, October 29, 1979.

Page 25
"A man is for all seasons . . ." Screen Actor's Guild Press Release, "Female SAG Members Work Less, Earn Less," January 25, 1980.

Pages 26–30
Principal demographics resources:
The National Institute on Aging.
The U.S. Bureau of the Census.
"Growing Numbers, Growing Force," A Report from the White House Mini-Conference on Older Women, Coordinated by Tish Sommers, President, Older Women's League; Published by the Older Women's League Educational Fund and the Western Gerontological Society, 1980.
"The Older Woman: Continuities and Discontinuities," Report of the National Institute on Aging and the National Institute of Mental Health Workshop, September 14–16, 1978; NIH Publication No. 79-1897, October 1979.
"The Status of Midlife Women and Options for Their Future," A Report with Additional Views by the Subcommittee on Retirement Income and Employment of the Select Committee on Aging, House of Representatives, 96th Congress, March 1980; U.S. Government Printing Office, Com. Pub. No. 96-215.

Page 30
"The more women become involved away from the household . . ." Robert N. Butler, M.D., Former Director, National Institute on Aging, "The 'E' in Elderly: Exercise," in *A Symposium of the National Conference on Fitness and Aging*, President's Council on Physical Fitness and Sports, September 10–11, 1981, p. 40.

Pages 31–32
Principal resource for discussion of midlife women working outside the home: "Vanished Dreams: Age Discrimination and the Older Woman Worker," Report by 9to5, National Association of Working Women, August 1980.

Page 32
Dracula Complex: Quoted from "Older Women at Work," Carol Hollenshead, *Educational Horizons*, Vol. 60, No. 4, Summer 1982, pp. 137–146.

Page 33
One of the most unique ongoing heart studies in the country: Framingham Heart Study, Framingham, Massachusetts. "Women, Work, and Coronary Heart Disease: Prospective Findings for the Framingham Heart Study," Suzanne G. Haynes, Ph.D., and Manning Feinleib, M.D., *American Journal of Public Health*, Vol. 70, No. 2, February 1980.

Page 34
Mental health studies of midlife women: Discussed in *The Second Stage*, Betty Friedan, 1981, pp. 76–77.

Page 34
"It's not responsibility that kills . . ." Estelle Ramey, M.D., Georgetown University Medical School, quoted in "Testosterone: The Bonding Hormone," Dianne Hales and Robert E. Hales, M.D., *American Health*, Nov./Dec., 1982.

Page 40

"swim against the current of senescence . . ." James F. Fries, M.D., "The Compression of Morbidity," Paper presented to Institute of Medicine, National Academy of Sciences, Washington, DC, October 20, 1982.

Page 42

"Such an old cell is very much like an old city . . ." Christian de Duve, "Cells Age," in *Aging Into the 21st Century*, Lissy F. Jarvik (ed.), 1982.

Page 58

Chart on sunscreens: Adapted from "A Guide to Sunscreens," in *Jane Brody's The New York Times Guide to Personal Health*, Jane Brody, 1982, p. 357.

Pages 78–79

Set point theory: Discussed in *The Dieter's Dilemma*, William Bennett, M.D. and Joel Gurin, 1982.

Page 90, footnote

Study of regeneration of cartilage: Robert Salter, M.D., Professor and Head of Orthopaedic Surgery, University of Toronto, discussed in "Joints Were Meant to Move—and Move Again," Pat Ohlendorf, *The Graduate*, Sept./Oct., 1980, pp. 6–9.

Pages 102–103

Dialogue from *The Mirror Crack'd*: From film script by Jonathan Hales and Barry Sandler, 1980, based on novel by Agatha Christie.

Page 107

Recommendation on calcium consumption: "How Diet Can Help Prevent Brittle Bones," Bess Dawson-Hughes, M.D., *Tufts University Diet and Nutrition Letter*, Vol. 1, No. 3, May, 1983.

Page 110

"If physicians were to prescribe calcium . . ." Joseph Lane, M.D., "Postmenopausal Osteoporosis: The Orthopedic Approach. An Interview with Joseph Lane," *The Female Patient*, Vol. 6, November 1981.

Page 111

"Age doesn't seem to be a major limiting factor . . ." Everett L. Smith, Ph.D., "Exercise for the Prevention of Osteoporosis: A Review," *The Physician and Sportsmedicine*, Vol. 10, No. 3, March, 1982.

Page 119

Everything You Always Wanted to Know About Sex, David Reuben, 1969.

Page 120

Feminine Forever, Robert A. Wilson, 1966.

Page 120

"Suppose that we had a menopausal woman president . . ." Edgar Berman, M.D., quoted in "What Is Menopause?" Louisa Rose, in *The Menopause Book*, Louisa Rose (ed.), 1977, pp. 3–4.

Page 121

"I guess I don't like being defined by the tense of my ovarian functions . . ." Grace Paley, "An Unsentimental Journey," *Ms.*, February, 1978, pp. 33–34.

Page 134

Discussion of experience of hot flash in South Wales: "Symptom Reporting at the Menopause," Pat Kaufert and John Syrotuik, *Social Science and Medicine*, Vol. 151, 1981, pp. 173–184.

Page 136

Recommendation on Vitamin E consumption: *Women's Health '82*, Vol. 1, No. 3, December, 1982.

Page 137

"Home-brew estrogen": Susanne Morgan, *Coping with a Hysterectomy*, 1982.

Page 137

Study on hormones and exercise. "Exercise and Reproductive Function in Women," David C. Cumming, M.D., and Robert W. Rebar, M.D., *American Journal of Industrial Medicine*, Vol. 4, 1983, pp. 113–125.

Page 139

Study on sweating and exercise: "Sweating Sensitivity and Capacity of Women in Relation to Age," Barbara L. Drinkwater, J. F. Bedi, A. B. Loucks, S. Roche, and S. M. Horvath, *Journal of Applied Physiology: Respirat. Environ. Exercise Physiol.*, Vol. 53, No. 3, 1982, pp. 671–676.

Page 139

The Menopause Clinic, Department of Reproductive Medicine, University of California School of Medicine at San Diego, La Jolla, CA 92093.

Page 145

Largest aging research project in the country: The Baltimore Longitudinal Study of the National Institute on Aging.

Page 147

"I am sixty years old and they say you never get too old to enjoy sex . . ." Quoted in "The Sexual Lives of Women Over 60," Carol Tavris, *Ms.*, July, 1977, pp. 62–65.

Page 147

"a myth perpetuated by our adult children . . ." Maggie Kuhn, Founder, Gray Panthers, quoted in

Breaking the Age Barrier, Elaine Partnow, 1981, p. 99.

Page 155
"Somewhere in my middle years . . ." Quoted in *Growing Older, Getting Better*, Jane Porcino, 1983, p. 171.

Page 169
"We concede that no simple equation can be derived . . ." P. A. Van Keep, W. H. Utian, and A. Vermeulen, *The Controversial Climacteric*, The Third International Congress on Menopause, Ostend, Belgium, June, 1981.

Page 171
"The emotional problems which may occur during the time of life associated with menopause . . ." Johanna Perlmutter, M.D., "The Estrogen Controversy," *Harvard Medical School Health Letter*, February, 1978.

Page 171
"Estrogens do not appear to prevent age-related changes in skin, hair and breasts.": National Institute on Aging, "To Be or Not to Be an Estrogen User?" Summary of Conclusions of the NIA Consensus Development Conference on Estrogen Use and Postmenopausal Women, September 13–14, 1979.

Page 171
"total hogwash . . ." Johanna Perlmutter, M.D., quoted in *Unfinished Business: Pressure Points in the Lives of Women*, Maggie Scarf, 1980, p. 442.

Page 172
"Although it was once hoped that estrogen would protect against heart disease . . ." National Institute on Aging, "To Be or Not to Be an Estrogen User?" Op. cit.

Page 173
"Currently, sufficient information is not available . . ." Howard L. Judd, M.D., "Estrogen Replacement Therapy: Indications and Complications," UCLA Conference, 1983 American College of Physicians, *Annals of Internal Medicine*, Vol. 98, 1983, pp. 195–205.

Page 176
"menostop": Susanne Morgan, *Coping with a Hysterectomy*, 1982.

Page 179
"There are more women . . ." Wulf H. Utian, M.D., Ph.D., *Menopause in Modern Perspective: A Guide to Clinical Practice*, 1980, pp. 8–9.

Page 233
"There is no drug in current or prospective use . . ." Walter M. Bortz, II, M.D., "Disuse and Aging," *Journal of the American Medical Association*, Vol. 248, No. 10, September 10, 1982.

Page 234
Breaking the Age Barrier studies:
Piro Kramar, M.D. and Barbara L. Drinkwater, Ph.D., "Women on Annapurna," *The Physician and Sportsmedicine*, Vol. 8, No. 3, March, 1980.

Sharon A. Plowman, Barbara L. Drinkwater, and Steven M. Horvath, "Age and Aerobic Power in Women: A Longitudinal Study," *Journal of Gerontology*, Vol. 34, No. 4, 1979, pp. 512–520.

Paul Vaccaro, Ph.D., Gail M. Drummer, Ph.D., and David H. Clark, Ph.D., "Physiological Characteristics of Female Masters Swimmers," *The Physician and Sportsmedicine*, Vol. 9, No. 12, December, 1981, pp. 75–78.

Page 236
"I returned from my three surveys . . ." Alexander Leaf, M.D., "Getting Old," *Scientific American*, 1973, Vol. 229, pp. 45–52.

Page 417
"ordeal of the imagination . . ." Susan Sontag, "The Double Standard of Aging," *Saturday Review of the Society*, September 29, 1972, p. 29.

ACKNOWLEDGMENTS

Thank you to the many who gave so generously of their time and expertise:

Evelyn Anderson, R.N., Ph.D., Co-Coordinator, The Menopause Clinic, University of California School of Medicine, San Diego, and Professor of Nursing, University of San Diego; Jeffrey Bland, Ph.D., Professor, Nutritional Biochemistry, University of Puget Sound; the Boston Women's Health Collective; Femmy DeLyser, R.N., Birth Educator and Director of the Pregnancy, Birth, and Recovery Program of Jane Fonda's Workout; Jay Fliegelman, Professor, Department of English, Stanford University; James F. Fries, M.D., Associate Professor of Medicine, Stanford University School of Medicine, and Director, Stanford Arthritis Clinic; James G. Garrick, M.D., Director, Center for Sports Medicine, Saint Francis Memorial Hospital, San Francisco; Sadja Greenwood, M.D., M.P.H., Min An Health Center, San Francisco; Sonia Hamburger, Co-Coordinator, The Menopause Clinic, University of California School of Medicine, San Diego; Henry G. Harter, D.C.; Michael F. Jacobson, Ph.D., Executive Director, Center for Science in the Public Interest; Gayle Kamer; Michael D. Lockshin, M.D., Professor of Medicine, Division of Rheumatology, Cornell University Medical College, and Attending Physician, Hospital for Special Surgery, New York; Judy Mahle Lutter, President, Melpomene Institute of Women's Health Research; Maryann Napoli, Center for Medical Consumers and Health Care Information, New York; the National Institute on Aging; the National Women's Health Network; Morris Notelovitz, M.D., Ph.D., Director, Center for Climacteric Studies, and Professor of Obstetrics and Gynecology, University of Florida; Maxine Ostrum, M.D.; Jane Porcino, Ph.D., Director, Gerontology Department, State University of New York at Stony Brook, and Co-Director, National Action Forum for Older Women; Aviva Rahmani, artist; Robert W. Rebar, M.D., Professor and Head, Reproductive Endocrinology and Infertility Section, Prentice Women's Hospital, Northwestern University; Tish Sommers, President, Older Women's League; and the Women's Equity Action League.

My appreciation and respect to Carol Garabedian, choreographer of the Prime Time Workout.

My love and gratitude to my wonderful stepmother, Shirlee Fonda.

My special thanks to Georges Borchardt, our literary agent, his wife and colleague, Anne, Fred Hills, our editor at Simon and Schuster, and to the unsung heroines Leslie Ellen, Debi Karolewski, Denise Kurtzman and Jennifer Robertson.

Mignon would like to give her personal thanks to Camille Wenzel, Kim McCarthy, Leslie McCarthy, Suzanne McCarthy, Colleen Di Pilla, Laura Seitel, Joyce Sachs, Dannielle Pellegrin, Mary Kushner, Mary Humboldt, Scott Altmann, and Bob Mulholland for their encouragement and support during the writing of this book; and a special thank you to Tootsie.

INDEX

Harvard Medical School Health Letter, 171
Hayden, Tom, 15, 69
HDL (high-density lipoproteins), 172, 201, 240
headaches, 175, 236
health records, 398–99
heart attacks, 130, 173, 175, 411
heart disease, 33, 48–51, 200, 204
  diet and, 188, 194
  estrogens and, 171–72
  risk factors in, 50–51
heart rate, training, 244–45, 246
height, loss of, 104, 105, 107
Hellman, Lillian, 40
Hepburn, Katharine, 40
herbs:
  fresh, 231
  for hot flashes, 137
  as natural diuretics, 160
high blood pressure, 50, 135, 148, 166, 173, 175, 194, 198–99
hiking, 248
  boots for, 254
  uphill, 245
hips, 90, 99
  injuries of, 104, 105
homemakers:
  Displaced Homemakers Network, 421
  "empty nest" and, 34–35
  health problems of, 33
honey, 197
hormones, 53, 105, 241
  adrenal, 137, 162, 163–66, 201
  defined, 124
  in meats, 188
  sex, 126, 127–28, 145, 194; see also estrogen
hormone therapy, 169–79, 411
  benefits of, 171–72
  false promises about, 169
  forms of drugs in, 170–71, 172
  guidelines for, 177–78
  for osteoporosis, 111–13, 171, 176
  other considerations for, 174–75
  overuse of, 169, 176
  research gaps on, 178–79
  risks of, 172–74, 411
  who should not use, 175
Hot Flash, 424, 425
hot flashes, 130, 133–41, 159, 197, 203, 209
  common-sense cool-downs for, 140–41
  estrogen therapy and, 171, 174
  exercise as alleviator of, 137–40, 241
  of men, 145
  pattern of, 135
Hospital for Special Surgery (New York), 111
hypertension, 50, 135, 148, 166, 173, 175, 194, 198–99
hypothalamus, 124–26
  hot flashes and, 134
hysterectomy, 171, 399–402, 426
  defined, 400–401
  second opinions and, 401–2

ice, for injuries, 92, 100
identity, age and, 23, 25
immortality, illusion of, 14
immune system, 46, 241
impotence, 146–47
income:
  of men vs. women, 32
  of single mothers, 29
infections:
  IUDs and, 130
  after menopause, 144
  urinary, 152–53, 197
  vaginal, 152–53
injuries, 247
  balance as prevention against, 238
  care for, 92–93
  exercise-induced, 238, 243, 247
  hip, 104, 105
  prevention of, 90–91, 97–101, 107–113, 238, 243, 251–57
  relaxation during stretching as prevention against, 243
  spinal discs and, 95, 96, 97
  walking and, 248
insomnia, 161, 163, 200
  remedies for, 161–62
insulin, 162, 196
intelligence, aging and, 47–48
iron, 191, 197, 201, 205, 218
IUDs, 130

Japanese women, breast cancer of, 410
Jewish Community Centers, 406
joints, 45, 46, 85–92
  care of, 90–92

ILLUSTRATION CREDITS

PHOTOGRAPHS

DRAWINGS

CARTOON